ELDERSPEAK

ElderSpeak

A Thesaurus or Compendium
of Words Related to Old Age

James L. Reynolds, MD

iUniverse LLC
Bloomington

ELDERSPEAK
A Thesaurus or Compendium of Words Related to Old Age

iUniverse books may be ordered through booksellers or by contacting:

iUniverse LLC
1663 Liberty Drive
Bloomington, IN 47403
www.iuniverse.com
1-800-Authors (1-800-288-4677)

ISBN: 978-1-4917-0510-0 (sc)
ISBN: 978-1-4917-0511-7 (hc)
ISBN: 978-1-4917-0512-4 (e)

Library of Congress Control Number: 2013916549

Printed in the United States of America

iUniverse rev. date: 01/07/2014

CONTENTS

DEDICATION

This book is dedicated to my wife, Liz, and children, Mary, Cathy, Jim, Jr., and Missy, whose company was sometimes forsworn in order to write, and to my elderly friends who are its inspiration.

PREFACE

ELDERSPEAK: AN OLD-AGE THESAURUS is a compendium of words that are useful to those interested in expanding their vocabulary applicable to the elderly. ElderSpeak's words are the antithesis of "elderspeak", a recent term for using babytalk, essentially, in communicating with the elderly on the assumption that they are cognitively impaired.

ElderSpeak fosters **gerontiloquence** (speaking among those *d'un certain agê*), and is helpful in translating ideas relating to the elderly into words. Knowing and keeping up with English words is difficult, as attested by the arrival on June 10, 2009, of our reputed millionth English word: "Web 2.0"—one not on the tip of many seniors' tongue. Paul J. J. Payack of "Million-Word March" made this millionth-word claim; he says it's only an estimate, but there's no doubt that the English vocabulary is gigantic. While the venerable Oxford English Dictionary lists some 600,000 words, the French lexis in Larousse is but some 100,000-odd words. ElderSpeak has about **2,000** words. They span a time frame from the current text-message *WOG* (<u>w</u>ise <u>o</u>ld <u>g</u>uy), to the archaic exclamation, **zounds**! (a contraction: by God's wounds!)

The word thesaurus (L, treasury, < G *thesaurus* storehouse) has three connotations: One, a book of word groups; two, a book of specialist vocabulary, i.e., words relating to a particular subject, a glossary; and three, a treasury: a place in which valuable things are stored. I hope that **ElderSpeak: A Thesaurus Or Compendium Of Old-Age-Related Words** fulfills each of those connotations.

The **ElderSpeak** lexicon selects only a soupçon of the million English words: those related directly, or primarily, to those in their **senium** (old age), notable not only for their historically-touted wisdom, but more recently, due to living generally much longer than their predecessors, for their deterioration, weaknesses, infirmities, stereotypical behaviors, personality traits, multiple problems, foibles, characteristics, and concerns peculiar to their age, e.g., **arthroxerosis** (chronic joint arthritis), **kainophobia** (fear of something new), **lethologica** (inability to remember words), **onomatomania** (preoccupation recalling a certain word), **sanctiloquence** (speaking solemnly or of sacred things), a tendency to **exheredate** or **forisfamiliate** (to disinherit), and to be **preterists** (those living in the past).

Usual, everyday, pedestrian words applicable to elders are generally excluded from this thesaurus unless too pertinent to ignore, e.g., the collation **senior moment**, and the words **magpie**, and **Alzheimer's**. The author hopes to find among the 645 meanings attributed to the ubiquitous verb "run" in the new—expected in 2137—Oxford English Dictionary one with its meaning germane to elders. **ElderSpeak** attempts to congregate into one easily accessible place unusual, exceptional, elder-related words that hitherto have been cached, in effect, by their narrow use and distribution.

The great majority of ElderSpeak's words are unusual. Churchill's dictum: "Short words are best and the old words when short are best of all.", is not generally followed. **Paro**, a hassle-free robo-seal pet, is an exception. Not infrequently the words in ElderSpeak are striking, medical, obscure, exotic, often marvelous; sometimes preposterous; they are apt to be obsolete or rare—even a **hapax legomenon** (< G "once said", a word of which supposedly only one use is recorded) is not shunned—and **gadzookary** (the use of archaic words or expressions) is embraced. **Epiolatry** (the worship of words) often occurs naturally as one ages. Some applicable foreign words and phrases are included.

German portmanteau holophrases, i.e., ideas expressed in one word, such as *Slimmsbesserung* (an improvement that makes things worse), *Torschlusspanik* (a sense of life passing one by), and *Opagefaengris* (a prison for elder men) are not neglected; nor are those in French and Latin, e.g., *abus de faiblesse* (taking advantage, usually financial, of an aged person who may be *non compos mentis* (not of sound mind).

Pleasant holophrases, i.e. words suggesting a whole idea or concept, such as **agerasia** (youthful appearance in an older person), **euphelicia** (healthiness resulting from having all of one's wishes granted), **eugeria** (a normal, happy old age)—eugeria is a worthy goal before the **eschaton** (the final end)—**evancalous** (pleasant to embrace), **dormition** (a peaceful and painless death), and **paleomnesia** (excellent memory for long-past events), are often offset by such unpleasantries as: **gerontopia** (post-presbyopic lens sclerosis causing myopia), **nocebo** (illness based on awareness of side effects), **nosomania** (irrational belief that one has a disease), **pathoneurosis** (neurotic preoccupation with true disease), **poliosis** (loss of hair color), **prosopolethy** (inability to remember faces), and **rhagades** (skin cracks and fissures: wrinkles).

Age-appropriate words of unusual etymology, e.g. **baragouin** (any jargon or unintelligible language), which is said to have originated in Breton soldiers' astonished utterances upon experiencing white bread for the first time, are esteemed. The origin of the word **termagant** (a shrew, a scold, a virago) is not only unusual, but of historic interest: It's from Old French *Tervagant*, an imaginary deity that medieval Europeans believed was worshiped by Muslims and was represented in morality plays as an overbearing, violent person in a long robe. Europeans, mistaking the robe for a dress, erroneously assumed the deity was a woman.

Mythologically based names, exemplified by **Medea's cauldron, Teiresias**, **Silenus**, and **Nestor**, are not disdained as outdated. In contrast, recent initialisms, **AAADD** (age-activated attention deficit disorder), **ADAM syndrome** (androgen deficiency in the aging male), **calcium CT** (computer tomography), and **FOX03A** (a long-life gene), as well as acronyms—properly, initialisms—often used by acronymists in emailing and *nouvelle-vague* text messaging, such as **CRAT** (Can't remember a thing.) or, indelicately, **CRS** (Can't remember s—t), **OBA** (old battle axe), and **WOG** (wise old guy) appear. Current words such as **donepezil** (a drug for treating Alzheimer's disease), **klotho** (a longevity gene named for Klotho, the Greek Fate who spun the thread of life), **resveratrol** (an alleged longevity agent found in red wine— now almost a **catholicon** {an all-purpose medicine})—**sulforaphane** (an immune-response stimulant), and **sundowning** (senile seniors' disruptive behavior apt to occur at sundown) keep the reader currently *au fait*. The word **gerocomical** (pertaining to treatment of the aged) is judged no laughing matter.

ElderSpeak's words may be roughly classified as follows:

I. Uncommon, unusual, rare, obsolete, archaic, etc., words specific to old age, the elderly.
II. Words that are old-age apt, but are not exclusively related to old age: **zaftig** (full-figured; pleasingly plump; buxom), *Schlimmbesserung* (an attempted improvement that makes

things worse), **sacchariferous** (containing sugar), **magpie, dormition** (sleeping; falling asleep).

III. Words that are everyday, common, but so senior specific that excluding them would be grievous: **senior moment, Alzheimer's disease, golden years, geezer**

IV. Words excluded:
    a. Those too well known: ancestors, grandparents, elders, dirty old man
    b. Those not old-age specific or apt enough: grobianism (rudeness, boorishness) or fidimplicitary (fully trusting someone).

The author confesses to a certain arbitrariness in including and excluding the thesaurus's words.

This lexicon should appeal to lexicographers—defined by Samuel Johnson as "harmless drudges"—lexicomanes, hyperlexics, lexies and wordies in general. William Safire's Norma-Loquendi types will predictably not be amused by words such as **rhonchisonant** (snoring), **oligophagous** (eating only certain foods) or **aconuresis** (urinary incontinence), but **lovertine** (addicted to lovemaking), **hyperprosexia** (excessive sexuality), **acedolagnia** (complete indifference to sex), **medomalacophobia** (morbid fear of losing an erection during love making), and **xeronisus** (inability to reach orgasm) may get their attention.

The author is not aware of other texts purporting to be a glossary or *omnium gatherum* of words relating to the elderly, a sort of idioticon of the aged. Such neglect does not square with the elderly being special, if not for their traditional wisdom—impugned more recently— but for their sheer number. The very words *elder* and *eldest* attest this singular status. Correct usage demands they be used only in relation to humans, usually in a family context, and that they be preceded by a definite or indefinite article in contrast to *older* and *oldest*, words that can apply to lower animals and things as well as **longevous** (long-lived) humans.

It is timely that the elderly be accorded their due: their very own onomasticon. After all, the U.S. population is going gray. Those over 65 years of age are predicted to double to 80 million in 30 years as baby boomers enter the older age group. Predictably, 20% of the U.S. population will be older than 65 in 30 years versus 12 percent now.

Women are living longer than men: In the U.S. for every 100 women age 85 and older, there are only 48 men (Source: U.S. Census). **Centenarians** worldwide are estimated to number 340,000, with most in the U.S. and Japan, although many Japanese, some 281 "centenarians", have recently been found missing: relatives have been spuriously collecting their government retirement checks—it's satisfying that this sort of chicanery goes on in Japan as well as in the U.S. Oldsters are the fastest-growing age segment of the population. Centenarians in the U.S., now 105,000, will number more than 601,000 by mid-century; this rapid advance is attributed to medical innovations, certainly, and also to improvements in diet and lifestyle. Worldwide, those older than 65 will, for the first time ever, soon outnumber children under five. ElderSpeak can't speculate on just when elders will peak at some future date. See the word **supercentenarian** for comment on the oldest living humans.

Thus, the elderly are both numerically important and meritoriously **macrobian** (long-lived) enough to have merited an old-age lexicon or idioticon (dialect dictionary) of sorts. The fastest growing age group in the U.S today are those who are age 85 and older: 5.3 million Americans. Elders over 65 vote more frequently and consistently than younger adults and constitute one-fourth of the electorate, even though they are only one-eighth of the population. Increasingly, the elderly cause **Stuldbrug** (1. the difficulties government social workers have with providing elders with continuing medical care, or 2. the paradoxical purpose of restricting so many pleasures enjoyed by the elderly in frantic efforts to prolong their life that it becomes unenjoyable.) The federal government increasingly insists that seniors conform to a healthy lifestyle: a lean diet and lots of walking and running in order to decrease Medicare expense. Government as **surbater** (one causing footsoreness) may risk engendering **lassipedes** (footsoreness) in its elderly subjects.

Perhaps the heretofore lexical omission, a glossary or gift of gab focused on the elderly, is due to Americans being unfavorably biased, according to researchers, more against the elderly than any other group, including those identified by younger age, race, or sexual orientation. Maybe if the elderly were to speak more learnedly using this dictionary's words, they would be better regarded . . . one hopes not ostracized for being misunderstood. Since only 35% of the elderly use the Internet—an index of **kainophobia** (fear of something new, novelty) and **tropophobia** (fear of making changes)—a dictionary in traditional book format should more easily be within their reach. ElderSpeak's definitions are, for the most part, copied—sometimes modified—from sources listed in the Bibliography.

Notably, this thesaurus's words are classified alphabetically into 48 broad categories: a Categorical List of Headwords & Phrases. These categories are then subcategorized, first, according to a curtailed definition, and, in certain larger categories, further sub-classified. Such taxonomy fosters locating an appropriate word, and facilitates word choice. If one can't recall a specific word (**lethologica**), or a synonym, but can categorize it, or have an idea in search of a word, finding it is facilitated—an *aide-mémoire* (a document, memorandum, note written as an aid to the memory) is always appreciated by the elderly.

Special attention is given to word origin, which aids greatly in remembering a word. For the word **frugalista** (one living frugally, but staying fashionable and healthy by swapping clothes, buying secondhand, growing one's own produce, etc.), e.g., Shakespeare's first use and meaning of the word "frugal" is noted. The Microsoft Encarta College Dictionary and the Oxford English Dictionary were my main etymologic sources, in addition to Stedman's and Dorland's Medical Dictionaries re: medical words.

Peter Mark Roget published his first thesaurus in 1875. His intent was to create much more than a book of synonyms, the first book of which was the work of Abbé Gabriel Girard, a French monk, who in 1718 published *La justesse de la langue françoise*, and in later editions called it *Synonymes François*. Roget in an 1805 unpublished manuscript had compiled such a synonym list, but he envisioned a much expanded revision, and a reverse dictionary as well, which he published in 1875: "The idea being given, to find the word, or words by which that idea may be most fitly and aptly expressed." His stated object was ". . . simply to supply and to suggest such [words] as may be wanted on occasion, leaving the proper selection entirely to the discretion and taste of the employer [user of his book]." Roget's thesaurus was non-prescriptive. It is to be noted that lexicographers tend to be obsessive-compulsive and depressed persons, as were Roget and our own colonial polymath, Noah Webster (American Dictionary of the English Language, 1828). Dictionary writing is arduous—more so than coal mining, e.g., suggested James Kelly in a recent Wall Street Journal review of "The Story of Ain't by David Skinner.

A diverse word is not only invigorating, but has connotative value, as increasingly recognized by politicians: Barak Obama uses "public" in lieu of "government", "sliding scale" rather than "free" to describe his health—scratch that—"insurance" reform, while conservatives use "death panels" in place of his "end-of-life choices". Elders' talk could benefit from more connotative disparity . . . or perhaps duplicity.

If ElderSpeak is helpful in expanding one's vocabulary, in translating an idea into a word—locating the *mot juste* for talking to or about the elderly—this **lipsanographer's** (one who writes about relics—fig., the elderly) intent and the book's mission shall have been fulfilled. Should one of ElderSpeak's **metaforgottens** (words outmoded, perhaps forgotten) reemerge causing reminiscence, that will be a bonus. There is always the nagging *tertium quid*, other words that should be included; it is hoped that others will add to ElderSpeak.

"By words the mind is winged."
—Aristophanes, dramatist (c. 448-385 B.C.)

"Stand up in the presence of the aged; show respect for the
elderly and revere your God. I am the Lord."
—Leviticus 19:32.

James L. Reynolds, B.S., M.D., FAAP, FACC
New Orleans, LA, 2013

USE OF THE THESAURUS

HEADWORDS

Headwords, i.e., main entries, which include phrases, and very common prefixes, are in bold type and are listed alphabetically. Pronunciation of a headword or phrase is indicated in parentheses ( ). A pronunciation key follows below. Syllabification is indicated by a hyphen, or by primary (') and secondary (") stress marks. The headword's part of speech is found next in abbreviated form—an abbreviation code is located on page 9. The headword's definition(s) follows. Sometimes a note about the word is added. Next, there may be a symbol, •, exemplifying the word's use in the aged. Etymology is indicated within brackets [ ]. Next, parts of speech related to the headword are given in bold type. Synonyms, or related words, and sometimes an antonym, follow, and are emboldened, also. Lastly, the headword is classified into one or more headword categories. Headword categories are emboldened and underlined. A list of the 48 headword categories by which headwords are classified is found on page 445.

PRONUNCIATION KEY

(Note: This Pronunciation Key is derived primarily from the Microsoft Encarta College Dictionary, Ed. 1, 2001)

I. Vowels

A. Simple Vowels

Symbol	Representation
a	the **short a** (ă) sound: **a**t = at, comb**a**t = kom'bat r**a**t = rat.
ay	the **long a** (ā) sound for certain words with **a**, **e**, or

aa	the **broad a** (a) sound: f**a**ther = faather, b**a**h! = baah.
aw	the **awe** sound in some **a**ll or **au** words: **a**ll = awl, c**a**ll = kawl, m**a**ll = mawl, m**au**l = mawl. (But c**a**lligraphy = kə-lig'grə- fee).
k;	c**a**se = kayss, conv**e**y = konvay, O**K** = ō-kay', k**a**le = kayl, **K**2 = kay"too'.

1

ə the **short multiple-vowel** the **schwa ə** sound for, **a**, **e**, **i**, **o**, & **u** in certain words: **a**bout = ə-bowt', apne**a** = ap'nee-ə, it**e**m = ī'təm, ed**i**b**l**e = ed'ə-bəl, comm**o**n =kom'ən, circ**u**s = sur'kəss,

e the **short e** (ĕ) sound for **e** or **ie**: **e**gg = egg, befri**e**nd = bi-frend', or the **indefinite e** (e) for a word such as **e**xsuccous (eks-suk'kəss). Note: the **silent e** at some word endings: writ**e** = rīt.

ee the **long e** (ē) sound for **e**, **ee**, **i**, or terminal **y**: m**e**dium, mee'dee-əm, **ee**l = eel, happ**y** = hap'pee.

i the **short i** (ĭ) sound for **i**, or sometimes **e**, or **hy**: **i**t = it, b**e**friend = bi-frend', rh**y**thm = rith'əm.

ī the **long i** (ī) sound for **i**, or sometimes **ey**: **I** = ī, **i**ce = īce, **ey**e = ī.

o the **short o** (ŏ) sound for **o**, or sometimes **a**: **o**dd = odd, **o**w! = ow!, w**a**sp = wosp, w**a**nt = wont.

ō the **long o** (ō) sound for **o** or **owe**: **o**h = ōh, **o**pen = ōpen, **owe** = ō; or for certain **oa** words: g**oa**t = gōt.

oŏ the **short vowel oŏ** sound in certain words with **oo**, **ou**, or **u**: g**oo**d = goŏd, f**oo**t = foŏt, c**ou**ld =coŏd, p**u**t = poŏt, f**u**ll = foŏl.

oo the **longer vowel oo** sound in certain words with **o**, **oo**, **ou**, & **u**: m**o**ve = moov, sch**oo**l = school, f**oo**d = food, b**ou**rse = boorss, r**u**de = rood.

u the **short u** (ŭ) sound in certain words with **o** and **u**: m**o**ther = muth'ər, t**o**n = tun, p**u**tt = put, **u**p = up, g**u**t = gut.

u: short For the **shorter u** (oŏ) sound: See preceeding oŏ.

u: long For the **long u** (ū) sound: See **yoo** under **B. Vowel Combinations**.

B. Vowel Combinations

Symbol	Representation
aaj/aazh: broad a + ge; sound = aaj	for certain words ending in -**age** camoufl**age** = kam'mə-flaaj, badin**age** = baa"dən-**aazh**'.

aar: broad a + r; sound = **ahr** — for certain **ar** & **arr** words: f**ar**m = faarm, st**arr**y = staar'ee.

air: short a (ă) + ir or er; sound = **air** — for certain **ar**, **are**, & **aer** words: sc**ar**ce = skairss, v**ary** = vair'ee, decl**are** = di-klair', **aer**ial = air'ree-əl, **aer**ate = air'rayt.

aw: the sound of **awe** — for certain words containing **al**, **all**, **au**, & **ou**: D**al**ton = Dawl'tən, **all** = awl, t**au**ght = tawt, t**au**tology = taw-tol'lə-gee, th**ou**ght = thawt.

awr: the sound of **awr** — if an "r" follows **o**, **oa**, **or**, or **ou** in certain words: **or**, **oar**, **orr**, & **our**: n**or**th = nawrth, st**ory** = stawry, b**oar**d = bawrd (or bōrd), h**or**rid = hawr'rid, s**our** = sawr, (but bourse = boors).

choo, chə: the sound of **chew** — for certain words containing **tu**: anfrac**tu**ous = an-frak'**choo**-əss, contemp**tu**ous = kon-temp'**choo**-əss expos**tu**late = exs-pos'**chə**-layt.

-əl word ending — for words ending in -**le**: tack**le** = tak'əl, gigg**le** = gig'gəl.

-əm word ending — for words ending in -**om**, -**um**: freed**om** = free'dəm, conundr**um** = kən-un'drəm.

-ən word ending — for words ending in -**on**: stati**on** = stay'shən.

ear & eer: the sound of **ear** — for certain words containing **ear** & **eer** words: b**eer** = beer, n**ear** = neer, w**eary** = weer'ee.

ənss — For words ending in-**ence**: presence = prez'zənss.

əndz — For certain words ending in-**ends**: cal**ends** = kal'ləndz or kay'ləndz.

-ənz — For words ending in -**ence**, -**ens**: desin**ence** = des'sin-ənz, senesc**ence** = sen-es'senz, mitt**ens** = mit'tenz.

-ər — For unstressed **er** words: sundown**er** = sun'down-ər. conve**r**sation = kon-vər-say'shən.

gwa-, gway, gwe-, gwek, gwes, gwi-, & gwī — For words with **gua**-, **gue**-, **gui**-, and **guae**: lan**gua**ge = lang'**gwi**j, lin**gua**cious = ling-**gway**'shəs, lapsus lin**guae** = lin'**gwī** lan**gui**d = lang'**gwi**d, lan**gue**scent = lang-**gwes**'sənt.

ir & ire: the sound of a.) **ir**, with a **short i** (ĭ) & b.) **īr** with a **long i** (ī) — a.) consp**ir**acy = kon-spir'rə-see. b.) v**iru**s = vī'russ, f**ire** = fīre, insp**ire** = in-spīr', **Ire**land = īr'lənd, des**ire** = di'zīr'.

jhə or **jee-ə**	For words ending in <u>gia</u>: apha<u>gia</u> = a-fay'**jha** or a-phay'**jee-ə**.
ow	For certain <u>ou</u> words: ab<u>out</u> = ə-b<u>ow</u>t', st<u>out</u> = st<u>ow</u>t.
owr, ow'r	For certain <u>owr</u>, <u>ow-r</u>, & <u>our</u> words: <u>our</u> = owr, fl<u>our</u> = flowr, d<u>owr</u>y = dow'ree.
oy	For <u>oi</u> & <u>oy</u> words: <u>oi</u>l = <u>oy</u>l, b<u>oy</u> = boy.
shən, sh'ən	For words ending in -<u>tion</u>: ambi<u>tion</u> = am-bish'**ən**, ammuni<u>tion</u> = am-yoo-ni'**shən**.
shənt	For words ending in -<u>cient</u>: somnifa<u>cient</u> = som"ni-fay'**shənt**.
shə, shəl	For some words ending in –<u>tia</u> or -<u>tial</u>: demen<u>tia</u> = dee-men'**shə**, reveren<u>tial</u> = rev-ver-ren'**shəl**.
shən/shənt	For words contain- ing <u>tien/tient</u>: cecu<u>tien</u>cy = cee-kyou'**shən**-see, balbu<u>tient</u> = bal-byoo'**shənt**,
shəs, shass	For certain words containing <u>tious</u>: fac<u>tious</u> = fak'**shəss**, frac<u>tious</u> = frak'**shəss**.
see-ō, shee-ō, shō	For certain words ending in -<u>cio</u>: braggado<u>cio</u> = brag"gə-dŏs'**see-ŏ**, **shee-ŏ**, or **shŏ**.

ur	For certain <u>ir</u>, <u>or</u>, & <u>ur</u> words, & <u>er</u> stressed words: f<u>ir</u>st = furst, b<u>ir</u>d = burd, w<u>or</u>st = wurst, <u>ur</u>ge = urge, b<u>ur</u>st = burst; v<u>er</u>bal = vur'bəl.
-(x)əss	For words ending in -(x)<u>ous</u>: fabu<u>lous</u> = fab'byə-**ləss**.
yawr, yər	For words con-taining -<u>ior</u> or ending in -<u>ior</u>: sen<u>ior</u>ity = seen-**yawr**'i-tee, sen<u>ior</u> = seen'**yər**.
yəs, yəss	For words with -<u>ious</u>: bil<u>ious</u> = bil'**yəss**. yoo For words with the (ū) sound of <u>long u</u>, or certain words with <u>you</u>: b<u>u</u>gle = b**yoo**g'əl, <u>u</u>nique = **yoo**-neek,' <u>you</u> = **yoo**, <u>you</u>'ll = **yoo**l, <u>you</u>rs = **yoo**rz (or yawrz)
-zee-ə, -zi-ə or -zhə	For words ending in -<u>sia</u>: apha<u>sia</u>: ə-fay'**zhə** (or ə-fay'**zi-ə**, or -**zee-ə**).
zī	For certain words with <u>si</u>: de<u>si</u>re = di-**zī**re'. (But vi<u>si</u>on = vizh'ən, q.v. under -<u>zhə</u>).

II. CONSONANTS

A. Consonants in General

a. The following **consonants** have the sound they usually have in ordinary spelling: <u>b</u> <u>d</u> <u>f</u> <u>g</u> <u>h</u> <u>j</u> <u>k</u> <u>l</u> <u>m</u> <u>n</u> <u>p</u> <u>r</u> <u>s</u> <u>t</u> <u>v</u> <u>w</u>

y & z. They are rendered thus (in bold): befriend = bi-frend', hug = hug, strap = strap, milk = milk, jazz = jaz, yes = yess, zwieback = zwee'bak", victor = vik'tər. Sometimes g followed by n, or w itself, is silent: gnu = noo, write = rīt. y is sometimes rendered as a short ĭ: Ayr = air, azygous (az'i-gəs).

b. Note: the consonants c, q, & x are not rendered phonetically by themselves, but by the following symbolic representation: hard c = k, and soft c = s: cot = kot, decide = di-sīd'; q = k or kw: quay = kee, queen = kween; x = eks, z, k, or ks: excess = eks'sess, Xanadu = zan'nə-doo, tax = taks, box = boks. See change in consonant pronunciation in consonant combinations below.

c. The following two-consonant combinations (consonantal digraphs) ch, th, & sh, q.v. under: II. Consonants, C. Consonant Combinations, have the sound they usually have in ordinary spelling.

d. For the si or su sound (voiced palatoalveolar fricatives), zh is used, qv. under: C. Consonant Combinations.

e. Doubling of consonants:
(1.) Double consonants are used phonetically when a word has a double consonant, or a consonant is preceded by the following primarily or secondarily stressed vowels: a, e, i, o, u, or oŏ and followed by either a vowel, or a schwa (the unstressed vowel ə), or by the letters: l, r, w, or y: happy = hap'pee.

(2.) ss is used at the end of syllables ending in s or (ss) to show that s not z is required: devious = dee'vee-əss, morass = mor-ass'(But bees = beez.). Terminal s is also doubled with voiced consonants: face = fass, miscue = miss-kyoo', mincer = minss'ər. But s is not doubled with voiceless consonants: discus = dis'kus, discinct = dis-inkt', discrimination = dis-krim"mə-nay'shən (But discriminating = diss-krim'mə-nay"ting; wasp = wosp, discretion = dis-kresh'ən.)

B. Simple Consonants

b, bb	but = but, ribbon = rib'bon
d, dd	do = do, ladder = lad'er
f, ff	fond = fond, differ = dif'fer
g, gg	go = gō, giggle = gig'gəl (Note: The hard g sound is rendered by g; the soft g sound is rendered by j. For silent g, see n below.)
h	hot = hot.
j, jj, soft g	For words with j or soft g: juice = jooss, pigeon = pij'jən.
k	For k, hard c, ck words, & for certain words with ch: key = key, cat = kat, thick = thik, chalazion = kə-lay' zee-ən, chiropodist = kir-op'pō-dist, choleric kol'ə-rik/ kə-ler'ik.
l, le, ll, & əl	let = let, silly = sil'lee. tackle = tak'əl, giggle = gig'gəl.

m, mm   mom = mom, hammer = ham'mer.

m word ending əm   rhythm = rith'əm, schism = ski-zəm.

n, nn: not = not, funny = fun' nee, gnu = noo, gnome = nōm, gnathic = na'thik. (Note: g before n is not pronounced except in initialisms: GNP = gross national product.)

p, pp   pen = pen, happy = hap'pee.

r, rr   road = rōd, hard = haard, carry = kar'ree.

s, ss   For certain words with s, ss, soft c, & ps: say = say, lesson = les'sən, yes = yess, molasses = mə-las'sez—see z, zz below—glass = glass, glassine = glas-seen', decide = di-sīd', psychic = sī'kik.

t   For words beginning with pt use t: ptyalism = tī'ə-liz-əm, pterygium = tur-rij'ji-əm.

-th'əm   For words ending in -thm use th'əm: rhythm = rith'əm.

v, vv   very = ver'ree, savvy = sav'vee, vague = vayg.

w   wet = wet, why = wī.

y   yes = yess, your = yawr or yoor (stressed), or yər (unstressed), young = yung.

z, zz   for words in z or zz, or certain words in s or ss: zoo = zoo, jazz = jaz, blizzard = bliz'zərd, glands = glanz, molasses= mə-las'sez.

C. Consonant Combinations

ch   For certain words: chin = chin, church = church. (See k under simple consonants for ch pronounced as k.)

-chə-   For certain words with -tu-: hirsutulous = hir-soo'chə-luss.

ks   For certain words with x: tax = taks, sex = seks.

ng   singing = sing'ing.

sh   For certain words with sh or ci: sheep = sheep, shop = shop, social = sō'shəl, facial = fay'shəl.

th   thin = thin, think = think, mother = muth'er, thing = thing, this = this.

zh   For certain words with si & su: vision = vizh'ən, concision = kən-si'zhən, pleasure = ple'zhər, measure = me'zhər.

III. FOREIGN NON-FRENCH RONUNCIATION

In occasional cases—particularly that of proper names—the following are used to indicate non-English sounds:

kh, ẖ as in Scottish lo<u>ch</u> = lokh,
       German Ba<u>ch</u> = Bakh, and
       Spanish Gi<u>j</u>ón = hee-hawn'/
       hee-hõn'
ö   as in German sch<u>ö</u>n = sh<u>ö</u>n.
ü   as in French r<u>ue</u> = r<u>ü</u>e, German
       gem<u>ü</u>tlich = gem-<u>ü</u>t'lik

IV. FRENCH PRONUNCIATION

(The International phonetic alphabet
is used for French words, except for
their nasal vowels: their IPA tilde is
placed rightward instead of above.
See wikipedia.org/wiki/ /IPA_chart_for_
French.)

A. Consonants

IPA	Examples	English Approximation
b	beau	beaud
d	deux	do
f	fête;	festival
	pharmacie	festival
g	gain; guerre	gain
k	cabas;	sky
	archaïque;	
	aquarelle;	sky
	kelvin	
l	loup	loop
m	mou; femme	moo
n	nous; bonne	no
ɲ	agneaux	± canyon
ŋ	parking	sing
p	passé	spy
ʁ	roue; rhume	guttural r
s	sa; hausse;	sir
	ce; garçon;	sir
	option; scie	sir
ʃ	chou; scheme	shoe

	shampooing	shoe
t	tout; thé	sty
v	vous; wagon	view
z	hazard; zéro	zeal
ʒ	joue; geai	measure

B. Semivowels

j	fief; payer;	yes
	fille; travail	yes
w	oui; loi;	we
	moyen;	
	web	we
ɥ	huit	between yet
	& wet	

C. Vowels

IPA	Examples	English Approximation
a	patte	± pat
ɑ	pâte; glas	bra
e	clé; les; chez;	pay
	aller; pied	pay
ɛ	mère; est; faite	
	best	
	abdomen	best
ɛ:	fête; maître	best
		(longer)

D. Nasal Vowels

ã	sans; champ;	nasalized
	vent;	[ɑ]
	temps; jean;	
	taon	
ẽ	pain; daim;	nasalized
	bien	[æ]
	Reims; plein;	
	vin	

œ̃	parfum; brun	nasalized [œ]	ɔ	sort; minimum	hot
ɔ̃	son; nom		u	coup	influence
			y	tu; sûr	± cute
			'	moyen	phrasal stress
Suprasegmentals				[mwa'jɛ~]	
ə	le; reposer	minor (elided)	.	pays	syll. boundary
i	si; île; y	beet (shorter)		[pe. i]‿ les agneaux	liaison
œ	jeune; sœur	± bird		[lez‿a'ɲo]	
ø	ceux; jeûne	± bird	'	hors	aspirate/mute
o	sot; bureau	mole		['ɔr]	
	haut; hôtel	mole			

SYLLABIFICATION

Syllables are indicated by a hyphen, -, or in the case of a stressed syllable, by a stress mark, ' (primary) or " (secondary).

STRESS

Primary stress is indicated by the symbol ', and secondary stress by ".

    a. Monosyllabic Words

Single-syllable words have no stress marks.

    b. Polysyllabic Words

In words of more than one syllable:

    (1.) The primary stress is indicated with an apostrophe, ', immediately after the stressed syllable.
    (2.) A secondary stress is indicated with an end-quote mark, ", immediately after the stressed syllable.

Unstressed syllables are indicated by a hyphen (-).

ETYMOLOGY

The etymology of headwords and others is indicated by brackets, [ ]. Language derivation throughout is usually indicated by the initial language stipulated, unless another specified language intervenes. If no derivation is specified for etymological components, the initial language specified applies to the components, also. If initial origin is Indo-European (I-E), it is usually omitted. Words and combining forms other than those in English are italicized.

Questionable or unknown—to the author or others—derivation is indicated by a question mark:?. Plus is indicated by the + sign. Knowing a word's etymology often makes the word more intelligible and more easily remembered. An apt example is the word **onology**, meaning foolish talk, which is derived from two Greek words: *onos*, meaning jackass, and *logos*, meaning word or talk.

ABBREVIATIONS

abbr. = abbreviation
abs. = absolute(ly)
A.D. = anno domini
adj(s). = adjective(s)
adj.phr(s). = adjective
    phrase(s)
adv(s). = adverb(s)
AF = Anglo-French
aff. = affix
alt. = alternative(ly)
ant(s). = antonym(s)
ANZ = Australia-New
    Zealand
arch. = archaic
c. = circa
C. = century
Cf. = compare
colloq. = colloquial
comb. = combining or
    combining form

FHW&P = Foreign Head
    Words & Phrases section
dat. = dative
dial. = dialect, dialectal
dim. = diminutive
Du = Dutch
E = English
ed. = editor or edition
e.g. or E.g. = for example
esp. = especially
F = French
f. = feminine
f.adj. = feminine adjective
fig. = figuratively
fl. = flourished
form. = formal
freq. = frequentative verb
fut. = future tense
Ger. = German
Gmc. = Germanic
Goth. = Gothic
gen. = genitive
gram. = grammar

G = Ancient Greek
H = Hebrew
hist. = historically
i.e., = that is
I-E = Indo-European
inf. = informal
int. = interjection
It = Italian
joc. = jocular(ly)
L = Latin
LG = Low German
lit. = literal(ly)
m. = masculine
m.adj. = masculine adjective
MD or MDu = Middle Dutch
ME = Middle English
   (1200-1500)
med. = medical, medicine
-moN = -*ment* in French (±
   -mawn in E).
MHG = Middle High German
MLG = Middle Low German
n(s). = noun(s)
N.B. = *nota bene*, (L) note
   well
neg. = negative
neut. = neuter
nf. = feminine noun
nm. = masculine noun
nm.&f. = masculine and
   feminine noun
nn. = nouns
n.phr(s). = noun phrase(s)
n.pl(s). = plural noun(s)
n.s. = singular noun
obs. = obsolete
OE = Old English
OF = Old French
OHG = Old High German
ON = Old Nors
OS = Old Saxon
pedant. = pedantic

phr(s). = phrase(s)
pl. = plural
pl.n. = plural noun
pp(s). = past participle(s)
ppl. adj. = participial adjective
prec. = immediately
   preceding
pref(s). = prefix(es)
prep.phr. = prepositional
   phrase
pres.p(s). = present
   participle(s)
pres.p.adj. =
   present-participle
   adjective
pref(s). = prefix(es)
prep. = preposition
priv. = privative
pr.n. = proper noun, noun
   phrase, or species name
prob. = probably
q.v.= *quod vide* = (L) which
   see
ref. = reflexive
rel. = related, related to
Rus = Russian
Sc = Scots, Scottish
Scand. = Scandinavian
sing. = singular
s.n. = singular noun
Sp = Spanish
suff (s). = suffix(es)
syn(s). = synonym(s) (for the
   head-word)
U.K. = United Kingdom
unk. = unknown
U.S. = United States, or
   loosely, American
v(s). = verb(s)
var(s). = variation(s),
   varient(s)
vbl.n. = verbal noun

v.i. = *vide infra* = (L) see below
vi.&vt. = both an intransitive and a transitive verb
vi(s). = intransitive verb(s)
viz. = *videlecit*, (L) namely

vs. = versus
v.s. = *vide supra* = (L) see above
vt(s). = transitive verb
Yid. = Yiddish

SYMBOLS

<   from, derived from; used as a separator in abbreviations; and as a period to end a sentence
=   stands for equals, is equal to
+   and, or plus, or questionable
?   questionable, questionably

~   stands for the headword under consideration
•   introduces exemplification of a headword.
/   ends a line of verse; separates like terms
[ ]   indicates etymology; or an insertion in a quotation
( )   parenthetical
{ }   sub-parenthetical

TYPE

Type style = Times New Roman. **bold** = vocabulary headwords, parts of speech of headwords, apropos of old age elements in definitions, and for antonyms & synonyms. *italicized* = etymologic foreign-source words, foreign words, and headwords illustrated in definitions by the symbol •. ***bold & italicized*** = foreign headwords. **<u>bold and underlined</u>** = headings of the 48 word categories, & letter and letter-combination pronunciation examples.

BIBLIOGRAPHY

A Word A Day: A Romp through Some of the Most Unusual and Intriguing Words in English. Anu Garg. John Wiley & Sons, Inc., Hoboken, New Jersey, 2003.

Another Word A Day: An All-New Romp Through Some of the Most Unusual and Intriguing Words in English. Anu Garg. John Wiley & Sons, Inc., Hoboken, New Jersey, 2005.

Bugaboos, Chimeras, & Achilles' Heels. John L. Dusseau. Prentice Hall, New Jersey, 1993.

Dickson's Word Treasury. A Connoisseur's Collection of Old and New, Weird and Wonderful, Useful and Outlandish Words. Paul Dickson. John Wiley & Sons, Inc., 1992.

Dictionary of Foreign Words And Phrases. Maxim Newmark, PhD. Dorset Press, New York, 1950.

Dimboxes, Epopts, And Other Quidams. David Grambs. Workman Publishing, New York,1986.

Dorland's Illustrated Medical Dictionary, ed. 27. Elizabeth J. Taylor, Ed. W.B. Saunders Co., Philadelphia, PA, 1988.

Forgotten English—A Merry Guide to Antiquated Words, Packed with History, Fun Facts, Literary Excerpts, and Charming Drawings. Jeffrey Kacirk. William Morrow & Co., Inc., New York, 1997.

Internet reference: http://wordsmith.org/awad/, Anu Garg, Ed. Various years.

Langenscheidt's Universal German Dictionary, revised ed. Langenscheidt, New York, 1993.

Larousse Concise French/English, English/French Dictionary. Marc Chabrier, Coordinating Ed., ed. 2, Larousse, Paris, 2006.

Larousse's French-English English-French Dictionary. Marguerite-Marie Dubois, Dennis J. Keen, Barbara Shuey, & Lester G. Crocker, Eds. Washington Suqare Press, Inc., New York, 1954.

Microsoft Encarta College Dictionary. Dr. Kathy Rooney, Editor-in Chief, St. Martin Press, New York, 2001.

Million-Dollar Words. More than 1,000 Words to Make You Sound Like a Million Bucks. Seth Godin and Margery Mandell. Running Press Book Publishers, Philadelphia, Pennsylvania, 1993.

More Joy of Lex. Gyles Brandreth. William Morrow & Co., Inc., New York, 1982.

Mrs. Byrne's Dictionary of Unusual, Obscure, and Preposterous Words. Josefa Heifetz Byrne, Ed. University Books, Citadel Press, New Jersey, 1974. (Republished as Word Lover's Dictionary. MJF Books, New York, 1994.)

On Language. A weekly column in the New York Times Magazine. William F. Safire. Various years.

1000 Most Challenging Words. Norman W. Schur. Facts On File Publications, N.Y., 1987.

Random House Webster's Pocket German Dictionary, ed.2. Random House, New York, 1996.

Reader's Digest Oxford Complete Wordfinder: A Unique and Powerful Combination of Dictionary and Thesaurus. The Reader's Digest Association, Inc. Pleasantville, N.Y,.1996. (Original text from The Concise Oxford Dictionary, ed. 8, R.E. Allen, Ed., 1990.)

Stedman's Medical Dictionary. The Williams & Wilkins Co., Baltimore, ed. 23, 1976.

The Bibliophile's Dictionary. 2,054 Masterful Words and Phrases. Miles Westley. Writer's Digest Books, Cincinnati, Ohio, 2005.

The Compact Edition of the Oxford English Dictionary: Complete Text, Reproduced micrographically, Vols. I & II, Oxford University Press, Glasgow, 1971.

The Concise Oxford Dictionary of Current English. H.W. Fowler and F.G. Fowler, Eds. Oxford University Press, London, ed. 5, 1964.

The Garden of Eloquence. A Rhetorical Bestiary. Willard R. Espy. Harper & Row, New York, 1983.

The Grand Panjandrum (Revised and Expanded). J. N. Hook. Collier Books, Macmillan, New York, 1980, 1991.

The Grandiloquent Dictionary. Russell Rocke. Prentice-Hall, Inc., Englewood Cliffs, N.J., 1972.

The Insomniac's Dictionary—The Last Word on the Odd Word. Paul Hellweg. Facts On File Publications, New York, 1986.

The Man Who Made Lists: Love, Death, Madness, And The Creation of Roget's Thesaurus. Joshua Kendall. Berkley Books, New York, 2009.

The Merck Manual of Geriatrics, ed. 3. Mark M. Beers, M.D. & Robert Berkow, M.D., Eds. Merck Research Laboratories, Waterhouse Station, N.J., 2000.

The Miracle of Language. Richard Lederer. Pocket Books, New York, 1991.

The New College Latin & English Dictionary. John C. Traupman, PhD. BantamBooks, New York, 1966.

The Penguin DICTIONARY GAME Dictionary. James Cochrane. Penguin Books, London, 1988.

The Superior Person's Book of Words. Peter Bowler. Laurel, 1979.

The Toastmaster's Treasure Chest. Herbert V. Prochnow & Herbert V. Prochnow, Jr. Castle Books, 2002.

There's A Word For It! Charles Harrington Elster. Scribner, New York, 1996.

They Have a Word for It—A Lighthearted Lexicon of Untranslatable Words and Phrases. Howard Rheingold. Jeremy P. Tarcher, Inc., Los Angeles, 1988.

Totally Weird and Wonderful Words. Erin McKean, Ed. Oxford University Press, Oxford, London, 2006.

Webster's New Twentieth Century Dictionary of the English Language (unabridged). Jean L. McKechnie, Ed. The World Publishing Co., Cleveland & New York, ed. 2., 1966.

Winged Words. Philip Howard. Oxford University Press, 1988.

Word Lover's Dictionary. Josefa Heifetz Byrne. MJF Books, New York, 1994. (First published as Mrs. Byrnes's Dictionary of Unusual, Obscure, and Preposterous Words. Josefa Heifetz Byrne, Ed. University Books, Citadel Press, New Jersey, 1974.)

Words That Make a Difference and How to Use Them in a Masterly Way—with Compelling Examples from The New York Times. Robert Greenman. Levenger Press, Delray Beach, Florida, 2000.

ALPHABETICAL LISTING
OF HEADWORDS & PHRASES
WITH THEIR DEFINITION,
ETYMOLOGY, & CATEGORIZATION

A

"All want to live longer, but not grow old."
—Benjamin Franklin

a dog in the manger (mayn'jər) n.phr. a person who tries to prevent somebody else from having or doing something that he or she can't have or do—a manger = a trough from which livestock eat. ● That **curmudgeon**, q.v., who had no cell phone, was *a dog in the manager* when other home residents tried to use theirs. [U.K. < OF *mangeoire* < *mangier* eat < L *manducare* chew < *mandere* eat; chew, champ; devour]. See **role**. See **mentality, mentation, behavior**.

AAADD n. an initialism: <u>a</u>ge-<u>a</u>ctivated <u>a</u>ttention-<u>d</u>eficit <u>d</u>isorder, not infrequently occurring with advancing age. It is a type of memory deficit manifested when an elder's intention to accomplish something is interrupted by something else needing more urgent attention or distracting his/her attention, then, due to the interruption, the original intention is forgotten. Such intervening interruptions, should they occur *seriatim*, result in nothing, or very little, being accomplished. [< analogy with ADHD, Attention Deficit Hyperactivity Disorder. ADHD, a true medical condition or disorder is found mainly in children]. See **memory**.

abasia (a-bay'zhə, -zhee-aa) n. inability to walk. [< G *a-*, priv., + *basis* step]. adj. **abasic** (-zik)/**abatic** (a-bay'tik). Cf. **astasia**, **astasia-abasia**, qv. See **standing, walking, wandering**.

abderite (ab'dər-rīt) n. a simpleton or dimwitted person inclined to scoff, laugh at everything. [< Democritus, a 5th C. B.C. Abderite, i.e., someone from Abdera in Thrace, philosopher, noted for his theory

17

of atoms, & called "the laughing philosopher"]. See **mentality, mentation, behavior**. See **intelligence**. See **role**.

abdominous (ab-dom'in-nəss) adj. fat, corpulent; having a large abdomen, protuberant belly, pot belly. (Elderly men are more obese than younger men and have higher waist-to-hip ratios than women.) [< L *abdomen* abdomen, belly; gluttony, greed + -ous, suff.]. syn. **ventricous**, q.v. Cf. **adipose, fubsy, lardy, pinguid, pursy**. See **physique, appearance**.

ablepsia (ay-blep'si-ə, -shə) n. blindness. [< G *a-*, priv., + *blepo* see]. syn. **amaurosis, cecity, cecutiency, occecation, purblind**, q.v. Cf. **hemeralopsia, idiopsia, nyctalopia**, q.v. See **eye**.

abuela (aa-boo-ayl'laa, -lə), *abuelo*(-ayl'lō) n. grandmother, grandfather. [Sp, grandmother, grandfather]. See **old woman, old man**.

abulia/aboulia (a-byool'li-ə) n. loss or impairment of the ability to perform voluntary actions or to make decisions; loss of will. [< G *a-*, priv., + *boule* will]. See **mentality, mentation, behavior**.

abus de faiblesse (aby də fɛblɛs) n.phr. exploiting frailty (of the aged). A legal term in France for elderly exploitation. [< F *abus* m. = abuse, misuse; error. *faiblesse* f. = weakness, feebleness, frailty]. See **intelligence**. See **tiredness, weakness**.

acanthosis verrucosa (ay-kan-thōs'siss ver-roo-kōs'sə) n. See **senile keratosis** (*keratosis senilis*). [acantho-, pref., denoting relationship to a spinous process, or meaning spiny or thorny, < G *akantha* thorn and L *verrucosa*, resembling a wart]. syn. = **actinic keratosis, senile** keratosis, q.v. See **skin**.

acarpous (ay-kaar'pəss) adj. fruitless, sterile. [< G *a-*, priv., + *karpos* < I-E gather (fruit)]. syn. = *agennesic*, **anandrious**, *apogenous*, q.v. See **sex, love**.

accumbent (ak-kum'bənt) adj. reclining, recumbent. • The more aged she becomes the more time she spends *accumbent*. [< L *accumbere* to take one's place at table < *ac-*, pref., = *ad-* (before c, k, & q) to, toward; near + *-cumbere* to lie down]. n. **accumbency**. See: **sleep, wakefulness**.

acedia (a-seed'di-ə) n. apathy, boredom, sloth, listlessness, carelessness; spiritual sluggishness or indifference; a state of depression (obs.). [< G *a-*, priv., + *kedos* care + < L & G *-ia*, a noun-forming suff., = a state or condition]. See **mentality, mentation, behavior**.

acedolagnia (ə-seed"dō-lag'ni-ə) n. complete indifference to sex. [< G *a-* priv., + *kedos* care + *lagneia* lust; coition]. adj. **acedolagnic**. Cf. **acokoinonia**, q.v. See **sex, love**.

acescent (ə-ses'sənt) adj. turning sour, rather sour (fig. & lit.); tending to turn acid. • The old dear became increasingly *acescent* with age. [< L *acescent-* < *acere* be sour + -ent]. See **emotion**.

acherontic (ak-ər-ron'tik) adj. cheerless, depressing. [< G mythology: Acheron, one of the rivers that ran through Hades]. See **emotion**.

achlorophyllaceous (a-klaw"rō-fil-ay'shuss) adj. colorless. • The old roué's failed humor was as *achlorophyllaceous* as his complexion. [< G *a-* priv., + *khloros* green + -phyll < *phullon* leaf + -aceous, -acean, suffs., resembling or related to, < L *-aceus*]. See **color**.

achrochordons (ak"rō-kor'donss) n.pl. skin tags: flesh-colored or pigmented lesions that are soft and often pedunculated—a benign skin tumor. They occur commonly on the neck, axillae, and trunk of the elderly. [G, *a-* priv., + *chroa* color + *chorde* cord]. See **skin**.

acokoinonia (ak"kō-koy-nōn'ni-ə) n. sex without passion or desire. [< G *akon* unwilling + *koinonia* community < *koinos* shared in common]. Cf. **acedolagnia**. See **sex, love**.

acolasia (a-kō-lay'zhə, zhee-ə) n. morbid sexual intemperance or lust. • Such *acolasia* qualifies him as a "dirty old man". [< G *akolasia* licentiousness]. See **sex, love**.

acomia (ay-kōm'mi-ə) n. baldness. [< G *a-*, priv., + *kome* hair] adj. **acomous**. See **hair**.

aconuresis (ak"kon-yoo-rees'siss) n. involuntary passage of urine, urinary incontinence. [< G *akon* unwilling + *ouresis* urination]. See **genitourinary**.

acopic(a-kop'pik) adj. relieving tiredness. [< G *a-*, priv., + *kopos* fatigue]. n. **acopic** something that relieves tiredness. See **tiredness, weakness**. See **therapy**.

acronyx (a-kron'nikss) n. an ingrown fingernail or toenail. [acr(o)-, pref., denoting relation to an extremity, top, tip, or summit, or to an extreme—G *akron*, tip, extreme—+ *onyx*, gen. *onychos*, nail]. See **joint, extremities, back**.

acrotism (ak'krō-tizm) n. absence or imperceptibility of pulsation, pulselessness. ● *Acrotism* confirmed the old codger's death. [< G *a-*, priv., + *krotos* a striking, or sound made by striking]. adj. **acrotic** (aa-krot'tik) = 1. pertaining to absence or weakness of the pulse. (2. affecting the surface. [< G *akros* extreme].) See **end-of-life, death**.

actinic keratosis (ak-tin'nik ker-ə-tōs'siss) n.phr. photo aging from chronic UV (ultraviolet) radiation: a dyskeratotic (premalignant) warty, scaly lesion occurring usually on the sun-exposed skin of face or hands in aged, light-skinned persons [< G *aktis* (*actin-*) a ray + *kerat(o)-*, pref., horn + *-osis*, suff., condition]. syns. **acanthosis verrucosa**; actinic or **senile elastosis**, q.v.; solar keratosis; senile keratoma or wart; verruca plana senilis; and verruca senilis. See **skin**.

acyesis (ay-sī-ees'siss) n. female sterility. [< G *a-*, priv. + *cyesis* pregnancy]. syn. = **atocia**, q.v. See **sex, love**.

ADAM syndrome n.phr. an initialism: Androgen Deficiency in the Aging Male, is associated with inadequate testicular androgen production resulting in a bioavailable testosterone level < 70ng/dL (2.4nmol/L), which can be associated with loss of libido, diminished muscle mass, and muscle strength, plus diminished energy and well-being. Testosterone declines with age by about 100 ng/dL/ decade after age 50, but bioavailable (unbound) testosterone declines far more dramatically, and testosterone-binding globulin increases with age. Loss of sperm quantity and quality can occur with age. Testosterone treatment may be indicated. (Merck Manual of Geriatrics). See **sex, love**. See **genitourinary**.

adamantine (ad-ə-man'teen, -tin) adj. 1. unyielding, firm. (2. like a diamond in hardness or luster.) ● He tried to get her to smile, but the *adamantine* **grimalkin** remained sour faced. [< G *adamas*, *adamantos*; untamable; *a-*, priv., + *daman* to conquer]. See **mentality, mentation, behavior**.

addle (ad'dəl) adj. 1. muddled, unsound (addlebrained, **addlepated**, q.v.). (2. empty, vain. 3. {of an egg} **addled**, q.v.) [OE *adela* filth, used as adj. then verb]. **addle** vt. to muddle, confuse. (**addle** vi.{of an egg} become addled.) See **addled** under **intelligence**.

addled (ad'dləd) adj. 1. muddled. (2. {of an egg} rotten, producing no chick.) See **addle**, adj., assimilated to pp. form. See **intelligence**.

addlepated (ad'dəl-payt'təd) adj. muddle-headed, confused. [OE *adela* filth, used as adj. then verb + pate (payt) n. (colloc. or joc.) 1. the top of the head. 2. the head, especially representing the seat of intellect; ME, origin unknown]. Syn. addlebrained. See **intelligence**.

adianoeta (aa-dī"ə-nō-et'tə) n. an expression that has an obvious meaning and an unsuspected secret one beneath. E.g., "I hear you have just published a new book; I'll waste no time in reading it." Or, re: the President Clinton-Monica Lewinsky affair: "It blows me away." adj. **adianoetic**. [< G *a-*, privative + *dianoetikos* of or pertaining to thinking]. Cf. *double entendre*, **subintelligitur**, q.v. See **talk**.

adipose (ad'di-poss) adj. containing fat; fatty; fat. **adipose** n. fat under the skin and surrounding organs; fat in the cells of adipose tissue. [< L *adiposus* fatty < *adip-*, stem of *adeps* fat]. n. **adiposity** (ad-di-pos'i-tee) n. **adiposeness**. syn. **fubsy**, **lardy**, **pinguid**, q.v. Cf. **abdominous**, **ventricous**; **pursy**, q.v. See **physique, appearance**.

adjunct (aj'junkt) adj. a thing added; not full time; secondary and not essential. ● Mr. Chips, now retired, continued as an *adjunct* professor at the college. [ad-, pref., < L *ad* to + *jungere* to join]. See **role**.

advesperate (ad-vess'pur-ayt) vi. to draw toward evening (obs.)— used fig.: approaching the end of life. [< L *ad-* to, toward + *vespera* evening < *vesper* evening star]. See **end-of-life & death**.

aesthetics/esthetics (es-thet'tikss) pl.n.—used singularly. (1. that branch of philosophy dealing with beauty.) 2. plastics, i.e., plastic surgery, aesthetic dentistry, and, more recently, aesthetic dermatology. (Plastic surgery is that branch of surgery having to do with the repair of defects, or the results of loss of tissue by direct union of parts, grafting, transfer of tissue from one part to another, etc.) (**Aesthetic physicians** do facelifts, nose jobs, breast augmentation; use Botox, a peripheral nerve blocker to erase wrinkles, **rugae** (temporarily); inject plastic fillers such as Juvéderm® and Restylane® for wrinkle abatement, skin depressions; employ laser treatments for skin blemishes, tattoos, etc.; perform chemical peels for skin smoothing; advertise facial rejuvenation; *et hoc genus omne*.) • *Aesthetics* is a branch of medicine appealing particularly to the aged. [< G *aesthesis* sensation. < G *plastikos* relating to molding]. adj. **aesthetic/esthetic**. Cf. **plastics**. See **therapy**. See **physique, appearance**.

aetate provectus (ī-taat'tay prō-wek'tuss) adj.phr. a collation meaning of advanced age, advanced in years. [< L *aetas, -atis* age + *provectus* advanced.]. Cf. **d'un certain age**. See **old**.

afforient (af-for'ri-ənt) n. & adj. a state of confusion, wandering. • The retirement home's occupants were not surprised by that particular lady's *afforient* behavior. [af-, pref., = ad- before f]. See **mentality, mentation, behavior**. See **standing, walking, wandering**.

agapism (aag'gə-piz-əm) n. The doctrine that exalts nonsexual (brotherly) love. [< G *agape* brotherly love]. See **sex, love**.

agathobiothik(ag"ə-thŏ-bī'ō-thik) n. the good life [< G *agatho* good + bio- pref., < G *bios* life +? suff. -*thik*?]. See **retirement**. See **work, activity**.

age (ayj) vi. show signs of advancing age; grow old; mature. [< L *aetas, -atis* age]. syns. become old, decline, deteriorate, develop, get old, get along (in years), grow old, grow up, mature, mellow, push, ripen, senesce, wane. See **old**. See **old age**.

aged (ayj'jəd) adj. (1. of the age of.) 2. having lived long, old. [probably < F *âgé*. See **age** vi.]. adv. **agedly**. n. **agedness**. syns. advanced in years, ancient, **antediluvian**, decrepit, elderly, getting along or on, gray, having or with one foot in the grave, **hoary**, immemorial, matured, mellowed, old, old as the hills, over the hill, ripened, **senescent, superannuated**. Syn. **sear**, q.v. See **old**.

ageism/agism (ayj'jiz-əm) n. 1. discrimination or prejudice against people of a particular age, especially of old people, and especially in employment. 2. the celebration of youth and good looks vs. the relative invisibility of older people, as seen, e.g., in advertising. ● Such aversive *ageism* is beneath you. [var. OF *aage* < L *aetat-*, pref., period of life; coined by Robert Butler, a Pulitzer Prize winner]. adj. **ageist**. See **old age**. See **mentality, mentation, behavior**.

agelast (aj'jə-last) n. a person who never laughs. [< F *agélast*, a neologism of Rabelais (C. H. Elster) < G *gelao* to laugh]. See **mentality, mentation, behavior**. See **role**.

agennesic (a-jən-nees'sik) adj. sterile; impotent. [< G *a-* priv. + *genesis* production]. n. **agenesia** (aj"jən-ee'zhə, -zee-ə) = sterility, impotency. [G, sexual impotence]. syn. = **acarpous**, **anandrious**, **apogenous**, q.v. See **sex**.

agerasia (a-jə-ray'zhə, -zhee-ə) n. youthful appearance in an older person, looking younger than one's age; not appearing to age. [< G eternal youth < *a-* priv. + *geras* old age]. syn. **neanimorphism**, q.v. ant. **geromorphism**, q.v. Cf. **paedomorphism**, q.v. See: **physique, appearance**. See **old age**.

ageing/aging in place n.phr. a collocation indicating a recent phenomenon: the preference of the elderly for remaining in their homes rather than moving to a retirement home or assisted living center. See **retirement**.

AGNES (ag'nes) an initialism: <u>a</u>ge <u>g</u>ain <u>n</u>ow <u>e</u>mpathy <u>s</u>ystem, an age-empathy suit. See **gray tech**.

agnosia (ag-nō'zhə, –zhee-ə) n. loss of the power to recognize the import of sensory stimuli. The varieties of agnosia correspond to the several senses and are distinguished as auditory or acoustic, visual, olfactory, gustatory, and tactile. (Other varieties of agnosia are: body-image ~ {autotopagnosia}: loss of body-image sense, finger ~: loss of ability to indicate fingers, ideational ~: loss of the spatial associations which make up the idea of an object from its component ideas, time ~: loss of comprehension of the succession and duration of events.) [G ignorance < *a-*, pref., priv. + *gnosis* knowledge]. See **health& illness**.

agomphious (a-gom'fi-əss) adj. toothless. [< G *a-* priv. + *gomphos* bolt, nail-peg & socket articulation, as a tooth in the alveolar socket]. syn. **edentate**, q.v. See **mouth, gums, & teeth**.

agonistes (ag-ō-niss'teez) adj. pertaining to one engaged in a struggle—this adj. is placed *after* the modified noun. • An apropos term for an elderly person engaged in a struggle with, e.g., osteoporosis or malignancy or Alzheimer's: Ronald Reagan *agonistes*. [G *agonistes* < *agon* struggle, contest. (The term refers to John Milton's "Samson Agonistes", a tragedy depicting the final phase of Sampson's life when he is blind and a captive of the Philistines.)]. n. **agonist** (ag'gən-ist). adj. **agonistic** (ag"gən-is'tik). adv. **agonistically**. See **mentality, mentation, behavior**. See **role**.

agrypnia (a-grip'ni-ə) n. insomnia. There is a recent medical device that induces slow brain and deep-sleep waves in sleeping patients by a technique called "transcranial magnetic stimulation"; it may restore deep sleep in patients with insomnia. [G, sleeplessness < *agreo* to hunt after + *hypnos* sleep]. adj. **agrypnic**. syns.: See **sleep & wakefulness**.

agrypnocoma (a-grip"nō-kōm'mə) n. an apathetic, lethargic state approaching coma. [< G *agrypnos* sleepless + *koma* coma]. See **sleep & wakefulness**.

agrypnotic (a-grip-not'tik) adj. sleepless: marked by, or suffering from insomnia. n. that which drives sleep away. [G *agrypnos* sleepless + -ic]. n. **agrypnode** = a drug that prevents sleep, drives sleep away. See **sleep & wakefulness**.

ahypnia (ay-hip'ni-ə) or **ahypnosis** (ay-hip-nō'siss) n. insomnia. [G < *a*- priv. + *hypnos* sleep]. adj. **ahypnic**. See **sleep & wakefulness**.

aide-mémoire (ɛd-memwar) (pl. **aides-mémoire** {ɛd-memwar}) n. 1. a note, memorandum written as a memory help, aid (esp. in diplomatic use). (2. revision notes {pl.}—for an examination.) See: **memory**.

aidoi(o)mania (ī-doy"yō-mayn'ni-ə) n. strong and/or abnormal sexual desire. [aidoi(o)- (alt. ede{o}-), pref., relating to the genitals, < G *aidoia* genitals + *mania* frenzy]. adj.

aidoi(o)maniacal (-mə-nī'ə-kəl). n. **aidoi(o)maniac**. syn. **edeomania**, q.v. Cf. **erotomania**, q.v. See **manias**. See **sex**.

akathisia (ayk"-ka-thi'zhə, -zhee-ə) n. a neurosis characterized by an inability to remain in a sitting position; motor restlessness and a feeling of muscular quivering. This can occur as a side effect of antipsychotic drugs, resulting in behavioral disturbances and awakening. [G -a, pref., priv. + *kathisis* a sitting]. syn. **acathisia, akathizia**. See **nerve, muscle, movement, touch**. See **sleep**.

alcoholomania (alk"kō-hawl"ō-mayn'ni-ə) n. abnormal interest in alcohol; dypsomania. [< Arabic *al* the + *kohl* a fine antimonial powder, the term being applied first to a fine powder, then, to anything impalpable (a spirit) + < G *mania* frenzy, madness, loss of reason < *mainesthai* to rage]. **alcoholomaniacal** (-mə-nī'ə-kəl). n. **alcoholomaniac**. syn. **dipsomania, methomania, posiomania**, q.v. Cf. **oenomania**. See **manias**. See **drink, food**. See **role**.

alector (ayl-lek'tor) n. a person who is unable to sleep. [< G *alektor* cock: it awakens one, keeps one awake]. See **sleep & wakefulness**. See **role**.

algophobia (al"gō-fōb'bi-ə) n. abnormal fear of or sensitiveness to pain. [algo-, pref., meaning pain, < G *algos* pain, + *phobos* fear]. adj. **algophobic**. n. **algophobe**. syn. **odynophobia**, q.v. See **phobias**. See **pain**.

alieni juris (al-i-ayn'nee yoŏr'riss) adj.phr. under the control of another because one is either mentally incompetent (or below legal age). [L, *alieni* of another's own + *juris* right, law]. ant. *sui juris* (soŏ'ī yoŏr'riss), q.v. See: **end-of-life, death**. See: **finance**. See **role**.

alieniloquent (ayl"li ən-il'lō-kwent) adj. speaking discursively or straying from the point. [< L *alienare* to estrange, make irrational + *loqui* to speak]. adv. **alieniloquently**. n. **alieniloquence**. See **talk**.

allochroous (al-lok'krō-əs) adj. multicolored; changing color. • Upon seeing her a second time, the elderly lady's allochroous hair attracted the detective's attention. [allo-, pref., other, different, alternate < G *allos* other < I-E other of more than two + < G *khroma* color + -ous, suff.]. See **color**. See **physique, appearance**.

alogism (al'lō-jiz-əm) n. an unreasonable, illogical statement or thought. [< G *a-*, pref., not. + *logos*, word, reason]. (n. **alogia** = inability to speak due to a central nervous system {brain} lesion.) See **talk**. See **mentality, mentation, behavior**.

alopecia (al"lə-pee'shə, al"lō-, -pee'shee-ə, -shee-aa) n. baldness, whether partial or complete. (This is the standard medical term for baldness, which recently has been found associated with two genes: one {labeled AR}, is on the X chromosome and is maternally inherited; if one's maternal grandfather was bald, one has a 50% chance of being bald. The other, a gene variation on chromosome 20, is neither dominant nor recessive, but additive; one inherits one copy of chromosome 20 from each of one's parents; inheriting the bald variation from both parents renders one 6.1 times more likely to show early hair loss—heir unapparent!) [< G *alopekia* a disease like fox mange < *alopex* a fox]. syns. **acomia**, **atrichia**, **calvites**, **depilous**, **phalacrosis**, **pilgarlic**, **poliosis**, **psilosis**, q.v. See <u>hair</u>.

alopeciaphobia (al"lō-pee'shee-ə-fōb'bi-ə) n. morbid fear of becoming bald. [G *alopecia* a disease like fox mange < *alopex* a fox + *phobos* fear]. syn. **peladophobia**, **phalacrophobia**, q.v. See <u>phobias</u>. See <u>hair</u>.

alphamegamia (al"fə-mə-gam'mi-ə) n. marriage between a young woman and an older man. (Should the wife be beautiful, she may recently be denominated a "trophy wife".) [< G, *alpha* the letter *a*, i.e., the beginning, the first + mega-, comb. form of G *megas* great + *gamos* marriage]. See <u>marriage</u>.

alter Kocker (awl'tər kok'kər) n.phr. "[a] canny stubborn old man who has been around but has ended up as an old fart. Or shrewd buzzard." (David Grambs); an old inept, forgetful over-the-hill guy. An *alter Kocker* may still be sexually active. [< Ger. < L *alter* other + Yid. < Ger. *Kocker*, lit., "old defecator"]. See <u>old man</u>.

Alzheimer's disease, dementia (altz'hīm-merz) n. a primary degenerative dementia of insidious onset and a gradually progressive course, occurring almost always after the age of 50; it's classified as presenile or senile onset depending on whether occurrence is before or after age 65. Alzheimer's disease is the most common form of dementia affecting the elderly; an estimated 5.3 million Americans have the disease. Some nine genes have been linked or associated with Alzheimer's disease. The pathology is usually of the Alzheimer's type, but occasionally of the Pick's type. What kills the brain cells in Alzheimer's disease has been blamed on five suspects: beta amyloid, found abundantly deposited; **ApoE4**, q.v.; N-APP, an amyloid cousin; neurofibrillary tangles; presinilin, two weakened proteins that usually help neurons function properly; and weakened mitochondria. A new suspect in causation is oxysteroids, i.e., cholesterol breakdown products, but which ones and how they operate are under study. Recently (April, 2010) a panel of experts from the National Institutes of Health reported "there are still no known preventive measures effective in halting Alzheimer's onset." The panel found no supplements, e.g., gingko biloba or fish oil, that are effective in prevention of the disease. The Alzheimer's Association points out that "most current research does link heart disease and hypertension with the increased risk of Alzheimer's.", and an Association spokesman stated, "Reduction of your risk of heart disease in middle life, even in late life, can help you reduce your risk of cognitive decline. Chronic diseases, such as diabetes and depression, and risk factors, such as smoking, are associated with increased risk of both Alzheimer's disease and cognitive decline." But, "studies have not yet demonstrated that these medical or lifestyle factors actually cause or prevent Alzheimer's disease or cognitive decline, only that they are related." Recently, levels of three substances found in spinal fluid are thought to be diagnostic of Alzheimer's: low amyloid, high phosphorylated tau, and low amyloid-beta.

Formal diagnosis is currently not possible until autopsy. A new plaque-imaging drug, Amyvid is being tested by Eli Lilly & Co. using proton-imaging tomography (PET) to "light up" areas of the brain containing beta amyloid; the diagnostic test is promising, and Lilly has obtained FDA approval for marketing the agent. Mental activity—reading, working crosswords—is likely to delay Alzheimer's onset, but once it occurs, its progress is more rapid in those mentally active. Being bilingual, for some reason, seems to stave off dementia's onset by, on average, four years by increasing "cognitive reserve", i.e., an ability to work even when a brain is stressed or damaged: The brain retains cognitive reserve, can stop paying attention to one thing while concentrating on something else. In mice, GSAP, the gene directing gamma-secretase-activating protein, which directs gamma secretase to produce the beta-amyloid plaques of Alzheimer's, can be blocked so that amyloid doesn't form; the mice stay healthy and plaqueless. There is no GSAP work done as yet in humans. An increased high-density cholesterol (HDL—"good" cholesterol) level in humans seems protective of Alzheimer's; an optimal level = 60mg/dl. "Five medications have been approved to treat the cognitive symptoms of Alzheimer's disease." Drugs used in treating Alzheimer's include Namenda (memantine), Razadyne (reminyl galantamine), **Exelon** (rivastigmine), q.v., **Aricept** (donepezil), q.v., Citicholine, Citicoline Cognizen (citicoline), and Cognex (tacrine). They may decrease certain symptoms especially early in the disease, but aren't effective for all and are not permanently curative. Angiotensin-receptor blockers are currently under review for treatment of Alzheimer's, as is electrical stimulation of the entorhinal cortex, which leads to the hippocampus, a memory center in the brain. A drug for treatment, crenezumab, is under study. [< Alois Alzheimer, German neurologist, 1864-1915]. See **APOE, donepezil, Rember®, CLU, PICALM**. See <u>intelligence</u>.

amadelphous (am-ə-del'fəss) adj. talkative, sociable, gregarious [< L *amator* lover < *amare* to love + < G *delphin* dolphin?]. See <u>talk</u>. See <u>mentality & mentation</u>.

amasesis (am-ə-sees'siss) n. inability to chew. [a- priv. + < L *mastico*, pp. –*atus* to chew]. See <u>mouth, gums, & teeth</u>.

amaurosis (am-aw-rōs'siss) n. blindness [< G *amauros* dark, obscure + -*osis* condition]. syn. **ablepsia, cecity, cecutiency**, q.v. See <u>eye</u>.

amaurosis fugax (am"maw-rōs'siss fyoog'gaks) n.phr. a transient episode of blindness or partial blindness lasting less than 10 min.; it may be due to transient retinal ischemia secondary to cerebral arterial disease, and popularly called "blackouts", (or to centrifugal force, e.g., "flight blindness", or visual blackout without loss of consciousness, in aviators.) [< G *amauros* dark, obscure + L *fugax* fleeting, swift, passing, transitory]. See <u>eye</u>.

ambagious (am-bayj'jəss) adj. 1. circumlocutory, circuitous, roundabout. 2. tortuous. [< L *ambages* winding, labyrinth; double-talk, evasion, digression; ambiguity; obscurity (*per ambages* = enigmatically]. adv. **ambagiously**. n. **ambagiousness**. See <u>talk</u>.

ambulophobia (amb"byoo-lō-fōb'bi-ə) n. morbid fear of walking. [< L *ambulare* to walk, travel, traverse + < G *phobos* fear]. adj. ambulophobic. n. ambulophobe. syn. **basiphobia** or **basophobia**, **basistasiphobia**, q.v. Cf. **stasibasiphobia, stasiphobia**, q.v. See <u>phobias</u>. See <u>standing, walking, wandering</u>.

AMD n. an initialism for <u>a</u>ge-related <u>m</u>acular <u>d</u>egeneration. A current experimental treatment is with a pea-sized telescope implanted in the cornea. It's estimated to help the macular blindness of one-fifth of those with the condition. (It is made by VisionCare Ophthalmic Technologies in Saratoga, CA, and awaiting full FDA approval.) (The initialism is one letter short of AMDG: Ad majorem Dei gloriam: To the greater glory of God, the Jesuit motto in Latin.) [L *macula*, a stain, spot, or thickening]. See: **eye**.

amnesia (am-nee'zhə) n. loss of memory. [G *amnesia*, alteration of *amnestia* forgetfulness < *amnestos* not remembered < *mnasthei* to remember]. See **memory**.

amnesiophobia (am-nee"zhə-fōb'bi-ə) n. fear of amnesia, forgetting. [G *amnesia*, forgetfulness + *phobia* fear]. adj. **amnesiophobic**. n. **amnesiophobe**. See **phobias**. See **memory**.

amphibology (am"fə-bol'lə-jee)/**amphiboly** (am-fib'ə-lee), n.pls. **–ogies/-olies**, n. ambiguous speech or wording; quibble; a phrase or sentence subject to dual interpretation due to grammatical construction—not due to hidden meaning, i.e. **adianoeta**, q.v., e.g. • At the nursing home Dick and Joe thought of asking Mary and *his* sister, Jane, to play bridge, but they decided against it. [< L *amphibologia* ambiguity < *amphibolia* < G *amphibolos* ambiguous < amphi-, pref., both, via L < G *amphi* on both sides + -*logia* speech]. (Note: "amphibole" {am'fə-bol"} is a mineral.) adj. **amphibological** (-bō- loj'ji-kəl). adj. **amphibolous** (am-fib'bə-ləss). adv. **amphibologically** (-loj'ji-kəl-lee) See **talk**.

amyous (am'mī-uss) adj. without strength. [< G a- priv. + *mys* muscle]. See **tiredness, weakness**.

an- pref. = **a-** before vowels or h, without; not, priv. [G, a- priv., without; not].

anabiotic (an-ə-bī-ot'tik) adj. apparently dead, but capable of being revived, resuscitative, restorative. n. a powerful stimulant, a revivifying remedy. n. **anabiosis** = resuscitation, return to life, after apparent death. [< G a reviving < *ana* again, toward + *biosis* life]. See **end-of-life, death**.

anaclitic (an-ə-klit'tik) adj. overly dependent on another. [< G *ana* toward, again + *klinein* to lean]. See **mentality & mentation**.

anacusis/anakusis (an'na-kus'siss) n. totally without hearing. syn. **anacusia**. [G *an-*, priv. + *akousis*, hearing]. See **hearing**.

anagapesis (an"nə-ga-pees'siss) n. lack of interest in former loved ones. [an-, priv., q.v., + G *agape* brotherly love]. See **mentality, mentation, behavior**. See **sex, love**.

anamnesis (an-am-nees'siss) n. 1. the act of remembering. 2. the previous, past medical history of a patient. [G, recollection]. See **memory**.

anamnestic (an-am-ness'tik) adj. 1. reminiscent; aiding the memory; mnemonic. 2. relating to the **anamnesis**, q.v. [< G *anamnesis* recollection]. See **memory**.

anandrious (an-an'dri-əss) adj. sterile. syns. *acarpous*, *agennesic*, *apogenous*, q.v. See **sex, love**.

anaphalantiasis (an"nə-fal"lən-tī'ə-siss) n. the falling out of the eyebrows, i.e. supercilia, < *super* above + *cilium* eyelid. [ana- < G *ana* up; toward; apart, again + *phalanx* a line or array of soldiers + -iasiss, a suff. meaning a process or the condition resulting therefrom < G *-sis* denoting an action, process or condition, and appearing in the suffixes *-asis*, *-esis*, *-iasis*, and *-osis*]. See **eye**.

anaphroditous (an-af'frō-dish'əss) adj. without sexual desire. [an-, q.v., + < G *aphrodisia* sexual pleasures < the goddess Aphrodite + -ous, suff., possessing, having or full of]. See **sex, love**.

anatripsis (an-ə-trip'siss) n. therapeutic use of friction, i.e., rubbing, with or without simultaneous application of a medicament. [G, a rubbing, < *ana* up, toward + *tribo* fut. of *tripso* to rub]. **See therapy**.

anautarchia (an-ow-taar'ki-ə) n. perpetual unhappiness. (Based on etymology lack of self-control would seem an alternative definition with unhappiness a predictable result.) [an-, pref., q.v., + < G *autarkhos* self governing]. See **anhedonia**. See **emotion**.

ancientry (ayn'shen-tree) n. (obs., rare) 1. the quality or state of being ancient or very old; ancientness, antiquity; old-fashioned style; seniority, priority. 2. ancient lineage. 3. a collective: ancients, elder people, elders. 4. antiquity. 5. pl. or collective: ancient things, relics, antiquities. (Shakespeare's shepherd in "The Winter's Tale" lamented adolescents "getting wenches with child, wronging the **ancientry**, stealing, fighting.") [< ancient + -ry, < F *ancien* < L *antianum* for *anteanum* former, previous < *ante* before + -(e)ry, suff., 1. activity or behavior, 2. collection of, 3. quality or character of, 4. state, condition]. See **old age, old person(s)**.

androgogy (an'drǝ-gō-jee) n. the science of teaching adults. • *Androgogy* should be an applied science in **gerontocomiums**, q.v. [< L *andro-* man + *agogos* guide]. adj. **androgogic** (an"drǝ—gōj'jik), adj. **androgogical** (an"drǝ—gōj'ji-kǝl). adv. **androgogically** (an"drǝ—gōj'). n. **androgogue** (an') = a teacher of adults. See **innovation, meisoneism**. See **work, activity**. See **role**.

andropause (an'drō-pawz") n. changes in older men such as loss of muscle mass, decline in bone-marrow density, loss of libido due to a decrease or deficiency in testosterone, i.e., late-onset hypogonadism—somewhat comparable to and a word borrowing from menopause. However, the relationship of testosterone level to andropausal symptoms, e.g., fatigue, weakness, depression, sexual problems, is problematic, controversial, as is replacement therapy, which has risks of its own. A drug recently approved by the FDA for testosterone replacement is Fortesta®, a 2% testosterone gel. Low testosterone level is not only associated with erectile dysfunction and infertility, but also with osteoporosis and muscle loss. [< L *andro-* man + < G *pauein* stop, cease]. adj. **andropausal**. Cf. **viripause**, q.v. syn. **male menopause**. See **sex, love**.

anecdotage (an'nek-dō-tej) n. (1. anecdotes, personally told stories, short accounts of an incident or event.) 2. (jocularly) garrulous old age. [< G *anekdota* things unpublished < *an-* not + *ekdidonai* to publish + –age, suff., condition < OF < assumed Vulgar L *-aticum* < *-aticus*, suff. forming adjs.]. See **old age**.

anemophobia (an"nǝ-mō-fōb'bi-ǝ) n. morbid fear of and sensitivity to wind, drafts. [< G *anemos* wind + *phobos* fear]. adj. **anemophobic**. n. **anemophobe**. See **phobias**.

anencephalia (an"nen-se-fal'li-ǝ) n. the condition of brainlessness (fig.). [an-, pref., q.v., + < G *encephal(o)-*, comb., indicating the brain or some relationship thereto + -ia, suff.]. adj. **anencephalic** = having no brain. See **intelligence**.

anencephalotrophia (an"nen-sef"fə-lŏ-trŏf'fi-ə) n. arophy of the brain, i.e., a wasting away of brain tissue. [an-, q.v., + < G *encephal(o)*-, comb., indicating the brain or some relationship thereto + *trophe* nourishment + -ia, suff.]. See **intelligence**.

anfractuous (an-frak'choo-əss) adj. circuitous; twisting; turning.
• With age her stories became increasingly anfractuous. [< L *anfractuosus* < *anfractus* bending]. n. **anfractuosity** (an"frak-choo-os'sə-tee), **-ties**. See **talk**.

angina (an'ji-nə) n. 1. sore throat. 2. a severe constricting pain, especially in the anterior left chest, and due to reduced coronary arterial blood flow: **angina pectoris**. adj. **anginal**. [L (via G *agkhone* strangling) spasmotic, choking, or suffocative pain, e.g., quinsy, i.e., severe sore throat, peritonsillar abscess, but now used almost exclusively to indicate chest pain due to heart, coronary arterial, disease, i.e., angina pectoris; pectoris < *pectoralis* < *pecttus* breast bone]. See **pain**. See **heart, rhythm**.

anginophobia (an"ji-nō-fōb'bi-ə) n. morbid fear of having a heart attack. [< G *agkhone* strangling + < G -phobia, suff., fearing < -*phobia* < *phobos* fear]. adj. **angiophobic**. n. **anginophobe**. Cf. **cardiophobia**, q.v. See **phobias**.

angioplasty (an"ji-ō-plas'tee, an"jee-ə-plas'tee) n. an angiographic (x-ray) procedure for elimination of areas of narrowing in blood vessels, often coronary (heart) arteries, using a balloon catheter. [angio-, pref., denoting relationship to a vessel, usually a blood vessel, < G *angeion* vessel + *plassein* to form]. adj. **angioplastic**. See **blood, circulation, & glands**. See **heart, rhythm**.

anhedonia (an-hi-dōn'ni-ə) n. the inability to be happy; absence of pleasure from the performance of acts that would ordinarily be pleasurable. [*an-*, pref., q.v., + < G *hedone* pleasure]. See **anautarchia**. See **emotion**. See **mentation, mentality, behavior**.

anhelation (an-hə-lay'shən) n. 1. panting, breathlessness; **dyspneic**, q.v. 2. a breathless or eager wanting, desire. (A new air-pump device exists that can effect breathing through the nose even for people unable to breathe on their own due to lack of control of respiratory musculature. The pump is controlled by the patient's soft palate that blocks and releases nasal air flow.) [< L *anhelatio* panting, puffing, difficulty breathing]. See **breathing**.

anicular (an-ik'kyoo-law) adj. old-womanish, weak; feeble minded. [< L *anilis* < *anus*, *-us* old woman, "venerable woman"; hag (N.B., *anus*, *-i* = ring, anus; rectum)]. See **old woman**.

anile (an'īl) adj. old-womanish; lacking in force, strength, or effectiveness; faltering; imbecilic. n. **anile** a woman of advanced years; in one's dotage, imbecile. n. **anility**, q.v. [< L *anilis* < *anus*, *-us*, old woman]. See **old woman**.

anililagnia (an-nīl"li-lag'ni-ə) n. love of a much older woman. [< L *anile* < *anus*, *-us*, old woman + G *lagneia* lust, coition—*lagneia furor* = extreme sex urge]. See **sex, love**.

anility (an-il'lə-tee) n. dotage, imbecility in an old woman. [< G *anus*, *-us* old woman]. See **intelligence**.

anilojuvenogamy (an"ni-lō-joov"vin-og'gə-mee) n. marriage between an older woman and a young man. [neologism of C. H. Elster: < L *anilis* of an old woman + *juvenis*, *-e* young man + < G *gamos* marriage]. (The counterpart is marriage of an older man to a young woman: **alphamegamia**, q.v. See **anisonogamia**.) See **marriage**.

animadversion (an"ni-mad-vur'zhən) n. a sensorious comment or adverse remark; criticism; reproach, reproof, blame, censure. [< L *animadvertere* to turn the mind toward < *animus* mind + *advertere* to turn toward < *vertere* to turn]. adj. **animadversional**. vi. **animadvert**. See **talk**.

anisonogamia (an-īs"sō-nō-gam'mi-ə) n. marriage between persons of unequal age, especially with a considerable age difference. [an-, pref., q.v., + < G *isonomos* < iso-, pref., equal, uniform < *isos* equal + *nomos* law + *gamos* marriage]. See **marriage**.

anisosthenic (an-īs"soss-then'nik) adj. of unequal force, strength. [< G aniso- < *anisos* unequal + *sthenos* strength]. n. **anisosthenia**. See **nerve, muscle, movement, touch**.

ankylosed (ang'ki-lōsd, -kə-) adj. fused or obliterated as a joint. [< G *ankylos* bent or crooked]. See **joint, extremities, back**.

ankylosis (ang-ki-lōs'siss, -kə-) n. (n.pl. **ankyloses**) stiffness or immobility and consolidation of a joint due to disease, injury, or surgical procedure. [G] See **joint, extremities, back**.

anomia (aa-nōm'mi-ə) n. inability to remember names. [a(n)-, pref., q.v., + < G *nomos* name]. syn. = **lethonomia**, q.v. Cf. **dysnomia**, q.v. See **memory**.

anorectic (an"ō-rek'tik) adj. 1. pertaining to lack of appetite. 2. a substance that decreases appetite. n. **anorexia** (-rek'see-ə). [< G *anorektos* without appetite for]. See **gastrointestinal**.

anosognosia (an-ōs"sog-nōs'si-'ə) n. unawareness or denial of a disease, or of one's disease, especially a neurological one. [< G *a-*, priv., + *nosos* disease + *gnosis* knowledge + -ia, L & G noun-forming suff. denoting a state or condition]. See **health, illness**. Cf. **agnosia**, **pathocryptia**, q.v.

anosmia (an-oss'mi-ə) n. loss or impairment of the sense of smell; olfactory anesthesia. [a(n)-, q.v., + < G *osme* sense of smell]. adj. **anosmic** (-mik). See: **nose & smell**.

anosodiaphoria (a-nōs"so-dī-ə-for'ri-ə) n. indifference, real or assumed, regarding the presence of disease, specifically of paralysis. [a(n)-, q.v., + < G *nosos* disease + *diaphoria* difference]. syn. **anosognosia**, q.v. See **mentality, mentation, behavior**.

anosognosia (an-os"sog-nō'zhə, zhee-ə) n. the lack of interest or belief in the existence of one's disease. [G a(n)-, q.v., + < G *nosos* disease + *gnosis* knowledge]. syn. = **anosodiaphoria**, q.v. See **mentality, mentation, behavior**.

anserine (an'sər-īne) adj. resembling or acting like a goose; silly; stupid. [< L *anserinus* < *anser* goose]. adv. **anserinely**. See **intelligence**.

antediluvian (an"ti-di-loov'vee-ən) adj., fig., utterly out of date, extremely old; lit., before the Biblical Flood, deluge. [< L *ante-* before + *diluvium* flood]. See **old**.

anticholinergic (an"ti-kol-in-ur'jik) adj. antagonistic to the action of parasympathetic or other cholinergic nerve fibers. (Many antihistamines, the mainstay of treatment for allergy, have anticholinergic properties that are especially prominent and worrisome in the elderly: sedation, dry mouth, orthostatic hypotension, constipation, urinary retention, confusion. Only **antihistamines**, q.v., without anticholinergic effect, e.g., astemizole, cetirizine, fexofenadine, and loratadine, should be used in the elderly (Merck Manual of Geriatrics). [anti-, pref., signifying against, opposing, < G *anti* against + choline (an organic chemical compound found in most animal tissues either free or in combination) < *chole* bile + < *ergon* work]. See **nose & smell**.

antihistamines (an"ti-his'tə-meenss) n.pl. drugs having an action antagonistic to that of histamine, and used in the treatment of allergic symptoms. These drugs (see **anticholinergic**) are used to treat the nasal congestion, obstruction, and rhinorrhea common in the elderly. See **nose & smell**.

antinomian (an"ti-nōm'mi-ən) n. & adj. a Christian believing—or Christian belief—that faith and divine grace alone will see one through eschatologically, i.e., through death, judgment, heaven, or hell. [< G *antinomia* < *anti-* priv. + *nomos* law]. n. **antinomianism** 1. a belief that Christians are not bound by established laws, especially moral laws, but should rely on faith and divine grace for salvation. 2. the belief that it is impossible to apply a universal moral code because it will have a different meaning for different people. See **mentality, mentation, behavior**.

antiquary (an'tee-kwair"ree) n. a collector, or scholar, or seller of, or dealer in antiques or antiquities. [< L *antiquarius* < *antiquus* old]. adj. **antiquarian** (an"tee-kwair'ri-ən). n. **antiquarian**. n. **antiquarianism**. See **role**.

antiquate (an'ti-kwāt) vt. 1. to cause something to become out of date or old by replacing it with something newer. 2. to **antique**, qv. • The arrival of these new-comers to the nursing home has *antiquated* us old-timers even further. [< L *antiquarius* < *antiquus* old].

antiquated (an'ti-kwayt"ted) adj. extremely out of date, or badly in need of updating or replacing. [< L *antiquatus* antiquated]. n. **antiquatedness** (an"ti-kway'ted-ness). See **old**.

antique (an-teek') n. 1. a valuable collectible old item, e.g., a piece of furniture, jewelry, china. 2. an art object, especially a classical one such as a painting, sculpture. adj. 1. made long ago, perhaps classical; old-fashioned (informal). vt. treat something, particularly something new, so that it looks antique or worn with time. adv. **antiquely**. n. **antiqueness**. [< L *antiquus* old]. See **old**.

antiquity (an-tik' kwə-tee) n. 1. the state of being very old or ancient. (2. ancient, especially classical, history. 3. an object, especially something collectible, decorative, valuable, or interesting that dates from a previous era. 4. the people of ancient civilizations, especially of ancient, classical Greece and Rome.) [< L *antiquitas* antiquity]. See **old age**.

antithalian (an-ti-thayl'li-ən) adj. against enjoyment. [< G *anti-* against + *Thalia*, the muse of comedy]. See **emotion**.

anxiolytic (ang-zī"ə-lit'tik) adj. serving to reduce anxiety. [circa 1960 < L *anxius* < *anx-* pp. of *angere* to torment, literally strangle + -lytic, suff., denoting lysis, i.e. cellular destruction, of the substance indicated by the stem to which it is affixed, < G *lutikos* able to loosen, dissolving < *luein* to loosen]. See **emotion**.

anypnia (an-ip'ni-ə) n. insomnia. [G *a-* = *an-* (usually before a vowel), priv, q.v. + *h)ypnos*, sleep]. adj. **anypnic**. syn. **aypnia**, q.v. **See sleep & wakefulness**.

apanthropy/apanthropia (a-pan'thrə-pee/ a-pan"thrə-pee'ə or ap'an-thrō'pi-ə) n. dislike of being with people; love of solitude; aversion to man, human society. [< G *apo* from + *anthropos* man]. ant. **monophobia**, q.v. See **mentality, mentation, behavior**.

aperient (aa-pee'ri-ent or a-pee'ri-ənt) n. & adj. laxative, causing evacuation of the bowels. [< L *aperient,* stem of *aperiens* opening, pres. p. *aperire* to open]. syn. **lapactic**, q.v. See **gastrointestinal**.

aperitive (aa-per'ri-tiv), n. 1. stimulates the appetite. 2. laxative. [L *aperiens* opening]. syn. **aperient**, q.v. See **gastrointestinal**.

aphanisis (a-fan'ni-siss) n. fear of losing sexual power. [< G *aphaneia* disappearance]. See **sex, love**.

aphasia (ə-fay'zhə) n. loss or impairment of speech, or of the power to understand written or spoken language. It is classified as expressive, receptive, and global. [G, speechlessness < a-, priv., not, without < G *alpha*, privative or negative, inseparable prefix, usually an- before a vowel + *phasis* speech]. syns. **logagnosia, logamnesia, logasthenia**, q.v. See **dysarthria**. See talk.

aphilophrenia (a-fil"lō-freen'ni-ə) n. a feeling that one is unloved or unwanted. [< G *a*-, priv. + *philo*- fond, loving + -phrenia, suff., < *phren* the mind, heart (as the seat of emotions, or alt., the diaphragm)]. See **mentality, mentation, behavior**.

apnea/apnoea (ap'nee-ə) n. a temporary suspension or absence of breathing. [< G *apnoia* not breathing < *pnein* breathe]. adj. **apneic** = related to or suffering from apnea. See **sleep apnea**. See breathing.

apocatastasis/apokatastasis (ap"pō-kə-tas'tə-siss) n. the state of being restored or saved, as in acquiring religion. [< G *apo* off, away + *kata* down + *stasis* standing, stoppage]. See therapy.

apodictic/apodeictic (a-pō-dik'tik/ -dīk'tik) adj. of clear demonstration; established; indisputably true. • With age he became increasingly *apodictic* in his pronouncements. [< G *deiktiknunai* to demonstrate < *deiknunai* to show]. adv. **apodictically/ apodeictically**. adj. **apodictical**. Cf. **thetic, thetical**, q.v. See **mentality, mentation, behavior**.

ApoE4/APOE -4 n. is a gene (apolipoprotein E-4 allele) variant—the first—considered to be a risk factor for late-onset Alzheimer's disease. however, non-carriers of the gene make up 40-70% of Alzheimer's patients. A more recently discovered gene in such patients is **CALHM1**, which controls levels of brain-cell calcium and amyloid-beta, a peptide found in Alzheimer-disease plaques. Two other Alzheimer-linked genes are **CLU**, q.v., & **PICALM**, q.v. Due to a recently discovered **TREM2** gene mutation the body's inflammatory system overreacts, thus preventing the body's immune system from dealing with amyloidal buildup. A new chemical marker, **FDDNP**, binds to the plaque and tangled brain deposits in Alzheimer's, and in ApoE4 carriers; it shows up in brain scans in medial, lateral, and especially frontal areas of the brain concerned with memory. Such scans may be predictive of Alzheimer's disease. Carriers of **ApoE3**, the most common variant of the gene—about two-thirds of Americans have it—don't get the disease, and **APOE2** appears to be somewhat protective. When APOE4 is inherited from both parents, the risk of Alzheimer's is raised at least five times. (APOE e4 is another name for APOE4.) Only a diligent acronymist can keep track of all these Alzheimer genes. See **TOMM40**. See intelligence.

apogenous (a-poj'jen-əss) adj. sterile; impotent. [< G *apo* away + *genesis* birth, origin, creation, production]. n. **apogeny** = loss of the ability to reproduce. syns. **acarpous, agennesic, anandrious**, qv. See **sex, love**.

apolaustic (ap-ō-laws'tik) adj. dedicated to pleasure; self-indulgent. [< G *apolaustikos* < *apolauo* enjoy]. See **mentality, mentation, behavior**.

apomnemoneumata (a-pom"nee-mon"yoo-maat'tə) n.pl. memoirs. [G]. See **memory**.

aponia (a-pōn'ni-ə) n. 1. non-exertion, abstention from labor. (2. Absence of pain.) [< a-, pref., without, not (privative), < G without, not, + < G *ponos* toil, pain]. adj. **aponic** = relating to aponia; (analgesic; relieving fatigue). See **work, activity**.

aponoia (a-pōn-oy'ə) n. amentia. [G, <*apo* away + *nous* mind]. See **mentality, mentation, behavior**.

apopemptic (a-pō-pemp'tik) adj. pertaining to farewell; sung as a farewell message (arch.). [< G *apopemptik, -os* < *apopempeiu* to send away]. See **end-of-life & death**.

apoptosis (a-pop-tō'siss, a-po-tō'siss) n. cell death occurring as a normal part of an organism's growth and development; cell deletion by fragmentation into membrane-bound particles that are phagocytosed (ingested) by other cells. [G, a falling or dropping off, < *apo-* off + *ptosis* a falling]. See **end-of-life & death**.

apositic (a-pō-sit'tik) adj. without appetite, distaste for food. [< G *apo* away + *sitos* food]. syn. **anorectic**, q.v. See **gastrointestinal**.

apraxia (a-prak'si-ə) n. 1. a disorder of voluntary movement, consisting in a more or less complete incapacity to execute purposeful movements, notwithstanding the preservation of muscular power, sensibility, and coordination. 2. a psychomotor defect in which one is unable to apply to its proper use an object which one is nevertheless able to name and the uses of which one can describe. (Apraxia can be evaluated by asking the person to draw intersecting pentagons. Inability to do so may suggest lesions of the parietal lobes, particularly the right lobe, as may occur with stroke or Alzheimer's disease.) [G a lack of acting, a want of success < *a-*, priv. + *pratto* to do]. adj. **apraxic** or **apractic** = marked by or pertaining to apraxia. See **verbal apraxia**. See **nerve, muscle, movement, touch**.

aprosexia (ap"prō-seks'see-ə) n. an abnormal inability to pay attention; near complete indifference to everything; inattention, due to ocular, aural, or nasal defects, or to mental weakness. [< G *a-* priv. + *prosexis* attention < *pros-echo* to hold to]. Cf. **hyperprosexia**, q.v., & **paraprosexia**, q.v. See **mentality, mentation, behavior**. See **intelligence**. See **sex, love**.

apud se (aa'poŏd-say) adj.phr. in one's senses. [L]. syn. *compos mentis*, q.v. See **mentality, mentation, behavior**. See **intelligence**. See **end-of-life, death**.

archaeolatry (aar"kee-ol'lə-tree) n. worship of anything archaic. [< G *arkhaios* old, ancient + *-latreia* worship]. See **old age**.

archaic (aar-kay'ik) adj. 1. ancient, belonging or related to a much earlier period. 2. outmoded, no longer useful or efficient. 3. describes a word or phrase that is no longer in general use but is still encountered in older literature and still sometimes used for special effect. [< G *arkhaikos* < *arkhaios* old, ancient < *arkhe* beginning]. adv. **archaically**. n. **archaism**. n. **archaist**. adj. **archaistic** (-is'tik). vt. **archaize** (-kay'-). n. **archaizer.** See **old**. See **old age**. See **role**.

arcus corneae/*arcus cornealis* (aar'koŏs kawr'nee-ī/ aar'koŏs kawr-nee-al'lis) n.phr. a white or gray opaque ring in the corneal margin. It can be present at birth, or appear later in life; it becomes quite frequent in those over 50. It results from cholesterol deposits in, or hyalinosis of, the corneal tissue and hyperlipemia. Syns. *arcus adiposus*, *arcus juvenilis*, *arcus lipoids corneae*, and **arcus senilis**, q.v., the last being applied particularly aptly in the elderly. [L, bow + L, *corneus* horny, *cornealis* corneal; *senilis* senile, old]. See **physique, appearance**. See **Eye**.

arcus senilis (aar'kuss se-nil'liss) (pl. = ***arcus senilium***) n.phr. arc, arch of old age. See ***arcus corneae, arcus cornealis*** for further information. (Also called ***arcus adiposus, arcus lipoides, gerontoxon***, and ***lipoidosis corneae***.) [L, *arcus*, a bow + *senile*, old]. See **physique, appearance**. See **eye**.

Ardipithecus ramidus (aar"di-pi'thə-kəs ram'mi-dəs) pr.n the genus and species name for the oldest known human ancestor, a female hominid, 4.4 million years of age, who has been reconstructed over several years from skeletal remains found in Ethiopia in the early 1990s. She is popularly known as "Ardi, being some million years older than, and has supplanted, "Lucy" (*Australopithecus afarensis*), who was, until Ardi's discovery, the oldest known human ancestor. [<Afar (a language) *Ardi* ground or floor + *ramid* root + < L m. suff. *-us*, thus Ardipithecus *ramidus*, literally, means "ground man-root"]. See **old woman**.

Aricept® (ar'ri-sept) n. the trade name for a drug, donepezil HCl (hydrochloride) used to treat Alzheimer's disease. **Donepezil HCl**, q.v., is a reversible inhibitor of the enzyme acetylcholinesterase, and is known pharmaceutically as E2020; it is made by Eisai, Inc. [?]. **Exelon®Patch**, q.v., is a more recent drug used to treat **Alzheimer's disease**, q.v. See **therapy**.

aristarchian (ar-is-taar'ki-ən) adj. extremely critical. [< *Aristarch*, who criticized Homer's poetry]. See **talk**.

arrect (a-rekt') adj. alert, intent. [L < *arrigo*, pp. of *arrectus*, to raise up: that which raises]. n. **arrectness**. See **mentality, mentation, behavior**.

arrière-garde (arjɛr-gard) (n.phr., lit. rear-guard.) adj. phr. old fashioned, old hat, passé. [F, < *arrière* rear, back part, stern + *garde* guard]. ant. = *avant garde*, fashionable. **See old**.

arteriosclerosis (aar-teer"ree-ō-sklə-rōs'siss) n. a group of diseases characterized by thickening and loss of elasticity of arterial walls. [< G *arteria* < *aer* air (arteries were supposed by the ancients to contain air, or < G *aeirein* to lift or attach + *skleros* hard + -sis, suff.]. adj. **arteriosclerotic**. See **atherosclerosis**, a form of arteriosclerosis. See **blood, circulation, glands**.

arthr(o) - pref. that denotes a joint or articulation of the skeleton. [< G *arthron* joint].

arthralgia (aar-thral'jə, -ji-ə) n. severe pain in a joint, especially one not inflamed. [arthr(o)-, pref., q.v., + < G *algos* pain]. alt. **arthrodynia** [*odyne* pain]. adj. **arthralgic**, alt. **arthrodynic** = relating to or affected with arthralgia or arthrodynia. See **joint, extremities, back**.

arthritis (aar-thrīt'tiss), pl. **arthritides** (aar-thrit'ti-dees), n. inflammation of a joint; state characterized by inflammation of joints. • About 50% of persons > 65 years of age have *arthritis*. [< G *arthron* joint, + -itis, suff., inflammation < G f. -*ites* inflammation]. adj. **arthritic** (aar-thrit'tik) = relating to arthritis. See **joint, extremities, back**.

arthrocele (aar'thrō-seel) n. 1. any swelling of a joint. (2. herniation of the synovial membrane through the capsule of a joint.) [arthr(o)-, q.v., + < G *kele* hernia]. See **joint, extremities, back**.

arthrodynia (aar"thrō-din'ni-ə) n. pain in a joint. [arthr(o)-, q.v., + < G *odyne* pain]. adj. **arthrodynic**. adv. **arthrodynicly**. See **joint, extremities, back**.

arthroendoscopy (aar"thrō-en-doss'kō-pee) n. examination of the interior of a joint with an arthroscope. [arthr(o)-, q.v., + < G end(o)-, pref., within, < *endon* within, + *skopein* to examine]. adj. **arthroendoscopic** (-doss-kaap'pik). adv. **arthroendoscopicly**. alt. **arthroscopy** (aar-thros'kō-pee). See **joint, extremities, back**.

arthrogryposis (aar"thrō-gri-pōss'iss n. persistent flexure or contracture or a joint. [arthr(o)-, q.v., + < G *gryposis* a crooking]. See **joint, extremities, back**.

arthroneuralgia (aar"thrō-nyoor"ral'jee-ə, -ral'jə) n. pain arising in or around a joint. [arthr(o)-, q.v., + < G *neuron* nerve + *algos* pain]. See **joint, extremities, back**.

arthropathy (aar-throp'pə-thee) n. any joint disease. [arthr(o)-, q.v., + < G *pathos* disease]. See **joint, extremities, back**.

arthroplasty (aar'thrō-plass"tee) n. plastic surgery of a joint or of joints; the formation of movable joints, e.g. total hip arthroplasty.

Arthroplasty's object is invigorated physical functioning. [< G *plassein* to form]. See **joint, extremities, back**.

arthrosclerosis (aar"thrō-sklə-rōs'siss) n. stiffening or hardening of the joints. [arthr(o)-, q.v., + < G *sklerosis* hardening]. adj. **arthrosclerotic** (-ot'-ik). See **joint, extremities, back**.

arthroscope (aar'thrō-skōp) n. an endoscope for examining the interior of a joint and for carrying out diagnostic and therapeutic procedures within the joint. [arthr(o)-, q.v. + < G *skopein* to examine]. adj. **arthroscopic** (ar-thrō-skop'pik). n. **arthroscopy** (ar-thros'kō-pee) = examining a joint with an arthroscope. syn. **arthroendoscopy** (aar"thrō-en-dos'kō-pee), q.v. See **joint, extremities, back**.

arthroxerosis (aar"thrō-zee-rōs'siss) n. chronic osteoarthritis. [arthr(o)-, q.v., + < G *xeros* dry, + -osis, suff.]. See **joint, extremities, back**.

artifact (aar'ti-fakt) n. 1. a man-made object, especially of archaeological or cultural significance. (2. something appearing to exist because of the way a thing, datum, or the like is examined or tested. 3. something in a biological specimen that is not present naturally, but has been introduced or produced procedurally.) 4. (fig.) someone extremely out date and out of touch with current affairs, practices, thought, etc. • (fig.) The octogenarian professor's 19th C. orientation made him feel an *artifact* among today's youth. [< L *arte*, a form of *ars* skill + *factum* thing made]. See **old man**. See **old woman**. See **role**.

asitia (a-sish'i-ə, -shə) n. anorexia; a loathing for food. [< G *a*- pref., privative, + *sitos* food]. See **gastrointestinal**.

asseverate (ə-sev'vər-rayt) vt. To state something earnestly or solemnly. [< L *asseverate*- pp. of *asseverare* < *severus* serious]. n. **asseveration** (-ray'shən). See **talk**.

assuetude (as'swee-tood) n. a custom or habit. • *Asuetude* plays a large part in elders' behavior. [ad- = as- before s, pref., < L *ad* to, increase, or mere intensification + *suetudo* < *suescere*, *suet*- to be wont + -tude, suff.].

astasia (as-tay'zha, zhee-ə) n. inability, through muscular incoordination, to stand. [< G *a-*, priv., + *stasis* step]. Cf. **abasia**, **astasia-abasia**, q.v. See **standing, walking, wandering**.

astasia-abasia (as-tay'zhə-a-bay'zhə) n. inability to either stand or walk normally; (Blocq's disease: attempting to stand or walk results in the person collapsing—a symptom of conversion hysteria.) [< G *a-*, priv., + *stasis* standing + *a-*, priv., + *basis* step]. See **standing, walking, wandering**.

asthenia (as-theen'ni-ə) n. loss of strength, weakness. [< G *astheneia* < *a-* priv. + *sthenos* strength]. adj. **asthenic** (-then'ik). See **tiredness, weakness**.

asthenophobia (as-theen"nō-fōb'bi-ə) n. morbid fear of weakness. [asthen(o)-, pref., denoting lack of strength or weakness, < G *asthenes* weak, < *a-* neg. + *sthenos* strength + *phobos* fear]. adj. **asthenophobic**. n. **asthenophobe** (-theen'nō-). See **phobias**. See **tiredness, weakness**.

astucious (as-too'shəss) adj. having keen perception; of astute and penetrating discernment; crafty; subtle. • "Why do Jews answer a question with a question?" "Why not?" asked {old} Marty, *astuciously*. (Russell Rock, The Grandiloquent Dictionary). [< F *astucieux* astute]. adv. **astuciously**. n. **astucity** (-too'si-tee) = astuteness. See **mentality, mentation, behavior**.

ataraxia (at"tər-aks'si-ə) n. imperturbability, utter calmness, peace of mind. [< G *a-* priv. + *taraktos* disturbed + -ia, suff.]. See **emotion**. See **mentality, mentation, behavior**.

ataxia/ataxy (a-taks'si-ə/a-tak'see) n. loss of muscular coordination. [< G *a-* priv. + *taxis* order]. adj. **ataxic**. syn. **ataxy, dysmyotonia, dyssynergia**, q.v. See **standing, walking, wandering**. See **nerve, muscle, movement, touch**.

athanasia (ath-ə-nay'zhə, -nay'zhee-ə) n. immortality; deathlessness [< Saint Athanasius's (293? – 373?) Creed, beliefs; he was bishop of Alexandria]. adj. **Athanasian**. See **end-of-life & death**.

atherosclerosis (ath"er-ō"skler-rōs'siss) n. an extremely common form of **arteriosclerosis**, q.v., in which deposits of yellowish plaques, atheromata, containing cholesterol, lipoid material, and lipophages are formed within the intima and inner media of large and medium-sized arteries. [ather(o)-, a pref. denoting fatty degeneration, or relationship to an atheroma, < G *athere* gruel]. See **arteriosclerosis**. See **blood, circulation, glands**.

athetise (ath'ə-tīz) vt. to spurn, reject. [a- priv. + the(o)-, comb. form, < G *theos* god, + -ise, suff.]. See **mentality, mentation, behavior**.

atocia (aa-tō'shə, -tō'see-aa, -tō-si-aa) n. female sterility. [< G *atokia* < a- priv. + *tokos* childbirth]. syn. = **acyesis**, q.v. See **sex, love**.

atony (at'tən-ee) n. 1. lack of normal muscular tone, strength; abnormal relaxation; lethargy. (2. lack of stress in a syllable.) [< G *atony* languor < a- priv. + *tonos* tension]. adj. **atonic**. n. **atonicity** (a"tə-nis'sə-tee). See **tiredness, weakness**.

atrabilarian (at"trə-bi-lair'ri-ən) n. a gloomy hypochondriac anxious to recount symptoms, the latest ache, long-term illness, etc., and his/her depression. [< L *atra* black + *bilis* bile]. See **emotion**. See **mentality, mentation, behavior**. See **role**.

atrabilious/atrabiliar (at"trə-bil'yəss)/(at"rə-bil'yər) adj. sad, melancholy; bad-tempered; morbid; dismal. [< L *atra* black + *bilis* bile (referring to one of the supposed four chief body fluids, humors, i.e., black bile)]. n. **atrabilarian** (at"trə-bi-lair'ri-ən), q.v. See **emotion**. See **mentality, mentation, behavior**. See **role**.

atrichia (a-trik'ki-ə) n. baldness. [< G a- priv. + *thrix* (trich-) hair]. syns. = **acomia, alopecia, calvities, depilous, phalacrosis, pilgarlic**, q.v. See **hair**.

atrophic laryngitis (a-trof'fik lar-in-jīt'tiss) n.phr. loss with old age of minor salivary gland moisture in the larynx, as well as fibrous support; muscle atrophies and squamous-cell metaplasia develops. A chronic tickling sensation occurs in the throat causing a recurrent clearing urge, and in elderly men, especially, development of a high, trembling voice with weakened amplitude and quality. [< G a- priv. + *trophe* nourishment, and laryng(o)-, pref., relating to the larynx, < G *larynx* + -*itis*, suff., inflammation]. See **talk**.

atrophic vaginitis (a-trof'fik vag-i-nīt'tiss) n.phr. changes in vaginal tissue due to decreased post-menopausal blood estrogen level: diminished vascularity, thinning, less acidic pH, and fewer rugae; the vagina becomes shorter and less elastic. Atrophic changes predispose the vagina to dryness, ease of infection, dyspareunia (difficult, painful intercourse), vaginismus (vaginal spasm). There is concomitant atrophic urethritis associated with decreased estrogen level. [G, L, a- negative + trophe nourishment, and L, vagina vagina + G, -itis (a f. adjectival termination agreeing with nosos disease, understood) inflammation]. See **genitourinary**.

atrophy (at'trə-fee) n. wasting away through imperfect nourishment; emaciation (fig. & lit.). **atrophy** vi & vt. • Atrophy, manifested by decreased thickness of the skin, is an age-related change. [< G atrophia < atrophos ill fed < a- not + trophe food]. See **physique, appearance**.

attenuate (at-ten'yoo-ayt) vt. to make slender, thin, weaken, less strong, reduced in value. • Age had so attenuated him that his former student almost failed to recognize him. [< L attenuare < tenuis thin + -ate]. adj. **attenuated**. n. **attenuation**. See **physique, appearance**. See **tiredness & weakness**.

attercop (ad'dər-kop) n. (British dialect or obs.) 1. a bad-tempered, malignant, venomous person. (2. a spider). [OE attercoppa < ator or attor poison + coppa < cop cup, vessel; in reference to the supposed venomous properties of spiders. Cf. also Du spinnecop spider and cob-web, formerly cop-webbe, whence probably the simple coppa was itself + spider]. See **mentality, mentation, behavior**. See: **role**.

aureate years (awr'ree-ayt, -ət) n.phr. golden years, end of life. [< L aureatus < aureus golden < aurum gold]. See **old age**.

auricular (aw-rik'kyoo-lər) adj. 1. pertaining to the ear, or sense of hearing. 2. spoken in the ear; private. 3. (formerly) pertaining to an atrium (upper chamber) of the heart. [< L auricular little ear < auris ear]. n. **auricula** = the portion of the external ear not contained within the head; the **pinna**, q.v. See **ear & hearing**. See **talk**.

aurist (awr'rist) n. an ear specialist. [< L auris ear]. syns. = **otiatrus**, qv., audiologist. (audiometrician = a technician specializing in audiometry). See **ear & hearing**. See **role**.

autognosis (aw-tog-nōs'siss) n. self-awareness, especially of one's emotional make-up. [<G *autos* self + *gnosis* knowledge]. Cf. the Delphic G aphorism: "Know thyself—*gnothi seauton.*" See **emotion**. See **mentality, mentation, behavior**.

autophobia (aw-tō-fōb'bi-ə) n. fear of oneself; fear of being alone; of loneliness. [<G *autos* self + *phobos* fear]. adj. **autophobic**. n. **autophobe** (aw'tō-fōb). syns. **eremophobia**, **isolophobia**, **monophobia**, **solophobia**, q.v. See **phobias**. See **emotion**. See **mentality, mentation, behavior**. See **loneliness, solitude, silence**.

autoptic (aw-top'tik) adj. based on one's own perception. (*Ipse dixit*: He himself said {it}.) [< G *autos* self + *optikos* optical, seen < *ops* eye]. See **mentality, mentation, behavior**.

aval (ayv'val, ayv'əl) adj. pertaining to grandparents [L *avus* grandfather; forefather, ancestor & *avia* grandmother]. See **old man**, **old woman**. See **old person(s)**.

avuncular (a-vun'kyoo-lər) adj. of or pertaining to an uncle, especially one who is friendly, helpful, or good humored. • The old man's *avuncular* manner made him a great hit with children. [< L *avunculus* mother's brother, maternal uncle. (diminutive of *avus* grandfather. *avunculus magnus* = great-uncle, *avunculus major* = great-great-uncle)]. See **old man**.

axiology (ak-see-ol'lə-jee) n. the study of the nature, types, and governing criteria of values and value judgments. [< G *axia* value + -logy, suff., speech, expression; science, study < *-logia* < *logos* word, study, speaking, reason]. See **religion, theology, morality**.

ayne (ayn) adj. (obs.) eldest, first born. [OF *aîné* first born, elder, heir apparent, earlier *aîsné*, *aînsné* < *aîns* + *né* born]. syn. **eigne**, q.v. See **old**.

aypnia (ay-ip'ni-ə) n. insomnia. [G *a-*, priv., q.v., + *(h)ypnos* sleep]. adj. **aypnic**. syns. **anypnia**, **insomnia**, q.v. See **sleep & wakefulness**.

azygophrenia (az'i-gō-free'ni-ə) n. a neurotic condition brought on by living a lonely single life. • *Azygophrenia* may result after the death of a spouse. [*a-*, priv. < G + *zygon* a yoke + *phren* mind]. See **mentality, mental state, behavior**. See **sex, love**.

azygous (az'i-gəs) adj. odd, unpaired; fig,. unmarried, widowed. [< G *a-* priv. + *zygon* a yoke]. See **sex, love**.

B

"We could certainly slow the aging process down
if it had to work its way through Congress."
—Will Rogers.

babushka (bə-boŏsh'kə) n. 1. a traditional Russian grandmother figure, old woman. syn. **beldam**, **biddy**, **crone**, **dowager**, **Ell**i, **matriarch**, q.v. (2. a headscarf folded and tied under the chin in the style of Russian peasant women.) [R, grandmother]. See **old woman**.

baby boomer (bay'bee boom'ər) n. (slang) someone born during a baby boom—particularly the one following the end of World War II—and soon to be old. The first baby boomers were age 65 in 2011. n. **baby boom** = a sudden large increase in the birthrate over a particular period, especially the 15 years after World War II. [U.S.]. See **old age**.

bacillophobia (ba-sil"lŏ-fōb'bi-ə) n. morbid fear of germs. [< L diminutive of *baculus* rod, staff (the microscopic appearance of some bacteria) + G *phobos* fear]. adj. **bacillophobic**. n. **bacillophobe** (-sil'lŏ-). syns. **bacteriophobia**, **microbiophobia**, q.v. Cf. **my**(or **i**) **sophobia**, **molys(o)mophobia**, q.v. See **phobias**.

bacteriophobia (bac-tee'ri-ŏ-fōb'bi-ə) n. fear of germs, bacteria. [bacterio-, pref., relating to bacteria < G *bakterion*, diminutive of *baktron* a staff + *phobia* fear]. adj. **bacteriophobic**. n. **bacteriophobe**. syns. **bacillophobia**, **microbiophobia**, q.v. See **phobias**.

badinage (baa"dən-aazh') n. the exchange of playful or joking remarks by people in conversation. ● The frequent *badinage* at the retirement home was a delight to old Mrs. Smith. [F, joking < *badin* fool, joker < assumed vulgar L *badare* to yawn, gape]. Cf. **persiflage**, **raillery**, q.v. See **talk**.

balbutient (bal-byoo'shənt) adj. stammering, stuttering. [< L *balbutiens*, *-entis* < *balbutire* to stutter]. syn. **lingual titubation**. See **talk**.

balderdash (bawl'dər dash) n. senseless or pointless talk or writing. [late 16th C.?]. Cf. **glossolalia, galimatia, idiolalia, jabberwocky, prate, prattle**, q.v. See **talk**.

balneal (bal'nee-əl), also **balnean** adj. of or pertaining to baths or bathing. • *balneal* facilities are important and extensive in a residence for the aged. [< L *balneum* a bath < G *balaneion* bathing room or bath]. See **therapy**.

balneology (bal"nee-ol'lə-jee) n. the study and practice of using baths as therapy. [< L *balneum* bath + -ology, suff., < -o- + -logy science, study < G -*logia* < *logos* word, reason]. See **therapy**.

bapineuzumab (bap'pee-nyooz"zoo-mab) n. a humanized monoclonal antibody to the toxic beta-amyloid nuropathologic plaques found clumped together in the brain of Alzheimer-disease patients. Wyeth manufactures the antibody and is engaged in experiments to determine if it is clinically useful in preventing or treating Alzheimer's disease. [origin uncertain, but the "-neu-" in the name = nervous system and "-zu-" = humanized monoclonal antibody]. See **Rember®**. See **intelligence**.

baragouin (baar'rə-gwin) n. any jargon or unintelligible language. [< F (Breton) *bara* bread + *gwenn* white, said to have originated in the Breton soldiers' astonished language on seeing bread that was white instead of the usual brown they experienced]. See **talk**.

bariatrics (bar"ree-at'rikss) n. that branch of medicine concerned with the treatment of obesity. [mid 20th C. < baro-, pref., pressure, weight < G *baros* weight + -iatrics, suff., a particular field of medicine < *iatros* doctor]. See **physique, appearance**.

basal-cell carcinoma (bays'səl sel kaar"sin-ōm'mə) n.phr. a pearly papule that left untreated develops into a superficial ulcer. It's derived from dermal basal cells, can be scaly or pigmented, is slow-growing, rarely metastasizes, and most likely (90%) occurs on the head and neck; it can invade underlying bone. Basal cell carcinoma is found 95% of the time in the 40-79-year-old age group. [< G *karkinoma* < *karkinos* crab, cancer +-*oma* tumor]. See **skin**.

basiphobia (bays'si-fōb'bi-ə) n. morbid fear of walking. [< basi(o)-, pref., denoting a relationship to a base or foundation, < G *basis* base, foundation support + *phobos* fear]. adj. **basiphobic**. n. **basiphobe**. syn. **ambulophobia, basophobia**, q.v. See **phobias**. See **standing, walking, wandering**.

basistasiphobia (bays"si-stas"si-fōb'bi-ə) n. morbid fear of standing and walking. [< G *basis* step + *stasis* standing still + *phobos* fear]. alt. **basostasophobia**. adj. **basistasiphobic**. n. **basistasiphobe**. syn. **stasibasiphobia**, q.v. See **phobias**. See **standing, walking, wandering.**

basophobia (bay'sō-fōb'bi-ə) See **basiphobia**. See **standing, walking, wandering**.

battologist (bat-tol'ə-jist) n. a person who annoyingly reiterates, repeats the same thing over and over. [< G *battologia* stuttering, said to be from Battos, a man who consulted the Delphic oracle about his defect of speech {See Herodotus iv. 155} + *legein*, to speak]. n. **battology** = futile repetition in speech or writing. adv. **battological**. syns. **obganiator, verbigerator**, q.v. See **talk**. See **role**.

befuddle (bee-fud'dəl) vt. to confuse, perplex somebody. [?]. n. **befuddlement**. adj. **befuddled**. syn. **fuddle**, q.v. See **talk**.

beldam (bel'dəm) n. old woman; an ugly old hag. [F *belle dame* beautiful woman—beldam is thus an antiphrasis: its meaning is antipodal]. syn. **rudas**, q.v. See **old woman**.

bemuse (bi-myooz') vt. to stupefy; to bewilder or **befuddle**, q.v., someone. • Her grandmother *bemused* the visitors with her inane commentary. [< be-, pref., adding the notion of thoroughness, excess to a vt., < OE *be-* about + *muse* < ME < OF *muser* to waste time]. adj. **bemused**. n. **bemusement**. adv. **bemusedly**. See **talk**.

benignant (bee-nīn'nənt) n. kind and gracious in behavior or appearance; kind especially to subordinates or inferiors. • His *benignant* behavior to caretakers at the retirement residence made him a favorite. [< L *benignus* kind hearted; mild; affable; liberal; favorable; bounteous]. n. **benignancy**. adv. **benignantly**. See **mentality, mentation, behavior**.

benign prostatic hypertrophy (BPH) (bee-nīn' pros-tat'tik hī-pur'trə-fee) n.phr. prostatic enlargement that is non-cancerous and occurs frequently in older men; it tends to progress with age and causes urinary frequency, urgency, and dysuria. [< L *benignus* kind + < *prostata* < G *prostates* one standing before < *pro* before + *states* < *sta-* stand + hyper-, pref., excessive, above the normal, < *hyper* above, over + *trophe* nourishment]. Cf. **prostatomegaly**, q.v. See **genitourinary**.

bibacious (bī-bay'shəss) adj. overly fond of drinking. [< L *bibere* to drink]. See **drink, food**.

bibliobibuli (bib"li-ō-bib'yə-lee) n.pl. (n.s. **bibliobibulus**) persons who read voraciously to the extent of becoming unaware of or oblivious to the real world. [biblio-, pref, book < G *biblos* book, diminutive, *biblion* small book, < *biblios* papyrus, scroll < Bublos, a Phoenician city from which papyrus was imported +? < L *bibulous* fond of drinking; absorbent; thirsty (for reading) < *bibere* to drink].

bibulous (bib'yoo-ləss) adj. (formal) tending too drink too much; addicted to alcohol. [< L *bibulus* < *bibere* to drink]. n. **bibulousness**. adv. **bibulously**. syn. **bibacious**, q.v. See **drink, food**.

biddy (bid'dee), pl. **biddies** (bid'deess) n. 1. an offensive term deliberately insulting a woman's behavior as being fussing or interfering (slang insult). (2. a chicken). [Early 17th C. < ?]. See **old woman**.

billingsgate (bil'lingz-gayt) n. coarse, abusive, foul language, invective for the purpose of vituperation, and vilification. [< Billingsgate, London, which, for hundreds of years, was the site and name of a fish market the personnel of which were noted for their very foul language; < the name of an early property owner, Billings, and near a gate in the old city wall (N.W. Schur)]. See **talk**.

biogerontologist (bī"ō-jer"ron-tol'lə-jist) n. a physician scientist who studies the biology of the aged, especially the damage that ageing does in order to reverse or prevent it so people can stay younger longer. [bio-, pref., life, biology, < G *bios* life, way of living, + gero-, geront-, geronto-, prefix relating to aging, old age < *geron*, old man, + *logos* word, study, discourse + -ist, suff., practicing a specific skill or profession, < -*istes*]. n. **biogerontology**. adj. **biogerontological** (-tō-loj'ji-kal or -jə-kal). adv. **biogerontologically**. See <u>role</u>.

biometry (bī-om'mə-tree) n. (1. the science of the application of statistics in biology, medicine, and agriculture.) 2. in life insurance, the calculation of the expectation of life. The Associated Press, on 4/30/10, reported that Icelandic men and Cypriot women are the longest lived worldwide; the study was recently published in the Lancet. Lancet researchers also found a widening gap between countries with the highest and lowest premature death rates in adults aged 15 to 60. [bio-, pref., life, biology < G *bios* life, way of living + *metron* measure]. adj. **biometric** (-met'trik). Cf. **longevity**, q.v. See **end-of-life, death**.

*birkie*n. See **old** *birkie*. See <u>old person(s), people</u>. See <u>role</u>.

blateroon (blat-ər-roon') n. (obs.) a constant talker, gabber, chatterbox, blabber, blabbermouth, prater, motormouth afflicted with **logorrhea**, q.v. [< L *blatera*, -*onem* blabber < *blaterare* to blab]. syn. **blatherer**, q.v. See <u>talk</u>. See <u>role</u>.

bleareye (bleer'rī) n. See syn. **lippitude**. See <u>eye</u>.

blepharitis (blef-faar-rī'tiss) n. eyelid inflammation, usually non-specific, but sometimes caused by staphylococcal infection of the lid margin and follicles. It can occur at any age, but is often more severe in old age. Signs are dilated blood vessels at the lid margins, scaling at the base of eyelashes, and loss of eyelashes. [blephar(o)-, pref., meaning eyelid < G *blepharon* eyelid + -*itis* inflammation]. See <u>eye</u>.

blether, **blather** (bleth'ər, blath'ər) vi. to talk loquacious nonsense.
• Alzheimer's disease has reduced his vocal communication to *blather*. n. to talk loquacious nonsense [< ME *blather* < ON *blathra* talk nonsense < *blathr* nonsense; *blether* is the Sc. form adopted form Burns, etc.]. n. **blatherer**. syns. **blateroon** (blat-ər-roon'), q.v. **blatherskite/blatherskate** = a **blithering**, q.v., person. See <u>talk</u>. See <u>intelligence</u>. See <u>role</u>.

blinkered (bling'kərd) adj. lit., pertaining to blinkers, i.e., blinders, put on a horse to obscure peripheral vision, but used fig. to indicate "blinding" someone to any except a sole or central idea without consideration of possible countervailing ideas or consequences. • The **sedens**, q.v., was *blinkered* by his provinciality. [< 13 C. blink, partly variant of blench (vi. to move back or away in fear) < OE *blencan* deceive, cheat < ?, and partly from MD *blinken* glitter]. See **mentality, mentation, behavior**.

blithering (blith'ər-ing) adj. senselessly talkative; consummate, as in ~ idiot; contemptible. [pres. p. of *blither*, a var. of **blether**, qv.]. See **talk**. See **intelligence**.

blood, circulation, glands: angioplasty, arteriosclerosis, atherosclerosis, bruit, CIMT, coronary arteriosclerosis/atherosclerosis, diabetes mellitus, dysarteriotony, dyscrasia, dyscrinism, dysdiemorrhysis, dysemia, dysendocrinism, dysglycemia, dyshematopoiesia/dyshematopoiesis, dyslipidosis, ecchymosis, epistaxis, hematoma, hypercholesterolemia, hyperglycemia, hyperlipidemia, hyperlipoproteinemia, immune scenescence, incruental, myxedema, peripheral arteriosclerosis/atherosclerosis, petechia, purpura, thrombophilia.

blood, circulation, glands: Subcategories

blood

I. Abnormal glucose (sugar) metabolism:
 1. Any abnormal glucose level: **dysglycemia**
 2. High glucose level: **hyperglycemia**
 3. High glucose level with illness: **hyperglycemia & diabetes mellitus**
II. Abnormal lipid (fat) metabolism:
 1. In general: **dyslipidosis**
 2. Increased blood lipids: **hypercholesterolemia, hyperlipidemia, hyperlipoproteinemia**
III. Blood disease:
 1. An undefined disease or abnormal condition of the body, especially of the blood: **dyscrasia**
 2. Any abnormal condition or disease of the blood: **dysemia**
 3. Imperfect formation of blood: **dyshematopoiesia/ dyshematopoiesis**

IV. Extravasated blood:
    1. In the skin (bruise): **ecchymosis, purpura**
    2 Localized mass: **hematoma**
    3. Minute skin or mucosal hemorrhage: **petechia**, pl. = **-ae**
    4. Nosebleed: **epistaxis**
V. Lack of Immunity:
    1. The progressive dysfunctioning of the immune system with age: **immune scenescence**
VI. Treatment:
    1. Correction of blood-vessel obstructions by use of a balloon catheter, possibly using a stent: **angioplasty**
VII. Without blood:
    1. Bloodless: **incruental**

circulation

I. Arterial disease:
    1. A sound heard by stethoscope indicating carotid artery obstruction: **bruit**
    2. Abnormal blood pressure (too high or too low): **dysarteriotony**
    3. Arterial-wall thickness ultrasound test: **CIMT.**
    4. Thickening and loss of elasticity of arterial walls: **arteriosclerosis**
II. A common type of arteriosclerosis with fat and fat-cell deposits in the two inner walls of medium sized arteries: **atherosclerosis**
    1. Arterial disease of the coronary arteries: **coronary arteriosclerosis**
    2. Arterial disease of the extremities: **peripheral arteriosclerosis/atherosclerosis** (PAD = peripheral arterial disease.)
    3. Clotting tendency:
        a. tendency of the veins to clot: **thrombophilia**
    4 Sluggish circulation:
        a. sluggish capillary circulation: **dysdiemorrhysis**
III. Inflammation of a vein with secondary thrombus formation: **thrombophlebitis**

glands

I. Abnormal endocrine glands in general: **dysendocrinism, dyscrinism**
II. Pancreas:
    1. Abnormally high blood sugar with illness: **diabetes mellitus**
III. Thyroid:
    1. Hypothyroidism with generalized edema (swelling): **myxedema**

bluenose (bloo'nōz) n. somebody excessively concerned with morals, morality. (dated, informal). [blue in the sense of puritanical]. syn. **wowser**, qv. See **mentality, mentation, behavior**. See **role**.

bodach (bod'dəck) n. an old man; a churl; a goblin or spectre. [Gaelic]. See **old man**.

borborygmus (bawr-bō-rig'məss), n.pl. **borborygmi** (-mī), n. the gurgling, rumbling sound, noise of flatulence, gas being propelled through the intestines. [L < G *borborygmos*]. n. **borborygm** (-rig'gəm). adj. **borborygmic** (-rig'mik). See **gastrointestinal**.

bots (botss) n.pl. (slang) robotic assist devices for care—cybercare— of the elderly. Such devices have been developed and are being tested as they become increasingly more accomplished and versatile in eldercare. Such robots decrease elder isolation, allow elders to remain at home longer rather than being institutionalized, improve elders' communication with family and care givers, assist with everyday tasks, provide interactive speech recognition, connect elders to the Internet and social networking, monitor their vital signs, provide videoconferencing, etc. One such advanced robot is called Kompai. It has a bowling-ball-sized head and "face", is on wheels, provides a touch screen on an easel, talks, understands speech, can navigate autonomously, and among other accomplishments, can play music. It uses Skype technology so the elder and family or caregivers can communicate visually via computer screen over long distance. Kompai uses ultrasonic sensors to detect an elder's location. Such robots assist with everyday tasks. Another elder-care robot is called CareBot (Gecko Systems in Congers, Ga.). It's on wheels and can remind users of daily tasks such as taking medications. Such robots can even assist with writing poetry and can read poems to the elderly. [bots = a contraction of robots, early 20th C. via Ger. < Czech < *robota* forced labor. It was coined by Karel Čapek in his play "R.U.R." (Rosum's Universal Robots) in 1920]. See **therapy**.

Bowen's disease (bō'wen) n.phr. is squamous cell carcinoma in situ or precancerous dermatosis; it is often due to arsenic exposure, but sun exposure is a probable contributing cause, and human papillomavirus may also be etiologic. The lesions are persistent, erythematous, scaly plaques with well-defined margins, and can occur anywhere on the skin or mucous membranes, singly or in multiples. Bowen's disease has the potential of becoming squamous cell carcinoma. The elderly, predominantly, are affected. [< John Templeton Bowen, an American dermatologist (1857-1941)].

bradycardia (brad"di-kaar'di-ə) n. slowness of the heart beat, usually defined as a rate, in adults, of less than 60 beats per minute. [brady-, pref., meaning slow < G *bradys* slow + *kardia* heart]. adj. **bradycardic**. See **heart, rhythm**.

bradylogia (brad"di-lōj'ji-ə) n. abnormal slowness of speech due to slowness of thinking, as in a mental disorder. [brady-, pref., meaning slow < G *bradys* slow + *logos* word]. syn. = **bradyphemia**, q.v. See **talk**.

bradyphemia (brad"di-feem'mi-ə) n. slowness of speech. [brady-, pref., meaning slow < G *bradys* slow + *pheme* speech]. syn. = **bradylogia**, q.v. See **talk**.

braggadocio (brag"gə-dōs'see-ō, -shee-ō, -shō) n. boasting, bragging vainglorious talk. n. **braggadocio** = a braggart. [< a character, *Braggadocchio*, in the Faerie Queen of Edmund Spenser (c. 1552-1599); *Braggadocchio* was a coward at heart. The n. brag < ME n. *bragg* & v. *braggen* & the suffix, -ade, indicate a noun of action. The It. suffix, -*occhio*, is an It. augmentative suffix]. syns. = **fanfaronade, gasconade, jactancy, & rhodomontade**, q.v. See **talk**. See **mentality, mentation, behavior**. See **role**.

brass-collar (brass' kol"lər) adj. unswervingly loyal to a political party, always voting a straight party ticket. [< the allusion to a brass collar of a faithful dog]. See **mentality, mentation, behavior**.

breathing: anhelation, apnea/apnoea, COPD, dysekpnea, dyspnea, emphysema, exsufflicate, orthopnea, pursive, pursy, rale, rhonchisonant, rhonchus, sleep apnea, sonorous, sough, stertorous, stridulous, suspirious, susurration, thixotropy training, wheeze, whiffle.

breathing: Subcategories

I. Abnormal breathing:
1. Air trapping, forcible expiration: **COPD, emphysema, exsufflicate**
2. Breathless, panting, short of breath: **anhelation, pursy**
3. Difficult breathing: **dysekpnea, dyspnea, pursive**
4. Difficult breathing when lying down: **orthopnea**
5. Makes whistling expiratory sounds while breathing, talking, or with activity: **wheezes**
6. Periodic suspension of breathing during sleep: **sleep apnea**
7. Temporary suspension of or absence of breathing: **apnea/apnoea**

II. Inspiration:
1. inspiratory training: **thixotropy training**

III. Abnormal Respiratory Sounds: **rale, rhonchisonant, ronchus, sonorous, sough, stertorous, stridulous, suspirious, sussuration, whiffle**

breviloquent (bre-vil'lō-kwent) adj. speaking briefly. [< L *brevis* short + < G *loqui* speak, talk, say, speak about, tell]. adv. **breviloquently**. n. **breviloquence**. Cf. **pauciloquent; omniloquent, polyloquent**, q.v. ant. **longiloquent, multiloquent, pleniloquent**, q.v. See **talk**.

Briareus (bri-air'ree-əss) someone who is in touch, and abreast with, and on top of everything, is *au fait* and *au courant*. [< *Briareus* < G mythology, a giant, also known as Aegaeon, who had 50 heads and 100 arms, a son of Gaia & Uranus, and one of three brothers (the other two were Cottus and Gyes), the Hecatoncheires. Briareus saved Zeus in a battle with the Titans (Titanomachia). Thetis later summoned Briareus to save Zeus again when some of the other Olympians were about to put Zeus in chains]. See **mentality, mentation, behavior**. See **role**.

bruit (brwee; if Anglicized: broo'ee, broot) n. 1. an auscultatory sound or murmur, i.e., heard on listening, especially through a stethoscope (by auscultation). Such sounds or murmurs are usually heard over the heart or in the carotid arteries of the neck, and, depending on the sounds themselves and their timing, can be indicative of carotid obstructive disease or cardiac structural abnormality. A bruit can be innocent, e.g., the venous hum. Besides the aneurysmal, carotid, and thyroid bruits, bruits are usually designated as "bruit de—", e.g., *bruit de canon, bruit de moulin, bruit de Roget, bruit de triolet*, etc. 2. (archaic) a story, true or not, that is passed around among people. • The elderly are plagued by carotid artery obstruction. A loud systolic (during cardiac contraction) *bruit* heard over the mid-lateral neck is a major sign of such obstruction, and if untreated, is predictive of a stroke. [15th C. OF, noise, sound < *bruire* roar. (Bruits, No.1.type, were named by Drs. Laënnec, Roget, Gallavardin, Bouilland, etc.)]. vt. **bruit** = to circulate stories, rumors, gossip. syn. **murmur**. See **heart, rhythm**. See **blood, circulation, glands**. See **talk**.

brumal (broom'mel) adj. relating to winter, wintry; fig. (arch.) the winter-period, i.e., the end of life. [< L *bruma* winter solstice; winter; winter's cold]. See **end-of-life & death**.

bruxism (bruks'is-em) n. an oral habit consisting of involuntary rhythmic or spasmotic nonfunctional gnashing, grinding, and clenching of teeth in other than chewing movements of the mandible, usually performed during sleep, which may lead to occlusal trauma. Causes may be related to emotional tension, repressed aggression, anger, fear and frustration. Bruxism is not uncommon in the elderly. Bruxism may be a clue to the existence of **sleep apnea**, q.v. [< G *brychein* to gnash the teeth]. Cf. **bruxomania**. syns. **clamping habit**, **clenching habit**. See **mouth, gums, teeth**. See **sleep, wakefulness**.

buccula (buk'kyoo-le) n. a double chin. [< L *buccula* little cheek < *bucca* cheek]. Cf. **dewlap**, **jollop**, **wattle**, q.v. See **physique, appearance**.

buffer (buf'fer) n. (obs.) an old person, particularly a man, and usually used with old: **old buffer**. (Unlisted are several other definitions not germane.) [origin obscure] syn. **fogy**, q.v. See **old man**, **old person(s)**, **old woman**.

burble (bur'bəl) vi. 1. to speak at length; babble. 2. make a bubbling sound. 3. simmer (with rage, mirth, etc.) vi.&vt. to speak or say something in a fast, excited way. n. 1. a gentle or bubbling sound. 2. a flow of fast, excited talking. [14th C. imitative, or < ME *burble* bubble]. n. **burbler**. adv. **burbly**. See <u>talk</u>. See <u>role</u>.

burdalone/burd-alone (burd'də-lōn) n. (obs.) a solitary person. [Sc, obscure]. See <u>loneliness, solitude, silence</u>. See <u>role</u>.

C

"Old man, exhausted by ordeal, detached from human
deeds, feeling the approach of the eternal cold, but always
watching in the shadows for the gleam of hope."
—Charles de Gaulle.

cacemphaton (kaa-kem'fə-ton) n. (obs., rare, rhetorical) 1. a scurrilous jest; a lewd allusion; *double entendre*. ● The old roué, a dirty old man now, was given to *cacemphaton*. (2. Sounds combined for harsh effect, e.g., ". . . thus, neither honour nor nobility, could move a naughty niggardly noddy." {Peacham, as sited by Lanham, R.A.}). [< G *kakemphaton* ill sounding, equivocal < G *kakos* bad + *emphainein* to show, indicate < *phainein* to show]. Cf. **adianoeta**, *double entendre*, q.v. See <u>talk</u>. See <u>sex, love</u>.

cache (kash) n. 1. a hidden store of things, especially things of value. 2. a secret place where stored things are kept. 3. an area of high-speed computer memory used for temporary storage of frequently used data. ● The forgetful old **grisard**, q.v., longed for a computer *cache* on which she could draw when confronted frequently by lapsed memory. [late 18th C. < F < *cacher* to hide, conceal]. vi.&vt. **cached**, **caching**, **caches** (1. to store a hidden supply of things.) (2. to store data in a cache.) alt. **cache memory**. See <u>memory</u>.

cache memory (kash mem'ō-ree) n.phr. = **cache**, q.v. See <u>memory</u>.

cachexia (kə-kek'see-ə) n. a condition marked by loss of appetite, advanced weight loss, muscular wasting, and general mental and physical debilitation caused by chronic disease. [< G *kakhexia* < *kakos* bad + *hexis* habit]. adjs. **cachectic**, **cachectical**, **cachexic**. Cf. **inanition**, q.v. See <u>gastrointestinal</u>. See <u>physique, appearance</u>.

cachinnation (ka-kin-nay'shən) n. loud, immoderate, or convulsive laughter. [< L *cachinnat-*, pp. of *cachinnare* an imitation of the sound]. n. **cachinnator**. vi **cachinnate**. adj. **cachinatory**. See **talk**. See **role**.

cacoethes carpendi (ka-kō'ə-thees kaar-pen'di) n.phr. a compulsion, ill habit, itch to criticize or find fault. [L *cacoethes* < G *kakoethes* neut. adj.< *kakos* bad + *ethos* disposition and L *carpendi* < *carpere* to carp at, criticize, take apart]. See **mentality, mentation, behavior**.

cacoethes loquendi (kaa-kō'ay-thees lō-kwen'dee) n.phr. compulsion, ill habit, itch to talk. [L *cacoethes* < G *kakoethes* neut. adj. < *kakos* bad + *ethos* disposition and < L *loquitari* to chatter away]. Cf. *cacoethes scribendi* = compulsion to write. See **talk**.

cacology (ka-kol'lə-jee) n. garbled diction or pronunciation; bad choice of words; incorrect pronunciation. [caco-, pref, bad, < G *kakos* bad + -logy, suff., science, study < *-logia* < *logos* word, reason]. adj. **cacologic** (-kō-loj'jik). adj. **cacological** (-kō-loj'ji-kəl). See **talk**.

cacosomnia (kak'-kō-som'ni-ə) n. bad, disturbed, unrestful sleep. [caco-, pref., meaning bad or ill < G *kakos* bad + *somnos* sleep]. adj. **cacosomnic**. n. **cacosomniac**. See **sleep & wakefulness**. See **role**.

caducity (ka doos'si-tee) n. 1. the weakness, feebleness of old age; **decrepitude**, q.v.; infirmity. 2. **senility**, q.v. 3. dropping or falling off. 4. the quality or state of being perishable; temporary. (5. the lapse of a will's legacy through the birth of an heir.) adj. = **caducous** (ka-doo'kəs) = 1. dropping off; 2. fleeting, uninduring; (3. in botany: falling off early, as some leaves.) [L *cadere* to fall]. See **tiredness, weakness**. See **old age**. See **physical appearance**.

caino(to)phobia See **kaino(to)phobia**.

calando (kə-laan'dō) adv., adj. a musical term: played with gradually decreasing volume and slowing tempo. Can be used fig. • The dowager's attention waned and her voice became perceptively *calando*. [< It, slackening]. See **talk**. See **nerve, muscle, movement, touch**.

calcium CT cardiac scan n.phr. 64-slice computerized tomography: an examination (scan) of the heart to detect calcium in the coronary-artery endothelium (inside lining of the coronary artery), an indication of plaque formation at that site; plaque rupture can result in plaque embolization with blockage of coronary flow to heart muscle. The report of the scan is indicated by a number, from 0 to 400, that indicates the risk of a coronary thrombosis (heat attack) within 2-5 years. Hypertension, smoking, diabetes, obesity, family history, etc., increase the risk of coronary disease. [tom(o)-, pref., denoting a cutting, or to a designated layer, as might be achieved by cutting or slicing, < G *tome* a cutting + < G *graphein* to write]. See **heart, rhythm**.

callidity(kal-lid'di-tee) n. slyness, craftiness. • The old roué's on-the-edge survival had engendered in him a noticeable degree of *callidity*. [< L *calliditas* skill; shrewdness; cunning, craft].

callosity(kal-los'si-tee), pl. **–ties**, n. a local thickening, hardening of the outer layer of the skin due to repeated friction or pressure. A corn. A **callus**. [< L *callosus* < *callus* hard skin]. syn. **callositas** = callosity; **clavus**, **keratoma**; **tyloma**, q.v. See **skin**. See **joint, extremities, back**.

calvities (kal-vish'ee-eez) alt. **calvity** (kal'vi-tee). n. baldness. [L baldness, alopecia < *calvus* bald]. adj. **calvous** (kal'vəs). syns. = **acomia, alopecia, atrichia, depilous, phalacrosis, pilgarlic**, q.v. Cf. **psilosis**; **alopeciaphobia, peladophobia, phalacrophobia; canescent, canities, poliosis**, q.v. See **hair**.

Calypso (kə-lip'sō) pr.n. (1. a sea nymph who was queen of Ogygia, an island upon which Ulysses wrecked.) 2. one who promises perpetual youth. (3. a small natural satellite of Saturn discovered in 1980.) 3. The European Union's program to help the needy go on holiday. The program especially targets the disabled, poor families, **senior citizens**, & "youth", i.e. those up to 30 years of age. [G, Calypso kept Ulysses for seven years on her island. She promised him perpetual youth and immortality if he would but stay with her forever; he refused]. (calypso = a spontaneously topical West Indian song; its origin is unknown.) See **youth, younger generation**. See **role**.

cancer, neoplasm, tumor: **cancerophobia, carcinomatophobia, dyskeratoma, dyskeratosis, keratoacanthomas, mesothelioma, Morton's neuroma**

cancer, neoplasm, tumor: Subcategories

I. Malignant tumor of pericardium, peritoneum, or pleura: **mesothelioma**
II. Morbid fear of cancer: **cancerophobia, carcinomatophobia**
III. Skin cancer with horniness: **dyskeratoma, dyskeratosis**
IV. Other: **keratoacanthomas, Morton's neuroma**

cancerophobia (kan"ser-ō-fōb'bi-ə) n. morbid fear of cancer. [L, cancer (also crab; the South; tropical heat.) (*Cancer* = Cancer, northern zodiacal constellation; sign of the zodiac) + -phobia, suff., = fearing < G -*phobia* < *phobos* fear]. adj. **cancerophobic**. n. **cancerophobe**. syn. **carcinophobia**, q.v. See **phobias**. See **cancer, neoplasm, tumor**.

canescent (kə-nes'sənt) adj. becoming white; tending to dull white, grayish, hoary. [< L *canescere* grow white < *canus* white, hoary]. See **color**. See **hair**.

canities (kan-ish'ee-eez) n. having grey or white hair; a hair coloration that is gray or white. [L *canus*, hoary, white]. Cf. **poliosis, canescent**, q.v. syn. **grizard**, q.v. See **color**. See **hair**. See **physique, appearance**.

cannabanoids (kan-nab'bin-noydss) n.pl. any of the principles of cannabis, the dried flowering tops of hemp plants, *Cannabis sativa*, which contain euphoric and halucinogenic principles. Cannabinoids are the active agents in marijuana and are pain relievers. In a 2009 survey by the Substance Abuse and Mental Health Services Administration < 1% of those > 65 years of age admits to smoking marijuana. Use in younger age groups is greater; use in the elderly is expected to increase. Marijuana is especially effective in curbing pain arising from nerve damage. Marijuana raises heart rate and lowers blood pressure. It may allow patients to decrease or eliminate narcotic use. Two cannabinoid treatment drugs are now available in the U.S., but only for treatment of nausea and appetite loss. Use in the elderly may risk falls, impaired cognition, and loss of memory and motor control; unsupervised use is risky. [< G *kannabis* hemp + -oid, suff., < G -*oeides* < *eides* form]. See **therapy**.

cantankerous (kan-tank'er-əss) adj. bad tempered, quarrelsome, perverse {perhaps < ME *contak* contention, on analogy with traitorous, rancorous]. adv. **cantankerously**. n. **cantankerousness**. See **talk**. See **mentality, mentation, behavior**.

capripede (kap'ri-peed) n. a **satyr**, q.v. • Affronted, she labeled him a *capripede*. [< L *caper* goat + *pes* foot]. See **sex, love**.

capromorelin (kap"rō-mor'rə-lin) n an investigational drug that increases growth hormone production leading to significant increases in lean body mass and improvement in physical function tests (Duke University & Pfizer Global Research) [?, perhaps < capr-, pref., goat, < L *caper* goat (from its smell) +?]. See **therapy**.

caprylic (ka-pril'ik) adj. having a rancid animal odor. [< L, *capr-* < *caper* goat: from its smell]. See **nose & smell**.

captious (kap'shəss) adj. 1. calculated to entrap or entangle; sophistical; tricky. 2. trivial, fault-finding; carping; caviling; fond of taking exception. • The elderly, perhaps out of boredom, lack of activity, often become *captious*. [< L *captiosus* deceitful; captious, sophistical; dangerous, harmful < *capere* to seize]. See **talk**. See **mentality, mentation, behavior**.

carcinophobia (kar"sin-ō-fōb'bi-ə) n. morbid fear of cancer. [< G *karkinos* cancer + -phobia, suff., fearing < G -*phobia* < *phobos* fear]. adj. **carcinophobic**. n. **carcinophobe**. syns. **cancer(o)phobia**, **carcinomatophobia**, q.v. See **phobias**.

carcinomatophobia (kar"sin-ō-mat"tō-fōb'bi-ə) n. morbid fear of cancer. [<G *karkinoma* < *karkinos* crab + -oma, suff. meaning tumor, < G *oma*, a noun-forming suff. + -phobia, suff., fearing, < G -*phobia* < *phobos* fear—from the crab-like pattern of a neoplasm's surrounding blood vessels]. adj. **carcinomatophobic**. n. **carcinomatophobe** (-mat'tō-). syns. **cancer(o)phobia**, **carcinophobia**, q.v. See **phobias**. See **cancer, neoplasm, tumor**.

cardiophobia (kar"di-ō-fōb'bi-ə) n. morbid fear of heart disease. [cardi(o)-, pref., relating to the heart (alt., the word, cardia, can refer to that part of the stomach immediately adjacent to the esophageal opening.) < G *kardia* heart + -phobia, suff., fearing < G -*phobia* < *phobos* fear]. adj. **cardiophobic**. n. **cardiophobe**. Cf. **anginophobia**, q.v. See **phobias**.

carminative (kaar-min'nə-tiv) n. 1. preventing the formation or causing the expulsion of flatus, farting, **crepitus**, q.v. 2. an agent that relieves flatulence. adj. **carminative** pertaining to prevention or relief of flatus. [< L *carmino*, pp. –*atus* to card wool;,. a special modern L use of the word = to expel wind]. syn. **physagogue**, q.v. See **gastrointestinal**. See **therapy**.

carphology (kaar-fol'lŏ-gee), alt. **carphologia** (kaar-fol-ŏj'ji-ə), n. involuntary picking at the bedclothes seen in grave fevers and in conditions of great exhaustion. Syns. **crocidismus, floccillation**, q.v. [< G *karphologia* a gathering of twigs < *karphos*, bits of wood, straw, wool, etc.; *karphologein* to pick bits of wool off a person's coat]. See **mentality, mentation, behavior**.

catachresis (ka-tə-krees'siss), pl. -ses (seez), n. the incorrect, improper use of words, e.g. mixing metaphors, [< G *katakhresis* < *katakhresthai* to misuse < cata-, pref., meaning down; wrongly < *kata* + *khraomai* use]. adj. **catachrestic** (-kres'tik). **catachrestical**. adv. **catachrestically** (-kres'ti-). See **talk**.

catamaran (kat'tə-mə-ran) n. 1. a nagging fishwife, quarrelsome scold, virulent virago, or shrill shrew. (2. a raft of two boats fastened side by side.) [1.? associated with cat. (2.< Tamil *katta-maram* tied tree or wood)]. syns. (**old**) **shrew, rixatrix, termagant, virago, Xanthippe**, q.v. See **old woman**.

cataphasia (kat-ə-fay'zhə, zhi-ə) n. involuntary, meaningless repetition of the same word. [cata-, pref., down, < G *kata* down, + *phasis* a saying]. See **talk**.

cataract (kat'tə-rakt″) n. an opacity, partial or complete, of one or both eyes, on or in the lens or its capsule, with the capability of impairing vision or causing blindness. There are a number of different forms. Cataracts are frequent in old age. (The Oxford Dictionary lists seven other definitions having nothing to do with the eye, including a floodgate, a waterfall, a portcullis, a brake for flax{obs.}, and a form of governor for single-action steam engines {obs.}.) [< L *cataracta* < G *katarraktes* waterfall, floodgate, portcullis—perhaps because an eye cataract and a portcullis are both obstructive]. ppl. adj. **cataracted** = having cataract(s). n. **cataractist** = a practitioner (ophthalmologist) who treats cataracts. adj. **cataractous** = affected with cataract(s). See **eye**. See **role**.

catarolysis (kat"tə-rol'li-siss) n. letting off steam by cursing. [< G *katarrassein* to dash down, dash headlong, rush or fall headlong < *kata* down + *arass-* or *arassein* to dash + *lysis* dissolution]. syn. **lalochezia**, q.v. See **talk**.

cathect (kə-thekt') vt. To invest mental or emotional activity in something: an idea, a person, a thing, an activity. • The old professor *cathects* the science of words, logology. [a back-formation < **cathexis**, q.v. < G *kathexis* a holding in, retention; the investment of emotional energy in something]. See **emotion**. See **mentality, mentation, behavior**.

cathexis (kə-thek'siss) n. a great deal of mental or emotional concentration on, attachment to, or investment in an idea or object. • The young man could not overcome his grandmother's *cathexis* that he head the family business. [< Freud, < G *kathexis* a holding in, retention; the investment of emotional energy in something]. vt. **cathect**, q.v. See **emotion**. See **mentality, mentation, behavior**.

catholicon (ka-thol'li-kən) n. a **panacea**; q.v., a cure-all. • Seniors, frustrated by their multitudinous health problems, search in vain for a *catholicon*. [< G *katholikos* general < *kata* according to, by + *holou* whole]. See **therapy**.

CCRC an initialism: <u>c</u>ontinuing <u>c</u>are <u>r</u>etirement <u>c</u>ommunity. CCRCs provide independent-living and skilled-nursing facilities to elders. There are currently about 1,850 CCRCs in the U.S. that have some 750,000 residents. "Entrance fees", sometimes quite large, are frequently charged to be domiciled, but are usually to some extent refundable upon departure or death under certain circumstances. Cf. **elder-care hostel**, **geriatric center**, **gerontocomium**, **hibernacle**, q.v. See **health, illness**. See **retirement**. See **therapy**.

cecity (see'si-tee) n. blindness. [< L *cæcus* blind]. See **eye**.

cecutiency (see-kyoo'shən-see) n. partial blindness; a tendency toward blindness; dim-sighted. [< L *cæcutient-* pres.p. stem of *cæcutire* to be blind < *cæcus* blind]. n. **cecutient** = a person with partial sight. adj. **cecutient**. Cf. **cecity**, **idiopt**, q.v. See **eye**. See **role**.

cenotaph (sen'nə-taf", sen-nō-) n. a monument erected as a memorial to a dead person or dead people buried elsewhere, especially those killed fighting a war. [< G *kenotaphion* empty tomb < *kenos* empty + *taphos* tomb]. adj. **cenotaphic**. See **end-of-life, death**.

centenarian (sen"ten-air'ree-ən) n. someone one hundred or more years of age; adj. = **centenarian** = 1. of 100 years; 2. of a centenarian. [< L *centenaries* containing a hundred < *centeni* hundred each < *centum* hundred]. See **old man, old woman**.

centenary (sen-ten'nə-ree) adj. 1. of a century, relating to or involving a period of 100 years. 2. once-a-century, occurring every hundred years. 3. **centennial**, adj., q.v. [L *centum* "hundred"]. See **old**.

centennial (sen-ten'ni-əl) adj., 1. relating to or involving a period of 100 years. 2. once a century, or occurring every 100 years. 3. of 100th anniversary, or marking an anniversary of 100 years. syn. **centenary**, q.v. n. the 100th anniversary, or a celebration held to mark a 100th anniversary. [< L *centum* hundred]. See **old**. See **old age**.

centophobia (sen"tō-fōb'bi-ə) n. morbid fear of novelty, something new; change. [< L *cento* a garment of patchwork, a piece of patchwork + -phobia, suff., fearing, < G -*phobia* < *phobos* fear]. n. **centophobe**. syn. = **neophobia**. See **phobias**. See **innovation, misoneism**.

Cerberus (sur'bər-əss) n. the fierce dog in Greek and Roman mythology that guards the gates of Hades by preventing those who have crossed the River Styx there from recrossing. Cerberus is pictured usually with three heads, but the number varies from one to 50. [< G *Kerberos*]. adj. **Cerberean** (sur-bə-ree'ən). See **end of life, dying**.

cerements (ser'rə-məntss) n.pl. burial clothes, shroud. ns. = 1. textiles; 2. cerecloth, i.e., cloth treated with wax for waterproofing.) [< L *cerare* < *cera* wax]. See **end-of-life & death**.

cereous (ser'ree-əss) adj. waxen. [< L *cera* wax]. See **skin**. See **physique, appearance**.

cernuous (sur'nyoo-əss) adj. bending, drooping, hanging down, like a flower. • The old duffer's *cernuous* posture professed his age. [< L *cernuus* with face turned toward to the earth, stooping forwards]. See **physique, appearance**. See **skin**.

cerumen (se-roo'men, sə-) n. earwax, the accumulation of which is more common among the elderly, and is a prominent cause of decreased hearing. (Ear wax is the ear's cleaning system: Wax entraps incoming dust, debris, bacteria and is gradually extruded by jaw movement—at about the same speed as fingernail growth. Wax's softness or dryness is genetically determined. Hardening causes impaction, which occurs in as many as 57% of seniors in nursing homes. In 2008 the American Academy of Otolaryngology published its guidelines for treating earwax.) [< L *cera* wax]. See **ear**.

chaetophorous (kee-tof'fawr-əss) adj. bristle-bearing; in need of a shave. • A seedy, *chaetophorous* appearance was not unusual in his later years. [L *chaeta* (= seta) < G *chaite* stiff hair + -phore, -phor(o), suff., carrying or bearing, < *phoros* carrying + -ous, full of, having the qualities of < L -*osus* and -*us*]. See **skin**.

chalazion (kaa-lay'zi-ən, ka-lay'), pl. **chalazia**, n. swelling, cyst, or sty—a chalazion that becomes painful—due to inflammation of a sebum-secreting gland (meibomian gland) at the edge of the eyelid: a meibomian sty, *hordeolum internum*. (Keeping the eyelids carefully cleansed is prophylactic, but sometimes neglected in the elderly. A persistent apparent chalazion can be a sebaceous-cell carcinoma.) [G, diminutive of *chalaza* a small lump or sty—meibaumian is < Hendrik Meibom, a Ger. anatomist (1638-1700), and hordeolum < L *hordeolus* a sty in the eye]. syn. **meibomian cyst**, q.v. See **eye**.

charlie/charley horse n. (informal, not capitalized) a severe, localized muscular cramp, contraction, or spasm especially in the upper anterior leg, or in the calf, sometimes following excessive muscular activity, possibly caused by fluid distention within the affected muscle's sheath. [unknown]. In the elderly, charlie horse is more common than in the young. [Origin uncertain, but the term is probably < U.S. baseball, possibly from a 19th C. pitcher named Charley who had the problem. (A Charley is an E term for a policeman.)]. See **nerve, muscle, movement, touch**. See **pain**. See **joint, extremities, back**.

cherry angioma (an-gee-ōm'mə) n.phr. small red-to-violaceous benign skin tumor in the form of papules, which usually occur on the trunk. They appear in early adulthood, are nearly universal by age 30, and increase in size and number with age. A synonym is **senile hemangioma**. [angi(o)-, pref., relating to blood or lymph vessels, < G *angeion* vessel + -*oma*, suff., tumor]. See **skin**.

chiropodist (kir-op'pō-dist) n. the former term for a **podiatrist**, q.v., = a foot doctor. [chir(o)-, pref., denoting relationship to the hand, < G *cheir* hand, + *pous* foot + -iatr(o), suff., denoting relationship to a physician or to medicine, < *iatros* physician]. See **therapy**. See **role**. See **joint, extremities, back**.

chiropody (kir-op'pō-dee) n. podiatry. Chiropody is an older term supplanted by **podiatry**, q.v. [chir(o)- meaning hand, < G *cheir* hand, + *pous* foot]. See **therapy**. See: **joint, extremities, back**.

chivvy (chiv'vee/**chivy**/**chevy**) (chev'vee) vt. to urge, pester, badger, or harass somebody, usually in order to make him or her do something, or do it more quickly. (U.K. to chase or hunt something. n. UK a chase, hunt, or pursuit.) [Probably < Chevy Chase, site of a 1388 battle in the Anglo-Scottish border wars]. See **talk**.

choleric (kol'lə-rik or kə-ler'rik) adj. easily irritated or angered, hot tempered. • His *choleric* disposition was the bane of the nursing home's staff. (Ancient physicians believed that four essential body fluids, i.e., body "humors", when in balance assured health. The four humors were yellow bile, < G *choler*, anger; blood, < L *sanguis*, sanguine, cheerfully optimistic; black bile, < G *melankolia* < *melas*, gen. *melanos* black, sad; and phlegm, G *phlegma*, heat < *phlegein* to burn, phlegmatic, lacking emotion. Each humor was associated with an element: air, water, earth, and fire, and a season. Humeral imbalance caused a change in temperament, or something more serious. [< G *cholerikos* < *chole* bile]. adj. **choler**. See **emotion**.

chronophobia (kron''nō-fōb'bi-ə) n. morbid fear of (the passage of) time. [chrono-, pref., relating to time, < G *khronos* time, + *phobos* fear]. adj. **chronophobic**. n. **chronophobe**. See **phobias**.

chthonic (thon'nik) adj. relating to the underworld as described in Greek myth. [< G *khthon* earth]. syn. **chthonian** (thōn'ni-). See **end-of-live, death**.

churlish (churl'ish) adj. pertaining to a person of low birth, a peasant; boorish; ill-bred; niggardly. n. **churl**. n. **churlishness**. adv. **churlishly**. [< OE *ceorl* man, cognate with carl(e), Sc, man, fellow]. See **mentality, mentation, behavior**. See **role**.

CIMT is an initialism for carotid intimal-medial thickness. CIMT is measured by means of a carotid-artery ultrasound test showing the thickness of the inner lining—both intimal and medial layers—of the carotid arteries in the neck as an indicator of **arteriosclerosis**, q.v., and its degree. Thickness can be expressed in percentage of normal and in probability risk, e.g., a 10% chance of having a heat attack in the next 10 years, or indicate a person's vascular (intima-plus-media thickness) age vs. the risk of someone that chronologic age, but perhaps10-20 years older with that vascular age, of having a stroke, heart failure, peripheral arterial disease, or hear-attack. There are software programs into which risk-factor numbers can be entered and customized therapeutic recommendations made to patients for their vascular-age improvement See **blood, circulation, glands**. See **heart, rhythm**.

cinerarium (sin"nə-rair'ree-əm), pl. -ree-a (-aa/ə), n. a place, e.g., an urn, where the ashes of a corpse are stored. [< L *ciner-* ashes]. See **end- of-life, death**.

cinerary (sin'ə-rair-ee) adj. pertaining to holding, or intended for, ashes, especially those of the cremated dead. [< L *cinerarius* of ashes < *cinis* ashes; ruin; death]. See **end-of-life & death**.

cinereous (sin-eer'ree-əss, sə-neer') adj. resembling or consisting of ashes. 2. of an ash-gray color. [< L *cinereus* < *ciner-* ashes + -ous, suff.]. See **color**. See **end-of-life, death**.

cinerescent (sin-ər-es'sənt) adj. ashen, grayish. [< L *cinereus* ashy < *cinis* ashes + -escent suff., resembling < L -*escent* pres. p. ending of verbs in -*escere*, expressing the beginning of action]. syn. = **cinereous**. See **color**. See **skin**.

circadian sleep dysrhythmia (sər-kayd'dee-ən sleep dis-rith'mee-ə) n.phr. sleep disorder, common in the elderly, and characterized by sleep and wakefulness out of phase with the conventional 24-hour sleep/wake cycle. [< L *circa* about + *dies* day]. See **sleep, wakefulness**.

circumforaneous (sir"kum-fə-rayn'nee-əss) adj. wandering from place to place. [< L *circumroaneus* < circum-, pref., around, < L *circus* circle + *forum* market]. adv. **circumforaneously**. See **standing, walking, wandering**.

claudicant (klaw'di-kənt) adj. relating to limping; lameness, having leg pain on walking. [< L *claudicare* limp < *claudus* gait-impaired]. n. one with **claudication**, q.v., intermittent claudication. See **pain**. See **role**. See **standing, walking, wandering**.

claudication (klaw-di-kay'shən) n. 1. limping or impaired gait, especially as a result of reduced blood supply to the leg muscles. 2. **intermittent claudication** (med.), i.e., intermittent leg pain, especially due to impaired blood supply to leg muscles. [L, *claudication* < *claudicare* to limp < *claudus* gait impaired}. See: **standing, walking, wandering**. See: **nerve, muscle, movement, touch**. See **pain**.

clavus (klayv'vus) pl. **clavi** (klayv'vee) n. 1. a corn [< L *cornu* horn], callosity [< L *callosus* thick skinned], **heloma**, q.v., or **tyloma**, q.v., as on the foot. Corns and calluses are caused by biomechanical factors: undue friction and pressure around a bony prominence, often due to tight or ill-fitting shoes. A soft corn = **heloma molle**, q.v., is usually found between the toes and is due to pressure from adjacent toes, in contrast to a **heloma durum** = a hard corn, which occurs over joints of the toes. (2. a severe pain in the head, sharply limited in area, as if caused by the driving of a nail. 3. a condition resulting from healing of a granuloma of the foot in yaws. A core falls out, leaving an erosion.) [L, a nail, wart, corn]. syns. **callosity**, **heloma**, **keratoma**, **poroma**, **tyloma**, q.v., & **callositas**. See **skin**. See **joint, extremities, back**.

cleptophobia See **kleptophobia**. See **phobias**.

climacophobia (klīm"ma-kō-fō'bi-ə) n. morbid fear of climbing or falling down stairs. [< G *klimax* ladder + *phobos* fear]. adj. **climacophobic**. n. **climacophobe**. See **phobias**. See **standing, walking, wandering**.

clinomania (klī-nō-mayn'ni-ə) n. excessive desire to stay in bed. [clino-, pref., slope, slant < G *klinein* lean + -mania suff., excessive enthusiasm for or attachment to, < G *mania* loss of reason]. adj. **clinomaniacal** (-mə-nī'ə-kəl). n. **clinomaniac**. See **manias**.

CLU n. the initialism of an Alzheimer's-disease gene that "appears to be involved in 'chaperoning' newly formed amyloid molecules and helping suppress their deposition in the brain." Another recently discovered Alzheimer gene is **PICALM**, q.v. The earliest known gene linked to Alzheimer's is **APOE**, q.v. [< clusterin, the name of the gene]. See **intelligence**.

clyster (klīs'stər) n. an enema; an injection into the rectum. [< G *klyster* a syringe]. See **gastrointestinal**. See **therapy**.

clysterize (klīs'ter-īz) vt. to treat with enemas, or with injections within the rectum. [< L *clysterizare* < G *klyster* a syringe]. See **gastrointestinal**. See **therapy**.

co- pref. together, with, jointly (used before a vowel instead of **con-** or **com-**, q.v). [L, short form of *com.*, prep., with, used in L only before vowels, h, gn, & (in the correct classical form) n, but in E as living pref. before any letter (The Concise Oxford . . .].

coacervate (kō-as'sər-vayt) vt. to accumulate, heap up, amass, in relation to money. (n. an aggregate of colloidal droplets bound together by electrostatic forces.) • His plan was seriously to coacervate his various properties during the next five years in order to retire at 70 years of age. [< L *coacervatio* piling up, accumulation < *coacervare* to pile up accumulate]. n. **coacervation**. See **finance**.

codger (coj'ər) n. (colloq.) a slightly queer, amusing, eccentric man of advanced age (artful codger = a pun based on Dickens' character, the Artful Dodger: Jack Dawkins in Oliver Twist). The term is sometimes preceded by the word, old. [18th C.? variant of "cadger", a carrier; itinerant dealer, street hawker, beggar, loafer]. See **old man**.

coetaneous (kō-ee-tayn'nee-əss) adj. of the same age or duration; contemporary. [< L *coataneus* < co- + aetas age]. syn. **coeval**, q.v. See **old**.

coeval (kō-eev'vəl) adj. of the same age, date of origin, duration, or contemporaty; equally old. n. a contemporary. • She's my *coeval* and we *coetaneous*, q.v., antiquarians have decided we need help with bathing and dressing. [< L *coaevus* < co- + aevum age < G *aion* age]. n. **coevality**. adv. **coevally**. syn. **coetaneous**, q.v. See **old**.

cogger (cog'gər) n. a phony male flatterer; offers compliments to mask a deception. Frequently the term is preceded by the word, old. • The old *cogger* dodged many questions. [? < the slang verb, cog, vi.&vt., to cheat in a gambling game by loading the dice]. See **old man**.

cogitabund (koj'jit-tə-bund) adj. pensive, musing, meditative, thoughtful (arch.). [< L *cogitabundus* thinking < *cogitare* to think]. n. **cogitabundation** (koj'it-tə-bund"day'shən) n. **cogitabundity** (koj'it-tə-bund'di-tee). See **mentality, mentation, behavior**.

cognition (kog-nish'ən) n. that operation of the mind by which we become aware of objects of thought or perception; it includes all aspects of perceiving, thinking, and remembering. (Cognition can be assessed quantitatively with, e.g., the Annotated Mini-Mental State Examination.) [< L *cognito* < *cognoscere* to know]. adj. **cognitive** (kog'ni-tiv), pertaining to cognition. (Experts differ about the value of cognitive screening for memory impairment, especially re: brief screening. The Alzheimer's Foundation of America {AFA} favors it and has a "National Memory Screening Day". A recent study in Nature found no evidence of cognitive transfer between specific mental tasks and general cognitive function—the Wall Street Journal's caption on this review (4/21/10) was "Study Finds Mental Exercise Offers Brain Limited Benefits"—it makes sense with or without a hyphen between Brain and Limited. See **intelligence**. See **mentality, mentation, behavior**.

cognitive dysfunction or impairment (cog'ni-tiv) n.phr. abnormality in perception, thinking, and memory. It occurs sometimes in the elderly after general anesthesia, and sometimes persists for several months. General anesthesia has been compared to sleep, but it is not sleep; rather it is functionally equivalent to brain-stem death. The electroencephalogram (EEG) in coma-recovery states can resemble an awake state, one of general anesthesia, or one of sleep depending on the degree of brain injury and the state of recovery. Cognitive impairment can be a precursor of Alzheimer's disease. (The term **cognitive dissonance** refers to a state of psychological conflict or anxiety resulting from a contradiction between a person's simultaneously held beliefs or attitudes, and is not to be confused with cognitive dysfunction.) [< L *cognitivus* < *cognoscere* apprehend, get to know < (g)*noscere* know]. Cf. **pump head**. See **intelligence**. See **mentality, mentation, behavior**.

coimetromania/koimetromania (coy-met"trō-may'ni-ə) n. 1. abnormal or morbid attraction, desire, or compulsion to visit cemeteries, graves, burial sites. [via OF *cimetiere* graveyard < LL *coemeterium* < G *koimeterion* sleeping place, dormitory < koiman to put to sleep < *keimai* I lie down + -mania, suff. connoting excessive enthusiasm for or attachment to, < G *mania* loss of reason, frenzy, madness < *mainesthai* to rage]. See **manias**. See **end of life, death**.

coimetrophilia/koimetrophilia (coy-met"trō-fil'li-ə) n. Special fondness, interest, or fascination for visiting cemeteries, seeing gravestones, sarcophagi, collecting tombstone epitaphs. [via OF *cimetiere* graveyard < LL *coemeterium* < G *koimeterion* sleeping place, dormitory < koiman to put to sleep < *keimai* I lie down + -phyla, suff. denoting love, fondness, affinity, craving for, < G *philos* fond, loving < *phileo* to love]. See **sex, love**. See **end of life, death**.

coimetrophobia/koimetrophobia (coy-met"trō-fō'bee-ə) n. fear, dread of cemeteries, graveyards, tombs. [via OF *cimetiere* graveyard < LL *coemeterium* < G *koimeterion* sleeping place, dormitory < koiman to put to sleep < *keimai* I lie down + -phobia, suff. < *phobos* fear]. See **phobias**. See **end of life, death**.

COLA (kōl'laa) an initialism: C̲ost O̲f L̲iving A̲djustment, which refers to an annual increase in Social Security (SS) benefit payments based on currency inflation and calculated by a formula set by law. (> 50 million people, mainly seniors, receive SS; there has been a COLA increase every year since 1975, with one of the highest increases in 2009 = 5.8%, but, due to recession, no increase is anticipated for 2010, and perhaps none until 2012. COLA law also caps part-B premiums of Medicare for certain of its beneficiaries. (Spending in 2008 on Social Security and Medicare was > $1 trillion and equal to one-third of the federal budget—New York Times article, 5/3/09.) See **finance**.

collyrium (kəl-lir'ee-əm), pl. **collyria/collyriums,** n. an eye salve or eyewash. [L, < G *kollurion*, dim. of *kollura* roll of bread]. See: **eye**.

color: achlorophyllaceous, allochrous, canescent, canities, cinereous, cinerescent, cretaceous, dealbate, dyschroia, dyschromia, erubescence, etiolate, feuillemorte, flavescent, fuliginous, hoarhead, hoary, icterical, luteolus, melanocyte, pallid, poliosis, sallow, Stygian, tenebrous, wan, whitebeard.

color: Subcategories

I. Abnormal color of the skin or hair: **dyschromia**
II. Brown & yellow:
   1. Yellow: **icterical**
   2. Yellowish brown, brown: **feuillemorte**
III. Dark, gloomy, sooty, dark gray, dull brown, black:
   1. Dark and gloomy: **Stygian, tenebrous**
   2. Gray: **cinereous, cinerescent, poliosis**
   3. Sooty, dark gray, dull brown, black, (fig.) mysterious: **fuliginous**
IV. Discoloration of the skin, a bad complexion: **dyschroia**
V. Light gray, white:
   1. Gray or white: **canescent, canities, hoarhead, hoary, poliosis**
   2. White: **cretaceous, dealbate, etiolate, hoary, whitebeard**
VI. Multicolored: **allochroous**
VII. Pale: **pallid, wan**
VIII. Pigment cell: **melanocyte**
IX. Redness: **erubescence**
X. Without color:
   1. Colorless: **achlorophyllaceous**
   2. Loss of hair color: **poliosis**
XI. Yellow:
   1. Pale yellow, yellowish: **flavescent, icterical, luteolus, sallow**
   2. Yellow, yellowish brown, brown: **icterical, feuillemorte**

colporrhaphy (kōl-pawr'-ə-fee) n. 1. a surgical procedure used in correcting female pelvic-organ prolapse. A recent substitute procedure is transvaginal polypropylene mesh-kit insertion, an operation that seems more successful, but complications, such as bladder perforation and pelvic bleeding, are more frequent. (2. repair of a vaginal rupture or tear, or suturing the vaginal wall to narrow the vagina.) [< colp(o)-, pref., denoting the vagina, < G *kolpos* any fold or hollow; specifically, vagina + *rhaphe* suture]. See **pelvic support disorders**. See **genitourinary**.

columbarium, (kol'ləm-bair'ree-əm), pl. **–ia** (-ee-aa), n. 1. a burial vault with niches for the placing of **cinerary**, q.v., urns. (2. a columbary, i.e., a dovecote.) [L, pigeon house < *columba* dove]. See **end-of-life & death**.

com- pref. together, with, jointly (used before b, p, n, or p, otherwise **con-**, q.v., or **co-**, q.v., before a vowel). [L].

combover (kōm'mōv-vər) n. (informal) a men's hairstyle designed to conceal baldness by allowing the hair to grow long on one side of the head and combing the long hair over the top. See **hair**.

comity (kom'mi-tee) n. mutual civility, friendliness, and consideration. • We strive for *comity* among the guests in this retirement community. [< L *comis* kind, courteous < *comitas* courtesy, friendliness]. See **mentality, mentation, behavior**.

commatic (kō-mat'tik) adj. having short, terse phrases or sentences; brief. [< G *kommatikos* consisting of short clauses < *komma* clause]. See **talk**.

commensal (kōm-men'səl) n.& adj.1. living and eating together. (2. pertaining to a relationship between organisms of two different species in which one derives food or other benefits from the association while the other remains unharmed and unaffected.) n. = **commensality** (-sal'lə-tee). adv. = **commensally** (-men'sal-lee). [< L *commensalis* at table together < *mensa* table]. See **togetherness**.

commentitious (kom-men-tish'əss) adj. (arch.) imaginary or fabricated. • The old biddy's stories were, for the most part, *commentitious*. [< L *commentum* invention < *comment-* pp. of *comminisci* to invent, literally, to think together]. Cf. **confabulation**, **mythopoeic**. See **talk**.

commorant (kom'mor-ənt) n. 1. a dwelling place; usual or temporary residence in a place. 2. a resident (especially at a university). [< L *commorans, -antis*, pres. p. of *commorari* to remain, abide < *mora* delay]. • Retired elderly *commorants* at universities are recently especially prevalent. adj. **commorant**. n. **commorancy**. See **togetherness**. See **end of life, death**.

commorient (kom-mawr'ri-ənt) adj. dying together. [com-, q.v., + < L *mors* death]. See **togetherness**.

comorbidity (kŏm"mor-bid'di-tee) n. the existence of two or more diseases or illnesses simultaneously; the presence of concurrent multiple chronic diseases. • Comorbidity is especially common in the elderly. [co-, pref., together, jointly < L short form of *com-* (*cum*, prep., with) used in L only before vowels, h, gn, & (in the correct classical form) n, + < L *morbus* sickness]. See **health, illness**.

comploration (kom-plawr-ay'shən) n. wailing and weeping together. [com-, q.v., + < L *complorare* to mourn for]. See **talk**. See **togetherness**.

compotation (kom-pō-tay'shən) n. drinking together. [com-, q.v., + < L *potare* to drink < G *symposion* drinking together]. n. **compotation** the drink itself. n. **compotator** a fellow drinker. See **togetherness**. See **role**.

compuphobia (com"pyoo-fōb'bi-ə) n. fear of computers or high technology. • *compuphobia* is particularly prevalent among the elderly. [< L *computare* reckon together < *putare* to reckon + < G *phobos* fear]. adj. **compuphobic**. n. **compuphobe**. syns. **cyberphobia**, **technophobia**, q.v. See **phobias**.

compursion (kom-pur'zhən) n. wrinkling one's face. • *compursion* is often a permanent feature in the elderly. [humorously, com-, q.v., + purse, v., a pursing together, < L alteration of late L *bursa* < G *byrsa* hide, wineskin]. See **skin**. See **physique, appearance**.

con - prefix together, with, jointly (**com-**, q.v., is used before b, p, n, or p, and **co-**, q.v., is used before a vowel.) [L, See **co-**].

conation (kō-nay'shən) n. mental effort having to do with desire, volition, striving. [< L *conation* < *conat-* pp. of *conari* try]. • The old duffer's *conation* failed to answer the riddle. See **mentality, mentation, behavior**.

concupiscence (kon-kyoop'pis-sənz) n. powerful feelings of physical desire. • The old geezer could not recall when *concupiscence* had last crossed his mind. [< L *concupiscere* to start longing for < *cupere* to desire]. adj. **concupiscent**. syns. **aidoiomania**, **edeomania**, **erotomania**, q.v. Cf. **prurience**, q.v. See **sex, love**.

confabulation (con-fab"byoo-lay'shən) n. The making up of tales, stories, recitals and a readiness to give a fluent answer, without regard whatever to facts to any question put; the act of replacing memory loss with fantasies: a symptom of **prepresbyophrenia**, q.v. [< L *confabulat-*, pp. *confabulari* to talk together < *fabula*, narrative]. n. **confabulator**. vi **confabulate** (-fab'-byoo-layt). adj. **confabulatory** (-fab'byoo-lə-tawr"ree). Cf. **commentitious**, **mythopoeic**, q.v. See **memory**. See **talk**. See **role**.

congener (kon'gen-ər) n. a person, animal, or thing of the same kind or nature as another. • Since you and I are *congeners*, we are both subject to the osteoarthritis of old age. [con-, q.v., + < L *genus* kind]. adjs. **congenerous** (-gen'ner-), **congeneric** (-ner'rik), & **congenetic** (-net'tik) = having a common origin. Cf. **coeval**, **coetaneous**, q.v. See **old** man. See **old** woman. *See* **old person(s), people**.

congruence (kon-groo'ənz) n. (1. agreement, consistency {of one with another, between two}). 2. a psychological term for the harmony, satisfaction felt, experienced when various aspects of one's life, such as motivation, achievement, expectation are in balance. • An amazing 96% of centenarians experience *congruence*: They say they are doing better than, or the same as, others of the same age. [< L *congruentia* < *congruere* to agree]. adj. **congruent**. See **mentality, mentation, behavior**. See **emotion**.

conservative (kon-sur'və-tiv) n. A supporter or advocative of traditional ideas, behavior, and often politics; a believer and supporter of conservatism. The number of conservatives increases with age. (Ambrose Bierce archly defined a conservative as "A statesman who is enamored of existing evils, as distinguished from the liberal, who wishes to replace them with others.") [< L *conservativus* < *conservare* to keep]. adj. **conservative**. adv. **conservatively**. n. **conservatism**. See **mentality, mentation, behavior**. See **role**.

conspue (konz-pyoo') vt. (rare) to spurn contemptuously; express detestation; clamor for the abandonment or abolition of person, policy, etc. • Most centenarians *conspue* today's liberal media. [< L *con*spuere to spit out, spit on]. See **talk**. See **mentality, mentation, behavior**.

consuetude (kon'swi-tyood) n. (archaic) established custom, tradition or usage. [con-, pref., with + < L *consuetudo* complete accustomedness < *suescere* become accustomed]. See **past, time**.

contabescent (kon-tə-bes'sənt) adj. wasting away, atrophied. [con-, q.v., + < L *tabes* a wasting away]. See **physique, appearance**.

contesseration (kon-tes"sə-ray'shən) n. the act of making friends; that act reinforced by some shared token of friendship. • The *contesseration* afforded grandma by a friend in the retirement home offset the loss of' her own cottage. [L < *contesserare* < *con* with + *tessera* to contract friendship by means of the **tessera hospitalis**, q.v., a square tablet, which was divided as a tally or token between two friends in order that they or their descendants might thereby ever afterwards recognize each other, + *tessera* a tally, token]. See **togetherness**.

conticent (kon'tis-sent) adj. silent. [L pres.p. of *conticere* to be silent or still < *con-*, pref., an intensive + *tacere* to be silent.]. • The retirement home's seniors were *conticent* despite the new director's hearty welcome. See **loneliness, solitude, silence**.

contubernial (kon"too-bur'ni-əl) adj. living together familiarly; pertaining to companionship. • The *contubernial* relationship in a retirement home facilitates companionship. [< L *contubernium* common war tent; military companionship]. alt. adjs. **contubernal** (-too'bur-), **contubernyal** (Chauser) ({-too'bur-}). See **togetherness**.

contumacious (kon"too-may'shəss) adj. stubbornly rebellious against authority; insubordinate; disobedient [< L *contumacia* stubbornness, defiance, willfulness; constancy, firmness]. n. **contumacy** (kon-too'mə-see). n. **contumaciousness**. n. **contumacity** (-ma'si-tee). adv. **contumaciously**. See **mentality, mentation, behavior**.

contumelious (kon"too-meel'lee-əss) adj. insolent, reproachful. [< L *contumeliosus* bringing dishonor; insulting, abusive; reproachful, insolent]. adv. **contumeliously**. **contumeliousness**. n. **contumely** (kən-too'mə-lee). ("For who would bear the whips and scorns of time,/Th' oppressor's wrong, the proud man's contumely?" William Shakespeare; Hamlet; c. 1600.) See **talk**. See **mentality, mentation, behavior**.

coot (koot) n. (pl. coots or coot) 1. (insult) somebody regarded as odd, eccentric, or unreasonably stubborn—often preceded by "old". (2. a water bird.) [13th C. <?]. See **old man**. **old woman**. **old person(s)**.

coparcener (ko-paar'sən-ər) n. a joint heir to an undivided property. [co-, pref., together, jointly + *parti(ti) onarius* < *partitionem* < *partiri* to part]. n. &. adj. **coparcenary, -ery** = joint heirship & pertaining to joint heirship, respectively. syn. **parcener**, q.v. See **finance**. See **role.**

COPD initialism = c̲hronic o̲bstructive p̲ulmonary d̲isease. See **health, illness**. See **breathing**.

coprolalia (kop-rō-lay'lee-ə, -rə-) n. the uncontrollable use of obscene language, especially as a result of an illness such as Tourette's syndrome. [copro-, pref., dung, excrement, < G *kopros* dung, + -lalia, suff., speech, speech disorder < G *lalia* talk < *lalein* to talk]. n. **coprology** (-prol'lə-jee, -lō-jee) = study of, or preoccupation with, excrement or obscene language. See **talk**.

coprolite (kop'prō-līt) n. a fossilized turd; can be used fig., offensively.
• That old *coprolite* has never had a kind word for anyone. [copr(o)-, pref., denoting relationship to feces < G *kopros* dung + *lithos* a stone]. syn. **coprolith**. See **gastrointestinal**. See **old man**.

coprostasia (kop-rō-stay'zhə) n. constipation; **costiveness**, q.v.; fecal impaction. [copro-, pref., meaning filth or dung, usually used in reference to feces, < G *kopros* dung, + *stasis* a standing]. adj. **coprostatic**. syn. **obstipation**, q.v. See **gastrointestinal**.

coprostasophobia (kop"prō-stas"sō-fōb'bi-ə) n. morbid fear of constipation. [copro-, pref., meaning filth or dung, usually used in reference to feces, < G *kopros* dung, + *stasis* a standing + *phobos* fear]. adj. **coprostasophobic**. n. **coprostasophobe** (-stas'-sō-). See **phobias**. See **gastrointestinal**.

coronary angiography (kor'ō-nay-ree an" ji-og'grə-fee) n.phr. roentgenographic (x-ray) visualization of the arterial blood vessels (coronary arteries) supplying the heart muscle with blood in order to detect their narrowing (stenosis) or blockage (thrombosis). This is accomplished by cardiac catheterization. The catheter, introduced percutaneously using a needle and sheath, is inserted usually into a femoral (upper leg at the groin) artery into the aorta, up this vessel, and, under fluoroscopic visualization, around its arch, thence into each of the two coronary arteries where a liquid angiographic medium ("dye") is injected. Its passage is recorded on cine (movie) tape or electronically. [< L *corona* < G *korone* crown + angio-, pref., blood vessel < *angeion* vessel, + *graphein* to record]. See **heart, rhythm**.

coronary arteriosclerosis (kor'rō-nay-ree ar-tee"ree-ō-skle-rōs'siss) a collocation indicating **arteriosclerosis**, q.v./ **atherosclerosis**, q.v., of the arteries that arise from the aorta to supply the heart muscle (myocardium). [< L *corona* < G *korone* crown + *arteria* < *aer* air (arteries were supposed by the ancients to contain air), or < *aeirein* to lift or attach + *skleros* hard + -sis, suff.]. See **blood, circulation, glands**.

cosset (kos'set) vt. to spoil by coddling or excessively pampering; to pet, pamper. • Grandmothers traditionally cosset their grandchildren. [perhaps OE *cotsæta* cot-sitter (i.e., an animal brought up in a home)]. See **mentality, mentation, behavior**.

costive (kos'tiv) adj. 1. slow or stiff in the expression of opinions, and in action and reaction generally. 2. constipated, i.e., infrequent stools, or stools that are dry, scanty, hard. Constipation is the most frequent gastrointestinal complaint in the elderly: As many as 60% of elderly outpatients report laxative use (Merck Manual of Geriatrics). [< ME *costif* < OF *costive* < a contraction of L *constipo* to press or crowd together < *constipare* to press or crowd together]. n. **costiveness** = constipation. syns. **coprostasia, dyschezia, obstipation**, q.v. See **talk**. See **gastrointestinal**.

crabbed (krab'bed, krabd) adj. 1. manifesting peevish, cross, or sour temper; irritable; fractious; perverse; grouchy. 2. difficult to understand (of handwriting); abstruse; perplexing. [< ME < OE *crabba* < MDu, MLG *krabbe* < ON *krabbi*, related to OS *krabit*, etc.]. adv. **crabbedly**. n. **crabbedness**. adj. **crabby** (sense no. 1. only). See **mentality, mentation, behavior**.

CRAFT a chat and text-message initialism = C̲an't r̲emember a̲n e̲ffing t̲hing. [See NetLingo.com]. Cf. **CRAT, CRS, CRTLA, OSIF, & SM**, q.v. See **Senior Texting Codes**, p. 429. See **memory**.

crambazzle (kram'baz-zəl) n. a worn-out, dissipated old man. [?]. See **old man**.

crapulence (krap'pyoo-lənz/-pyəl- lənz) n. overindulgence, especially in alcoholic drink, or due to excess in eating or drinking. ● *Crapulence* is the etiology of obesity in many of the elderly, especially in men. [< L *crapulentus* drunken, very drunk, < G *kraipale* drunken headache]. adj. **crapulent**. See **crapulous**. See **drink, food**.

crapulous (krap'pyəl-ləss) adj. regularly overindulging in food and, especially, in alcoholic drink. [< L *crapulentus* drunken, very drunk, < G *kraipale* drunken headache]. n. **crapulousness**. adv. **crapulously**. See **crapulence**. See **drink, food**.

crassilingual (kras-si-ling'gwəl) adj. thick-tongued; indistinct, distorted pronunciation due to a thickened tongue (lit.), or to some (fig.) other speech impediment producing similar sounds. [< L *crassus* thick + *lingua* tongue]. See **talk**. See **mouth, gums, & teeth**.

CRAT a chat and text-message initialism = <u>C</u>an't <u>r</u>emember <u>a</u> <u>t</u>hing. [See NetLingo.com]. Cf. **CRAFT, CRS, CRTLA, OSIF,** & **SM**, q.v. See **memory**.

cremains (kree-maynz') n. the ashes of a cremated body. [< a blend—a portmanteau word—of cremate < L *cremare* to burn & remains < *remanere* < *manere* to stay]. See **end-of-life & death**.

crepitus (krep'pi-təss) n. 1. a noisy discharge of gas from the intestine: a fart, noisily passing gas, or breaking wind. (2. {med.} = crepitation: a crackling noise or vibration.) [< L *crepo* to rattle]. adj. **crepitant**. Cf. **carminative, eructation, flatus, physagogue**, q.v. See **gastrointestinal**.

cretaceous (kre-tay'shəss) adj. chalky, grayish white; of the nature of chalk. ● Her use of rice powder made the **rudas's**, q.v., mien appear *cretaceous*. [< L *cretaceous* < *creta* chalk + -aceous, suff., used to form adjs.< -aceus comparative adj., formative]. See **color**.

cretomania (kree"tō-mayn'ni-ə) n. excessive, uncontrollable sexual desire in a man. [< L *Creta* Crete {*creta*, chalk, white clay} + < G *mania* frenzy, madness, i.e., Cretan mania]. adj. **cretomaniacal** (-mə-nī'ə-kəl). n. **cretomaniac**. syn. **erotomania, gynecomania, satyriasis, satyromania**, q.v. See **manias**. See **sex, love**.

crine (krīn) vi. to shrink, shrivel up. [< Gaelic *crion* to wither < *crion* dry, withered]. See **physique, appearance**.

crocidismus (krō-see-diz'məss) n. the plucking of the nap of a woolen blanket or garment. bedclothes. [< G *korkydismus* or *krikidos* < *krokys* the nap of cloth]. syn. **carphology, floccillation, floccilegium, tilmus**, q.v. See **mentality, mentation, behavior**.

crone (krōn) n. 1. an offensive term that deliberately insults a woman's (old) age, appearance, and temperament. 2. a woman aged over 40 (approving; used by one woman to another) [< F *carogne* withered old woman, literally carrion < L *caro* flesh]. See **old woman**.

crony (krō'nee), pl. -ies, n. a close friend, especially one of long standing. It is used frequently with "old", although tautological. [mid 17ᵗʰ C., < G *khronios* long lasting < *khronos* time]. See **old man**. See **old woman**. See **old person(s), people**.

crotchet (kro'chət) n. 1. a whim; peculiarity; idiosyncrasy; perverse idea, notion, or opinion. (2. a small hook or hook-like instrument. 3. U.K. music = quarter note.) ● The elderly seem predisposed to *crotchets*. [F *crochet* little hook < *croche* hook]. adj. **crotchety**. Cf. **maggot**, q.v.

CRS an indelicate chat and text-message initialism = <u>C</u>an't <u>r</u>emember <u>s</u>—t. [See NetLingo.com]. Cf. **CRAFT, CRAT, CRTLA, OSIF, & SM**, q.v. [See NetLingo.com]. See **memory**.

CRTLA a chat and text message initialism = <u>C</u>an't <u>r</u>emember <u>t</u>he <u>t</u>hree-<u>l</u>etter <u>a</u>cronym. [See NetLingo.com]. Cf. **CRAFT, CRAT, CRS, OSIF, & SM**, q.v. See **memory**.

crusty (kruss'tee) adj. 1. gruff, curt, and candid in speech. ● He's a *crusty* old goat. (2. with a crisp crust.) [< L *crustosus* < *crusta* shell]. n. **crustiness**. adv. **crustily**. Cf. **feisty**, q.v. See **talk**.

cryptomnesia (krip-tom-nee'zhə, neez-zee-ə) n. the phenomenon of "created" images, stories, etc., that one doesn't actually invent, but rather remembers subconsciously from some earlier experience; one is not consciously aware of the phenomenon's origin. [crypt(o)- pref. < G *kryptos* hidden, concealed; without apparent cause + *mneme* memory]. See **memory**.

cuggermugger (kug'gər-mug"gər) n. whispered gossiping. [?] See **talk**. See **role**.

curmudgeon (kur-mud'jən) n. a mean-spirited, humorless, irascible, ungenerous, churlish, miserly, cantankerous, crotchety, irritable person, typically an old man. adj. **curmudgeonly** [sic]. n. **curmudgeonry**. [16th C., origin unknown]. syn. **gnof**, q.v. See **old man**. See **mentality, mentation, behavior**. See **role**.

cyberphobia (sī"bər-fōb'bee-ə, -bur-) n. pathological fear of computers and informational technology. [cyber-, pref., computers and informational systems, e.g., cybernetics, cyberspace, c. mid-20th C., < G kubernetes steersman < kubernan to steer + -phobia, suff., an exaggerated or irrational fear < G phobos fear]. adj. **cyberphobic**. n. **cyberphobe**. syns. **compuphobia**, **technophobia**, q.v. See **phobias**.

cyclothyme (sī'klō-thīm) n. someone with prominent mood swings: vacillates in emotion, behavior between being bright and elated onetime, one moment to being depressed the next. [cyclo-, pref., relating to a circle or cycle < L cyclicus cyclic < G kyklos circle, + < G thymos mind, emotions]. adj. **cyclothymic**. n. **cyclothymia**. See **role**. See **emotion**.

D

"Ours seems to be the only nation on earth that asks its teenagers what to do about world affairs, and tells its goldenagers to go out and play."
—Julian Gerow.

dacryagogue (dak'ree-ə-gōg") n. 1. an agent that induces a flow of tears. (2. a lachrymal duct.) [dacry(o)-, pref, denotes a relationship to tears < G dakryon tear, + -agogue, suff., an agent that leads or induces, < agogos leading, inducing]. adj. **dacryagogic** (-goj'jik) = pertaining to a dacryogogoue. See **eye**. See **emotion**.

dacrygelosis (dak"ri-jel-lōs'siss) n. the condition of alternating crying and laughing. [< L dacry-, dacryo- combining forms relating to tears, tear duct or sac + G gelasma a laugh < gelao to laugh + -osis a G suff. = a process, condition or state]. See **eye**. See **emotion**.

dacryocystitis (dak" kri-ō-sis-tīt'tiss) n. a chronic recurrent infection of the lachrymal punctum (tear duct opening) and sac. • *Dacryocystitis* is more common in the elderly. [dacry(o)-, pref., relating to tears or to the lachrymal sac or duct, < G *dakryon* tear + kystis sac, + *-itis* suffix, inflammation]. See **eye**.

dacryogenic (dak"kree-ō-jen'nik) adj. promoting the secretion of tears. [dacry(o)-, pref, denotes a relationship to tears < G *dakryon* tear + -genic, suff., producing or productive of < *gennan* to produce]. See **eye**. See **emotion**.

daphnean (daf'nee-ən) adj. timid, bashful. (According to Greek mythology, Apollo fell in love with Daphne, a nymph and sworn virgin. He chased her to the Arcadian River Ladon where she prayed to the river god and was turned into a laurel tree.) [G, *Daphne* laurel (Victors at the Pythian Games were crowned with a laurel wreath.)]. See **emotion**.

Darby and Joan (daar'bee & jōn) n. a name for old-people's clubs in the U.K. Darby and his wife Joan were an 18th-C. devoted old couple leading a quiet, uneventful life. They inspired a poem that appeared in "The Gentleman's Magazine" (London, 1735): "Old Darby, with Joan by his side,/ You've often regarded with wonder:/He's dropsical, she is sore-eyed,/ Yet they're never happy asunder . . ." Henry Woodfall, a printer's apprentice, was inspired to write this ballad about his boss John Darby and his wife Joan after Darby's death. The poem inspired follow-up poems and eventually Darby and Joan became a metaphor. In the UK, clubs for old people in the U.K. are still called Darby and Joan clubs. (After Anu Garg {words at wordsmith.org}).

darraign, **-rain, -raine, -rayne, -rein, -reine, -reyne,** etc. (da-rayn')/ **deraign** (dee-rayn') vt. & vi. (obs.) to settle an argument (law). (darrain {da-rayn}{obs.} = to prepare for battle; to deploy troops.) [< OF *déraisnier* to render a reason or account of, to explain, to defend, etc.]. See **talk**.

dealbate (dee-al'bayt) adj. a botanical term meaning covered with a filmy white powder. • The **beldam's** *dealbate* visage, covered in rice powder, came as a surprise. [-de, pref., down, away; completely, < L *de*, adv. & prep., + *albatus* dressed in white < *albere* to be white]. See **color**. See **skin**.

deblaterate (dee-blat'tər-rayt) vi. to babble. [-de, pref., down, away; completely, < L *de-* pref., down, apart, away, + < L *blatire* to babble]. See **talk**.

débrouillard (debrujar, ard) nm., nf. an ever-capable and self-reliant person, who is independent, competent, resourceful, not in need of help; sorts things out, clears things up, follows up and sees things through. American equivalent = a go-getter. • Even at age 80 he continued to manifest the qualities of a *débrouillard*. [F, < *débrouiller*, to disentangle, clear up, sort out; *se débrouiller* to manage, to see it through]. See **role**.

decrepit (di-krep'pit) adj. in poor condition, especially old, overused, or not working efficiently. [< L *decrepitus* < *crepitus*, pp. of *crepare* crack, creak]. See **physique, appearance**. See **tiredness, weakness**. See **old**.

decrepitude (di-krep'pi-tood) n. the condition of being old, worn out, or in poor working order. (John Updike's golfer, Farrell, was said to be poking his way "down the sloping dogleg of decrepitude.") [< de- pref. < L *de-*, *dis-* apart, away, + *decrepitus* < *crepitus* pp of *crepare* crack, creak]. vi.&vt. **decrepitate**. n. **decrepitation** (-tay'shən). (See **physique, appearance**. See **tiredness, weakness**.

decubital (dee-kyoob'bi-təl) adj. pertaining to or resulting from lying down, i.e. < **decubitus**, q.v. [< L *decumbo* to lie down]. See **skin**. See **sleep, wakefulness**.

decubitus (dee-kyoob'bi-təss) (pl. = decubitus, i.e., 4th, not 2nd, declension.) n. 1. an act of lying down, or the position assumed when lying in bed. 2. a bedsore: decubitus or pressure ulcer. The elderly have less fat and muscle to dissipate pressure. [L, a lying down]. See **skin**. See **sleep, wakefulness**.

dedentition (dee-den-ti'shən) n. loss of teeth. [< L *de-* pref., from, away + *dentitio* to teethe]. See **mouth, gums & teeth**.

deipnosophist (dīp-nos'sə-fist) n. a skillful dinner conversationalist. [G, < *Deipnosophistai* of Athens who sparked the dinner conversation of smart men]. adj. **deipnosophistic** (-nos"sə-fis'tik). See **talk**. See **drink & food**. See **role**.

deisidaimonia (dee"si-dī-mōn'ni-ə) n. morbid fear of supernatural powers. [< L *deus* god, deity, divine being + < G *daimon* divine power, guiding spirit + -ia, suff.]. Cf. **theophobia**, q.v. See **phobias**. See: **religion, theology, morality**.

delassation (dee-las-say'shən) n. fatigue, tiredness. [< L *delassare* to tire out, weary]. See **tiredness, weakness**.

delirament (dee-lir'rə-ment) n. a raving; a foolish story. [< L *deliramentum* nonsense, absurdity < *delirare* to be off the beam, be crazy, be mad; to drivel]. See **talk**.

delirium (dee-leer'ri-əm), pl. **deliria** (-ri-aa), n. an acute, reversible, organic mental disorder characterized by reduced ability to maintain attention to external stimuli and disorganized thinking, as manifested by rambling, irrelevant, or incoherent speech; there are also a reduced level of consciousness, sensory misperceptions, disturbance of the sleep-wakeful cycle, and level of psychomotor activity, disorientation to time, place, or person, and memory impairment; confusion with hyperactivity. Too much or prolonged sedation in an intensive-care unit can result, particularly in the elderly, in delirium and in long-term cognitive impairment and decline. [de-, pref., signifying down or away from, < L *de* away from, down from, + *lira* a furrow or track, i.e., "off the track"]. Cf. **senile delirium**, q.v. See **nerve, muscle, motion, touch**.

Delphic (del'fik) adj. ambiguous, equivocal, oracular. [< G oracle (of Apollo) at Delphi]. syn. **dilogical**, q.v. See **talk**.

dementia (dee-men'shə) n. an organic mental disorder characterized by a general loss of intellectual abilities involving impairment of memory, judgment, and abstract thinking as well as changes in personality. (Nothing currently has proven to be effective in staving off dementia except exercise. Smoking in middle age more than doubles the risk of dementia later in life according to a recent {2010} study. The worldwide cost of dementia is estimated {by Alzheimer's Disease International} to cost $604 billion in 2010.) [de-, pref, remove; reduce; down or away from < L, away from; down from, down + *mens* mind]. See **intelligence**.

démodé, e (demɔde) adj. old-fashioned, out-of-date. [F] See **old**. See **past, time**.

demulcent (dee-mul'sent) adj. softening, soothing. n. something that soothes. • Treatment of **actinic keratosis**, q.v., of the elderly demands a moisturizing and *demulcent* cream. [< L *de-mulceo*, pp. – *mulctus* to stoke lightly, to soften]. See **therapy**.

dentigerous (den-tij'jər-əs) adj. having teeth. • Being fully *dentigerous* at his advanced age is an accomplishment. [< L *denti-* teeth + *-gerous* bearing, from *gerere* to bear.] syn. = **dentulous**. See **mouth, gums, teeth**.

dentulous (den' choo-ləs) adj. having teeth. [< a back formation of **edentulous** (toothless), q.v., < ex-, pref. (out of), q.v., + < L *dens* tooth. (Earliest recorded use = 1926—Anu Garg.)]. syn. = **dentigerous**. See **mouth, gums, teeth**.

dentophobia (den"tō-fōb'bi-ə) n. morbid fear of dentists. [< dent-, denti-, dento-, pref., relating to the teeth < L *dens* tooth + -phobia, suff., fearing, < G *-phobia* < *phobos* fear]. adj. **dentophobic**. n. **dentophobe**. See **phobias**. See **mouth, gums, teeth**.

deosculate (dee-os'kyoo-layt) vi. (obs.) kiss affectionately. [< L *de-* pref., away, apart + *oscula*, little mouth, dim. of *os* mouth]. See **sex, love**.

depilous (dee-pil'ləs) adj. without hair; bald. [de-, pref., negative sense; away from, < L *de-*, pref., down, apart, away from, + < *pilus* hair]. syn.= **acomia, alopecia, atrichia, calvities, phalacrosis, pilgarlic**, q.v. See **hair**.

desiccated (des-si-kayt'təd) adj. 1. dried out; sometimes pulverized, also. (2. used to describe something, especially a literary work, lacking in energy or vitality.) [< L *desicat-*, pp. of *desiccare* dry out < *siccus* dry]. vt. **desiccate** = to remove moisture from. n. **desiccation**. adj. **desiccative** = removes moisture from. n. **desiccator** = something that or someone who removes moisture, dries out. See **physique, appearance**. See **role**.

desinence (des'in-ənz) n. an ending, termination. • Although he was 90, his death was sudden and unexpected; such *desinence* greatly affected his friends and admirers. [via F < L *desinentia* < *desinens*, pres.p. of *destinere* to put down, leave < *de-* down + *sinere* to allow]. adj. **desinence** = terminal, final, describing anything that puts an end to, or constitutes the end of something: often used in reference to a poem, sequential novel, word ending or suffix. See **end-of-life, death**.

desipient (dee-sip'pi-ənt) adj. silly, foolish. [< L. *desipiens* silly, foolish < *desipere* to be silly, act foolishly]. n. **desipience**. See **intelligence**.

desquamate (des'kwa-mayt) vi. to shred, peel, or scale off, as the casting off of the epidermis in scales or shreds. n. **desquamation** (des"kwa-may'shən). (This, along with **elastosis**, q.v., occurs in the elderly due to **actinic keratosis**, q.v.) [L *desquamare*, pp. -*atus* to take the scales off, skin (fish); (fig.) to peel off]. See **skin**.

desuetude (des'swi-tood or -tyood) n. disuse; the state of disuse or neglect; outmoded. [< L *desuetudo* disuse, lack of use]. See **old age**.

detumescence (dee-tyoo-mes'ənz) n. to cease or subside from swelling. • A state of permanent *detumescence* rendered the **ogygian**, q.v., incapable of vaginal penetration. [< L *detumescere* < *de-*, pref., opposite, reverse, oppose, remove + *tumescere* to begin to swell]. See **health, illness**. See **sex-love**.

deuterogamist (doo-tər-og'gə-mist) n. a widow or widower who remarries; one who remarries a second or another time. [< G *deutero* second + *gamos* marriage]. n. **deuterogamy**. (triterogamist = thrice married < G *tritos* third?) Cf. **digamist**, q.v. See **marriage**. See **role**.

devorative (dee-vawr'rə-tiv) adj. capable of being swallowed whole. • Due to esophageal obstruction in this eighty-year-old, her food was not *devorative*, but had to be minced. [<L *de-* pref., away, from + *vorare* to swallow, devour]. See **gastrointestinal**.

dewdropper (dyoo'drop"pər) n. (slang) one who sleeps by day and plays by night. See **sleep & wakefulness**. See **role**.

dewlap (doo'lap) n. 1. a loose fold of skin on somebody's throat, usually forming later in life. (2. a loose fold of skin hanging from the neck of certain animals such as cows.) [< obs. *dewe* <? + lap < OE *læppa* flap of a garment; lobe; loose piece]. Cf. **jollop, buccula**, q.v. See **physique, appearance**.

dextrophobia (deks"trō-fōb'bi-ə) n. morbid fear of the right or things on the right. • His politics were *dextrophobic*. [< dextro-, pref., meaning right, or toward or on the right side, < L *dexter* right, + < G *phobos* fear]. adj. **dextrophobic**. n. **dextrophobe**. ant. **levophobia**, **sinistrophobia**, q.v. See **phobias**.

diabetes mellitus (dī-ə-beet'teez mel'li-təss) n.phr. a syndrome characterized by hyperglycemia (high blood glucose {sugar}) with fasting blood glucose levels > 125 mg/dL, or any postprandial (shortly after a meal) level > 200 mg/dL, and resulting from absolute or relative impairment of insulin secretion and/or insulin action. (*diabetes insipidus* = chronic excretion of large amounts of urine {polyuria, hydruria}, also common in diabetes mellitus, of low specific gravity and due usually to inadequate output of pituitary antidiuretic hormone. The word diabetes, when used without qualification, = diabetes mellitus.) [G, *diabetes*, a siphon (or a compass) < *dia* through + *bainein* to go + L, *mellitus* sweetened with honey]. adj. **diabetic**. n. **diabetic** = a person with diabetes. See **blood, circulation, glands**. See **role**.

DIAPPERS (dīp'pərss) (diapers with an extra p) a mnemonic that is useful for remembering the reversible causes of transient urinary incontinence, common in the elderly: Delirium, Infection (symptomatic urinary tract infection), Atrophic urethritis (in women and with vaginitis), Pharmaceuticals, Psychiatric disorders (especially depression), Excessive urine output (e.g., from hyperglycemia, as in diabetes), Restricted mobility, and Stool impaction. See **genitourinary**.

dicacity (dī-kas'si-tee) n. oral playfulness; talkativeness. [< L *dicacitas* wittiness, sarcasm]. • His *dicacity* increased with age. Cf. **logodaedaly**, q.v., **paronomasia**. See **talk**.

digamous (dig'gə-məss) adj. married a second time. [< G *di-*, pref., two + *gamos* marriage]. Cf. **deuterogamist**, q.v. See **marriage**.

dilogical (dī-loj'ji-kəl) adj. having a double meaning; ambiguous. [< G *di-*, pref., two + *logos* word]. syn. **Delphic**, q.v. Cf. **dittology**, qv. See **talk**.

dimbox (dim'bokss) n. someone who smoothes things over, gets a compromise, settles disputes amicably, gets others to make up their differences. [?—probably not related to dimbulb, American slang (1930-'35) for one who is stupid, a dimwit]. Cf. **irenicist**, q.v. See **role**.

dinic (din'nik) adj. pertaining to dizziness, vertigo. [< G *dine* an eddy, whirlpool]. n. **dinic** a remedy for dizziness. See **standing, walking, wandering**. See **therapy**.

dipsomania (dip"sō-mayn'ni-ə) n. alcoholism. [< G *dipsa* thirst + *mania* madness, frenzy]. adj. **dipsomaniacal** (-ma-nī'ə-kəl). n. **dipsomaniac**. syn. **alcoholomania**, **methomania**, **posiomania**, q.v. Cf. **oenomania**, q.v. See **manias**. See **drink, food**. See **role**.

diremption (di-remp'shən) n. violent or final separation. [< L *diremptus* separation < *dirimere* to take apart, separate, divide; to break off, disturb, interrupt; to put off, delay, to break off, end, bring to an end; to nullify, bring to naught]. See **work, activity**.

dis- pref. having the same force as the original Latin preposition, *dis* to undo; do the opposite; opposite or absence of; to deprive of; to remove from; not; to free from; completely. [L, *dis-*, an inseparable particle denoting separation, taking apart, sundering in two]. (Note: dis- is not to be confused with the prefix **dys-**, q.v.)

disability measures n.phr. refers to medicolegal grading of disability in order to quantify loss of function and earning power in the disabled. Disability scales are applied in the elderly in an attempt to provide objective and/or measurable assessment of physical functioning and activity, depression, and quality of life. The most common scales are: 1. Katz Activities of Daily Living (ADL) Scale, which measures the ability to perform 6 basic activities, e.g., bathing, dressing without assistance. 2. Rosow-Breslau Functional Health Scale, which measures 3 aspects of gross mobility, e.g., climbing a flight of stairs without assistance. 3. Nagi Scale, which measures difficulty performing 5 types of physical activity, e.g., stooping or crouching, walking two or three blocks, lifting objects weighing up to 10 lbs. 4. Center for Epidemiologic Studies Depression Scale, which has a yes/no response format and yields a score of 0-10. 5. Health-Related Quality of Life, which requires four items that are self-rated by examinees. See **work, activity**.

discalceate (dis-kal'see-ayt) vt & i. to take the shoes off. • As her Alzheimer's disease progressed she discalceated frequently and was unconcerned with her toilet and personal appearance. [< dis-, pref., q.v., + < L *calcaetus* shoe, sandal]. adj. & n. **discalceate**. adjs. **discalceated**, **discalced** (-kalst') = barefooted or only sandaled (as a friar or nun). See **joint, extremities, back**. See **physique, appearance**. See **role**.

discinct (dis-sinkt') adj. belt less, dressed loosely. [dis-, pref., q.v., + < L *cinctus* belt, sash]. See **physique, appearance**.

disequilibrium (diss"ee-kwi-lib'bree-əm) n. any derangement of proper balance. [dis-, pref., q.v., + < L *aequilibrium* equal balance < *aequus* equal + *libra* balance]. See **standing, walking, wandering**.

disespoused (diz-es-powzd') adj. left, broken off; divorced. [dis-, pref., q.v., + < L *spons-*, comb., < OF < L *spondere* pledge]. See **marriage**.

distrait, **e** (distrɛ, ɛt) adj. inattentive or absentminded distracted. [F < OF < L *distractus*, pp. of *distrahere* to distract]. See **mentality, mentation, behavior**.

dittology (dit-tol'ə-jee) n. a dual interpretation, meaning. [< Tuscan *ditto* said < L *dictus* pp. *dicere* say + < G *logos* word, reason < *-logos* speaking]. Cf. **dilogical**, **Delphic**, **equivoke**, **subintelligitur**, q.v. See **talk**.

diurnal (dī-urn'nəl) adj. daily; pertaining to daytime; (living one day); active in daytime. [< L *diurnus* of the day, by day, day, daytime; daily, of each day; day's, of one day < *dies* day]. See **work, activity**. See **past, time**.

diurnation (dī-ur-nay'shən) n. the habit of sleeping or being dormant during the day. Cf. **dewdropper**, q.v. [< L *diurnus* daily, < *dies* day]. See **sleep, wakefulness**.

diuturnal (dī-yoo-tur'nəl) adj. pertaining to long duration. [< L *diuturnus* long, long lasting]. See **past, time**.

divagate (dīv'və-gayt, div'və-gayt) vi. 1. to wander, wander around, stray. 2. digress; deviate, wander from the subject. [< L *divagatus* pp. of *divagari* to wander around, off < dis-, pref., + *vagari* wander. Earliest documented use:1599]. n. **divagation** = wandering off, straying from the point. See **talk**. See **standing, walking, wandering**.

diversivolent (dīv"vər-siv'vō-lənt) adj. looking for trouble or an argument. [< L *diversus* pp. of *divertere* to separate < *verteri* turn + *volens* willing, permitting; ready; favorable]. See **talk**.

dixit (diks'it) n. an unconfirmed, sometimes dogmatic statement. [L, he said < L *dicere* to say]. n.phr. *Ipse dixit* (ip'say diks'it) = he himself said (it); the master himself has spoken—a dogmatic assertion. See **talk**.

doctiloquent (dok-til'lō-kwent) adj. speaking learnedly on some subject. [< L *doctor* teacher < *doceo* pp.of *doctus* to teach + *loqui* to speak]. adv. **doctiloquently**. n. **doctiloquence**. See **talk**.

dolorifuge (də-lor'i-fyooj) n. something that cures or alleviates grief. [< L *dolor*, pain, grief, sorrow < *dolore* to feel pain + -fuge, suff., denoting an agent that drives away or banishes, < *fugare* to put to flight]. See **therapy**.

donepezil hydrochloride (HCL) (don"e-peez'zil hī"drō-klor'īdə) n. a drug used in treating mild-to-moderate **Alzheimer's disease**, q.v. It is a centrally-acting acetylcholinesterase inhibitor and sometimes results in modest benefits in cognition and/or behavior. Donepezil is marketed as **Aricept®** and used in a dose of one 5mg tablet per day. It is sometimes used in combination with memantine, a newer agent. Memantine is marketed by various trade names: Namenda®, Axura®, Akatinol®, Ebixa®, Abixa®, and Memox® by various pharmaceutical companies. Memantine acts on the glutamatergic system by blocking NMDA (N-methyl-D-aspartic acid) glutamate receptors. See **therapy**.

dormition (dawr-mi'shən) n. 1. sleeping; falling asleep. 2. a peaceful and painless death. 3. (fig.) death (of the righteous). [L, < *dormire* to sleep + -tion, suff., of nouns indicating action or condition, < L –tionem, suff., < pp. stems in -t- + -ion]. See **end-of-life & death**. See **sleep, wakefulness**.

dotage (dō'tij) n. an offensive term for the lack of strength or concentration sometimes believed to be, or is, characteristic of old age; senility. [< dote, vi.< ME & MD *doten* be silly]. adv. **dotingly**. See **old age**. See **intelligence**.

dotard (dōt'taard) n. one in his/her **dotage**, q.v.; an old, feeble-minded person. syn. = **twichild**, q.v. (L = *senex delirus*). n. **dotardness**

(dō'taard-ness). [<ME & MD *doten* be silly]. See **old man**. See **old woman**. See **old person(s)**. See: **role**.

dotation (dō-tay'shən) n. an endowing or endowment. [< L *dotoare* vt. to endow]. See **finance**.

dott(e)rel (dot'trel, dot'ter-el), n.pl. –**els** or –**el**, 1. a silly, gullible person; a senile person. (2. a reddish brown bird of the plover family with white markings on the head and neck.) [< MDu *doten* to be silly: the bird is easily caught]. See **old person(s)**. See **role**. See **intelligence**.

dotty (dot'tee) adj. 1. (colloq.) shaky of gait; mentally unbalanced, feeble-minded, half idiot; eccentric, unconventional. (2. dotted about, sporadic, marked with dots.) [< Sc *dottle* fool < ME *doten* to dote < OE *dott* head of boil + -y, suffix-forming adj., < OE -*ig*, full or having the qualities of]. See **intelligence**. See **standing, walking, wandering**.

double entendre/double entente (dubl ãtãdr/dubl ãtãt) n.phr. an expression with two meanings, one often indelicate. • The old rake frequently adverted to *double entendre* when cornering and conversing with a lady in their retirement home. v. *entendre* (ɑ~ɑ~dr) = to understand. n. *entente* (ɑ~tɑ~t) understanding. prep.phr. à *double entente* (dubl ɑ~tɑ~t) = with a double meaning. [F]. See **talk**. See **sex, love**.

double stance/double support n.phr. the standing position during walking when both feet of a person are simultaneously on the ground; the center of gravity is then in stable position between the feet. Double-stance time increases from 18% in young adults to 26% or more in the elderly. This elderly increase reduces gait momentum and thereby less time for the swing leg to advance; this results in a shorter step length, i.e., smaller steps. Increased double stance reduces gait velocity. Impaired balance will increase double-stance time The time spent in double stance excellently predicts both step length and gait velocity. adj. **double-stance**. See **standing, walking, wandering**.

douceur (doo-sur') n. 1. a sweet or charming manner. (2. a gift; a tip; a bribe; a reward). • The doyenne's *douceur* belied her innate intelligence. [F, sweetness, mildness, gentleness, pleasure]. See **mentality, mentation, behavior**.

dowager (dow'wə-jər) n. 1. a rich-looking or respected woman of advanced years. 2. a woman who has inherited a title or property from her deceased husband. [< F *douagere* < L *dos* dowry]. See **old woman**. See **role**.

doyen (doy'yən or doy-en') n. a man who is the most senior or experienced and respected member of a group or profession. [F, < L *decanus* person in charge of ten others]. The F m. & f. = *doyen/doyenne*, q.v. See **old man**. See **role**.

doyen/doyenne (dwajɛ̃/dwajɛn) nm./nf. a man/woman who is the most senior or experienced and respected member of a group or profession. [F < *doyen* < L *decanus* person in charge of ten others]. See **old man**. See **old woman**. See **role**.

draconic (drə-kon'nik) adj. of or like a dragon. [< L *draco* < G *drakon* snake]. adv. **draconically**. See **physique, appearance**.

dragon (drag'gon) n. 1. a woman who is regarded as fierce and formidable (insult; often collocated with old). (2. a large and usually ferocious fire-breathing creature in myths, legends, and fairy tales that has green scaly skin, a long tail, and wings. 3. a large lizard.) [< L *draco* < G *drakon* snake]. See **old woman**. See **role**.

drimble/drumble (drim'bəl/drum'bəl) vi. (obs.) to act sluggishly; to drone or mumble. [?]. See **talk**. See **mentality, mentation, behavior**.

drink, food: alcoholomania, bibacious, bibulous, crapulence, crapulous, deipnosophist, deipnosophistic, dipsomania, dysmetabolism, ebriection, ebrious, edacious, fuddle, *lécheur*, manducable, methomania, nephalism, oenomania, oligophagous, oligotrophia/oligotrophy, opsomania, osophagist, parorexia, piddle, pingle, poltophagy, posiomania, potatory, pultaceous, sacchariferous, toper, trophic, ventripotent.

drink, food: Subcategories

drink

I. Abstinence:
    1. Alcoholic abstinence: **nephalism**

II. Drink content:
2. Containing sugar: **sacchariferous**
III. Positive attitude toward drinking:
1. Abnormal interest in, mania for, wine: **alcoholomania, dipsomania, oenomania, posiomania**
2. Alcoholic over-drinking: **crapulence, crapulous, ebrious, fuddle, posiomania,**
3. Alcoholic over-drinking with mental breakdown: **ebriection**
4. Drinkable: **potatory**
5. Given to drink: **potatory**
6. Love of drinking, over-drinking (See no. 2., also.): **bibacious, bibulous, methomania**
7. One who loves drinking: **toper, dipsomaniac, methomaniac, oenomaniac, posiomaniac**

food

I. Appetite:
1. Love of eating: **ventripotent,** *lécheur*
2. Picky eater; lack of interest in food, eats little: **osophagist; oligophagous, piddle, pingle**
3. Oovereating: **crapulence, crapulous, edacious**
4. Perverted appetite: **parorexia**
5. Particular food craving: **opsomania**
II. Content:
1. Containing sugar: **sacchariferous**
2. Re: pulpy food: **pultaceous**
III. Conversation:
1. Dinner conversationalist: **deipnosophist**
2. Re: dinner conversation: **deipnosophistic**
IV. Edibility:
1. Re: edible: **manducable**
IV. Malnourishment: **oligotrophia/oligotrophy**
V. Metabolism: **dysmetabolism**
VI. Over-chewing of food: **poltophagy**
VII. Re: nutrition: **trophic**

dromomania (drō-mō-may'ni-ə) n. compulsive traveling or longing for travel. [drom(o)-, pref., denotes connection to conduction, to running or to speed, < G *dromos* a course, race, + *mania* madness]. adj.

dromomaniacal (-mə-nī'ə-kəl). n. **dromomaniac**. Cf. **philobat**, q.v. See **manias**. See **role**.

dropsy (drop'see) n. swelling of the body tissues with fluid; the abnormal accumulation of serous fluid in the cellular tissue or in a body cavity. [< L *hydrops* dropsy < G *hydror* water]. syn. **edema** (a more current term). See **physique, appearance**. See **skin**.

dudgeon (duj'jən) n. resentment; feeling of offence; sulky displeasure; aggrieved humor—usually used as the collocation: **in high dudgeon**. [origin unk.]. See **emotion**. See **mentality, mentation, behavior**.

duffer n., as in the phrase **old duffer**, q.v. See **old man**. See **old woman**. See **old person(s)**.

dulciloquy (dul-sil'lə-kwee) n. (obs.) softness of speaking. [< L *dulcis* sweet + *loquitari* to chatter]. See **talk**.

d'un certain age (d' œ̃ sɛrtɛ̃ aʒ) adj. phr. a polite (*poli*) way of saying someone, especially a woman, is elderly, old. [F, lit., of a certain age]. See **old**.

Dupuytren's contracture (dyoo-pwee-trens, -trawN) n.phr. nodular proliferation of the palmar fascia leading to fascial contracture with some degree of permanent flexion of the fingers—especially the fourth and fifth—of one or both hands. It is a common autosomal dominant disorder with variable penetrance, more common in elderly men, and of unknown causation. [< Guillaume Dupuytren, a F surgeon and surgical pathologist. (1777-1835)]. See **joint, extremities, back**.

durance (door'əns) n. (archaic or literary) long confinement; forcible confinement or imprisonment. ● He felt his habitation in a retirement home was an intolerable *durance*. [< L *durus* harsh, tough, rude, cruel < *durare* to harden]. See **work, activity**.

dwaible/dwaibly (dway'bəl/ dway'blee) adj. unstable; weak and shaky. [Sc]. See **standing, walking, wandering**.

dys- (dis-) pref. conveying the idea of bad; abnormal; impaired; difficult; disordered. [< G *dus-* bad, impaired, abnormal]. (Note: not to be confused with the particle **dis-** q.v.)

dysacusis (dis-ə-kyoos'siss) n. 1. any impairment of hearing not primarily due to loss of ability to perceive sound, but to a discriminative loss in distinguishing words, syllables, phonemes, pitch. 2. pain in the ear due to sound. [dys-, q.v., + G *akousis* hearing]. syns. **dysacousia**, **dysacusia**, **dysacousma**. See **ear, hearing**.

dysania (dis-ayn'ni-ə) n. having a hard time awakening in the morning. [dys-, q.v., +?]. ant. **euania**, q.v. See **sleep, wakefulness**.

dysaphia (dis-af'fi-ə) n. impairment in the sense of touch. adj. **dysaphic**. [dys-, q.v., + < G *haphe* touch]. See **nerve, muscle, movement, touch**.

dysarteriotony (dis"awr-tee-ri-ot'tə-nee) n. abnormal blood pressure: either hypertension (too high) or hypotension (too low). [dys-, q.v., + arteri-, arterio-, pref., artery < L *arteria* artery, < G *arteria* < *aer* air, + *terein* to keep (i.e., to contain air—so the Greeks thought) or *aeirein* to lift or attach + *tonos* tension]. See **blood, circulation, glands**.

dysarthria (dis-aar'three-ə) n. difficulty in speech articulation due to lack of muscle control caused by damage to the central nervous system. [dys-, q.v., + < G *arthron* joint]. (Dysarthria types are: **dysarthria literalis** {li-ter-aal'liss} = stammering, **dysarthria syllabaris** {sil-laa-baar'ris} = syllabic stammering, and **dysarthria spasmodica** {spas-mot'ti-kə} = stuttering). A more recent classification of dysarthria divides it into six types: ataxic, flaccid, hyperkinetic, hypokinetic, spastic, and mixed (Merck Manual of Geriatrics, ed. 3). adj. **dysarthric**. See **verbal apraxia**. See **talk**.

dysbasia (dis-bay'zhə or –bayz'zee-ə) n. difficulty in walking. [dys-, q.v., + < G *basis* a step]. See **standing, walking, wandering**.

dysbulia (dis-byool'li-ə) n. loss, weakness, or uncertainty of will power. adj. = **dysbulic**. [dys-, q.v., + < G *boule* will]. See **mentality, mentation, behavior**.

dyscalculia (dis"kal-kyool'lee-ə) n. impairment of the ability to do mathematical problems because of brain injury or disease. [dys-, q.v., + < L *calculare* to calculate]. See **intelligence**.

dyscheiria (dis-kīr'ri-ə) n. inability to distinguish which side of the body has been touched, but absent a loss of touch. adj. = **dyscheiral** (-kīr'/ **dyschiral** (-kir'). [dys-, q.v., + *cheir* hand]. See **nerve, muscle, movement, touch**.

dyschezia/dyschesia (dis-keez'zee-aah, -keez'zee-ə/ -kee'zhə, -kee'zee-aa) n. difficult or painful defecation, i.e., evacuation of feces from the rectum. [dys-, q.v., + < G *chezein* to defecate, to go to stool + -ia, suff.]. See **gastrointestinal**.

dyschroia (dis-kroy'ə)/ **dyschroa** (-krŏ'ə) n. a bad complexion; discoloration of the skin. [dys-, q.v., + < G *chroia, chroa* color]. See **skin**. See **color**.

dyschromia (dis-krōm'mi-ə) n. any abnormality in the color of the skin or hair. [dys-, q.v., + < G *chroma* color]. See **hair**. See **skin**. See **color**.

dyscinesia (dis-si-nee'zhə, -neez'zee-ə) n. = **diskinesia**, q.v. See **nerve, muscle, movement, touch**.

dyscoimesis (dis-koy-mees'siss) n. a form of insomnia marked by difficulty in falling asleep. [dys-, q.v., + < G *koimesis* a sleeping < *koimao* to put to sleep]. syn. **dyskoimesis**, q.v. See **sleep, wakefulness**.

dyscrasia (dis-kray'zhə, -zee-ə) n. an undefined disease or abnormal condition of the body, especially one of the blood—a term formally used to indicate an abnormal mixture of the ancient "four humors". [< G *dyskrasia* bad temperament]. n. **dyscrasy** (dis'krə-see) = **dyscrasia**. adj. **dyscrasic** (-kray'sik), **dyscratic** (-kray'tik). Cf. **dysemia, dyshematopoiesis**, q.v. See **blood, circulation, glands**. See **health, illness**.

dyscrinism (dis-krīn'niz-əm) n. (obs.) a condition resulting from an altered secretion of any of the glands, especially of the endocrine glands. [dys-, q.v., + < G *krino* to separate, secrete + -ism, suff.]. Cf. **dysendocrinism**, q.v., syn. (obs.) **pathocrinia** (path"ō-krīn'ni-ə). See **blood, circulation, glands**. See **health, illness**.

dysdiadochokinesia (dis"dī'əd"dō'kō-kīn-nee'zhə or –neez'zee-ə) n. inability in, or impairment of, moving a limb in opposite directions, as those of flexion and extension. adj. = **disdiadochokinetic** (-kīn-net'tik). [dys-, q.v., + < G *diadochos* working in turn + *kinesis* movement]. (**disdiadochokinesia** = **dysdiadochocinesia**.) See **standing, walking, wandering**. See **nerve, muscle, movement, touch**.

dysdiemorrhysis (dis"dī-ee-mor'ri-siss) n. sluggishness of the capillary circulation. [dys-, q.v., + < G *dia* through + *haima* blood + *rhysis* a flowing]. See **blood, circulation & glands**.

dysekpnea (dis-ek'nee-ə) n. the clinical state of protracted or difficult expiration, as in, e.g., asthmatics, those with **COPD**, q.v., or **emphysema**, q.v. [dys-, q.v., + < G *ek* out + *pnoia* breathing]. See **breathing**.

dysemia (dis-eem'mi-ə) n. any abnormal condition or disease of the blood. [dys-, q.v., + < G *haima* blood]. Cf. **dyscrasia**, **dyshematopoiesia**, q.v. See **blood, circulation & glands**.

dysendocrinism (dis-en'dō-krin-iz"zəm), alt., **dysendocrinia** (-do-krin'ni-ə) & **dysendocriniasis** (–nī'ə-sis) n. faulty or deficient action of the endocrine glands, and the disorders resulting therefrom— all these terms are now obs. and superseded by terms referring to specific endocrine glands. [dys-, q.v., + endo-, pref., indicating within, inner < G *endon* within + *krino* to separate]. See **blood, circulation & glands**.

dyseneia (dis-een'nee-ə) n. defective articulation, i.e., speaking distinctly and connectedly, secondary to deafness. [dys-, q.v., + < G *ania* bridle; *dysenios* refractory]. Cf. **dysarthria**, q.v. See **ear & hearing**. See **talk**.

dyserethism (dis-er'ree-thiz"zəm) n. impairment of sensibility to stimuli; a condition of slow response to stimuli. [dys-, q.v., + < G *erethismos* irritation]. syn. = **dyserethesia** (dis-er'ree-thee'zhə, -thee'zee-ə). syn. **dysesthesia** (dis'es-thee'zhə, -thee'zee-ə), q.v. See **nerve, muscle, movement, touch**.

dysergia (dis-er'ji-ə) n. a lack of harmonious action between the muscles concerned in executing any definite voluntary movement. [dys, q.v., + < G *ergon* work]. Cf. **dysmetria**, q.v. See **standing, walking, wandering**. See **nerve, muscle, movement, touch**.

dysesthesia (dis-es-thee'zhǝ, -theez'zee-ǝ) n. 1. impairment of the senses, any sense, but especially that of touch. 2. an unpleasant abnormal sensation produced by normal stimuli. [dys-, q.v., + < G *aesthesis* perception]. adj. **dysesthetic** (-the'tik). syns. **dyserethism**, **dyserethesia**, q.v. See **nerve, muscle, movement, touch**.

dysfluency (dis-floo'en-see), pl. -ies, n. lack of ease, smooth easy flow, fluency, especially in speaking. • Her speech *dysfluencies* were the result of a stroke. [dys-, q.v., + < L *fluentia* < *fluere* flow]. See **talk**.

dysgenesia (dis"jen-nee'zhǝ, -neez'zee-ǝ) n. impairment of the powers of procreation. [dys-,q.v., + < G *gennan* to generate + -ia] See **sex, love**.

dysgenic (dis-jen'nik) adj. applying to factors that have a detrimental effect upon hereditary qualities, physical or mental. [dys-, q.v., + < G *genesis* production]. n. **dysgenesis**. ant. = **eugenic**. See **sex, love**.

dysgeusia (dis-jyooz'zee-ǝ, -jyooz'zhǝ) n. impairment or perversion of the gustatory sense. Some elderly suffering the decreased **ofaction**, q.v., of old age, experience an unpleasant taste in their mouth, dysgeusia, or **dysosmia**, q.v., i.e., an unpleasant smell. [dys-, q.v., + < G *geusis* taste]. See **gastrointestinal**. See **nerve, muscle, movement, touch**.

dysglycemia (dis"glī-seem'mee-ǝ) n. any derangement of the sugar content of the blood. [dys-,q.v., + < G *glykys* sweet]. See **blood, circulation & glands**.

dysgnosia (dis-nōs'zee-ǝ, -nō'zhǝ) n. any cognitive disorder, i.e., any mental disorder or disease. [G *dysgnosia* difficulty of knowing < dys-, q.v., + gnosos knowledge]. See **intelligence**.

dysgonesis (dis-gōn'nee-siss) n. a functional disorder of the genital organs. [dys-, q.v., + < G *gone* seed + -sis, G suff. of action]. adj. **dysgonic** (dis-gon'nik). See **sex, love**.

dysgrammatism (dis-gram'mǝ-tiz"zǝm) n. partial impairment, because of brain injury or disease, of the ability to speak grammatically. [dys-, q.v., + < G *gramma* written character, letter + -ism, suff., unusual or unhealthy state < G -ismos, a noun-forming suffix]. See **talk**.

dysgraphia (dis-graf'fee-ə) n. 1. impairment of writing ability due to brain injury, disease. 2. writer's cramp. [dys-, q.v., + < G *graphe* writing]. See **nerve, muscle, movement, touch**.

dyshematopoiesia/dyshematopoiesis (dis-heem'ma-tō-poy-ees'si-ə)/(-ee'siss) n. imperfect formation of blood. [dys-, q.v., + < G *haima* blood + *poiesis* making]. adj. **dyshenatopoietic** (-poy-et'tik). Cf. **dysemia, dyscrasia**, q.v. See **blood, circulation, glands**.

dyshepatia (dis"he-pay'shə, -pay'shee-ə, -pay'shee-aah) n. disordered liver function. [dys-, q.v., + < G *hepar* liver]. See **gastrointestinal**.

dyskeratoma (dis"ker-ə-tŏm'mə) n. a skin tumor showing **dyskeratosis** (-tōs'siss), i.e., a defect in keratin formation in which some cells (keratinocytes) of the epidermis (outer skin layer) undergo premature or atypical keratinization (horniness). Dyskeratoma may be benign or malignant. A warty dyskeratoma is benign, usually solitary, typically a flesh-colored-to-brown elevated papule with a depressed and crusted center containing a keratotic (horny) plug, occurring in association with the pilosebaceous (hair and sebacious {fat & skin-cell debris} gland) unit, especially on the scalp, face, neck, and axilla, and principally seen in older men. [dys-, q.v., + kerato-, a comb. form denoting relationship to horny tissue, or the cornea < *keras*, gen., *keratos* horn + -oma, a suff. meaning tumor or neoplasm < -*oma* denoting result]. adj. **dyskeratotic**. syn. **isolated dyskeratosis follicularis**. **dyskeratosis**, q.v. See **cancer, neoplasm, tumor**. See **skin**.

dyskeratosis (dis"ker-ə-tōs'siss) n. See **diskeratoma**. See **cancer, neoplasm, tumor**.

dyskinesia (dis"kī-nee'zhə, -neez'zee-ə; dis"ki-) n. difficulty in performing voluntary movements. [dys-, q.v., + < G *kinesis* movement]. adj. **dyskinetic** (-kī-net'tik). syn. = **dyscinesia**, q.v. See **nerve, muscle, movement, touch**.

dyskoimesis (dis-koy-mees'siss) n. difficulty in getting to sleep. [dys-, q.v., + G *koimesis* sleeping]. syn. **dyscoimesis**, q.v. See **sleeping & wakefulness**.

dyslalia (dis-lay'li-ə) n. disorder of articulation due to structural abnormalities of the articulatory organ—not central nervous system, i.e., **dyslogia**, q.v.—or impaired hearing. [dys-, q.v. + < G *lalia* talking]. Cf. **dysarthria**, q.v. See **talk**.

dyslexia (dis-leks'si-ə) n. incomplete **alexia**; a level of reading ability markedly below that expected on the basis of the individual's level of overall intelligence or skillful ability. [dys-, q.v., + < G lexis word, phrase]. See **work, activity**.

dyslipidosis (diss"lip-i-dōs'siss), pl. **dyslipidoses** (-dō'seez), n. a general designation applied to a localized or systemic disturbance of fat metabolism. [dys-, q.v., + lip(o)-, comb. form denoting relationship to fat or lipid, < G *lipos* fat + -osis, suff.]. syn. dislipoidosis (dis-lip"poi-dō'sis), pl dyslipoidoses (-dō'seez). syn. **dyslipidemia** = a disorder of lipoprotein metabolism. See **blood, circulation, glands**.

dyslogia (dis lōj'ji-ə) n. 1. impairment of the power of speech in consequence of a central nervous system lesion. 2. impairment of the reasoning faculty. [dys-, q.v., + < G *logos* speaking, reason]. Cf. **dysarthria, dyseneia, dyslalia, dysphasia, dysphrasia**, q.v. See **talk**. See **intelligence**.

dyslogistic (dis-lōj-jis'tik) adj. unfavorable; antagonistic; uncomplimentary; belittling. [dys-, q.v., < G *dus-* bad + *logos* word; witticism; speaking; reason +-ic]. ant. = **eulogistic**. See **talk**.

dysmasesis (dis-ma-see'siss) n. difficulty in mastication. [dys-, q.v., + < G *masesis* chewing]. See **gastrointestinal**.

dysmentia (dis-men'shi-ə) n. a disturbance in intellectual functioning that may be temporary. [dys-, q.v., + < L *mens* (*ment-*) mind]. See **intelligence**.

dysmetabolism (dis"me-tab'bō-liz-əm) n. defective metabolism. [dys-, q.v., + < G *metaballein* to turn about, change, alter]. See **drink, food**. See **gastrointestinal**.

dysmetria (dis-met'tri-ə) n. a form of **dysergia**, q.v., in which the subject is unable to arrest a muscular movement at the desired point. [dys-, q.v., + < G *metron* measure]. See **standing, walking, wandering**. See **nerve, muscle, movement, touch**.

dysmimia (dis-mim'mee-ə) n. impairment of the power of expressing thought by gestures. [dys-, q.v., + G *mimia* imitation]. See **nerve, muscle, movement, touch**.

dysmnesia (dis-nee'zhə, -nee'zee-ə) n. a naturally poor or impaired memory. [dys-, q.v., + < G *mneme* (in compounds *mnesi-*) memory]. adj. **dysmnesic**. Cf. **chrysomnesia**, **paramnesia**, q.v. See **memory**.

dysmorphobia (dis"mor-fōb'bi-ə) n. a morbid fear of deformity. [dys-, q.v., + < G *morphe* form + *phobos* fear]. adj. **dysmorphobic**. n. **dysmorphobe**. See **phobias**.

dysmyotonia (dis"mī-ō-tōn'ni-ə) n. abnormal muscular tonicity, either hyper- or hypo-. [dys- + < G *myo* muscle + *tonos* tension, tone]. See **nerve, muscle, movement, touch**.

dysnomia (dis-nōm'mee-ə) n. partial nominal aphasia, difficulty in remembering names. [dys-, q.v., + < G *onoma* name]. syns. **anomia**, **dysnomia**, **nominal aphasia**, q.v. See **memory**.

dysnystaxis (dis-nis-taks'siss) n. light sleep; a condition of half sleep. [dys-, q.v., + < G *nystaxis* drowsiness]. See **sleep & wakefulness**.

dysonogamia (dis"sō-nō-gam'mi-ə) n. marriage between persons of unequal age, especially with a considerable age difference. [dys-, q.v., + < G *nomos* law + *gamos* marriage]. syn. **anisonogamia**, q.v. ant. **isonogamia**, q.v. Cf. **anilojuvenogamy**, **nomogamosis**, **opsigamy**, **sororate**, q.v. See **marriage**.

dysopia (dis-ōp'pi-ə) n. impaired sight. [dys-, q.v., + < G *opsis* vision]. syn. **dysopsia** (dis-op'si-ə). See **eye**.

dysorexia (dis"sō-reks'si-ə) n. diminished or perverted appetite. [dys-, q.v., + < G *orexis* appetite]. See **gastrointestinal**.

dysosmia (dis-oz'mi-ə) impaired sense of smell. [dys-, q.v., + < G *osme* smell]. Cf. **anosmia**, **hyposmia**, q.v. See **nose & smell**.

dyspareunia (dis"pə-roon'ni-ə) n. painful (for the female) intercourse or pain with attempted intercourse; difficult or painful coitus. About one-third of sexually active women > age 65 years of age report dyspareunia (Merck Manual of Geriatrics). Causation is variable;

age-related atrophic (a wasting away, diminution in the size of a cell, tissue, organ, or part) vaginitis, with inadequate lubrication, is a frequent cause. [G *dyspareunos* badly mated < dys-, pref., q.v., + *pareunos* lying beside < *para* beside + *eune* a bed]. See **sex, love**. See **genitourinary**.

dyspepsia (dis-pep'see-ə) n. 1. impairment of the power or function of digestion; usually applied to epigastric discomfort following meals, indigestion. 2. having a bad temper; gloomy; irritable. [dys-, q.v., + < G *peptos* digested < *peptein* to digest]. adj. **dyspeptic**. See **gastrointestinal**. See **mentality, mentation, behavior**.

dysphagia (dis'fay'jhə or -jee-ə) n. difficulty in swallowing. [dys-, q.v., + < G *phagein* to eat]. adj. **dysphagic**. syn. **dysphagy**. See **gastrointestinal**.

dysphasia (dis-fay'zee-ə, -fay'zhə)/ **dysphrasia** (dis-fray'zhə, -fay'zee-ə) n. lack of coordination in speech and failure to arrange words in an understandable way; it is related to cortical (brain) damage. [dys-, q.v., + < G *phases/phrases* speaking]. syn. = **dysphrasia**. [dys- + < G *phrasis* speaking]. Cf. **dysarthria**, **dyseneia**, **dyslalia**, **dyslogia**, q.v. See **talk**. See **nerve**.

dysphemia (dis-feem'mi-ə) n. disorder of phonation, articulation (e.g., stammering), or hearing due to emotional or intellectual deficit. [dys-, q.v., + < G *pheme* speech]. See **talk**. See **ear & hearing**. See **emotion**. See **intelligence**.

dysphemism (dis'fə-miz"zəm) n. an unpleasant or derogatory word or phrase substituted for a more pleasant or less offensive one; such a substitution. [late 19th C. < dys-, q.v., + *pheme* speech; after euphemism]. n. **dysphemist**. adj. **dysphemistic**. adv. **dysphemistically** (dis"fem-is'tik-kal-lee). ant. **euphemism**. See **talk**. See **role**.

dysphonia (dis-fōn'ni-ə) n. hoarseness; difficulty or pain in speaking. [dys-, q.v., + < G *phone* voice]. adj. **dysphonic** (-fon'-ik). See **talk**.

dysphoria (dis-for'ri-ə) n. a generalized feeling of physical and mental discomfort, unpleasantness. [G, *dysphoria* discomfort, excessive pain, anguish, agitation < dis-, q.v., + *pherein* to bear]. adj. **dysphoric**. ant. = **euphoria**. [*eu-*, pref., good]. See **mentality, mentation, behavior**.

dysphoriant (dis-fōr'ree-ənt) n. 1. producing a condition of dysphoria. 2. an agent that produces dysphoria. • Frequent disruption of elevator service in the high-rise retirement home was a *dysphoriant*. [dys-, q.v., + G, *dysphoria* discomfort, excessive pain, anguish, agitation < *pherein* to bear]. See **dysphoria**. See **mentality, mentation, behavior**.

dysphylaxia (dis"fī-laks'si-ə) n. 1. a form of insomnia marked by too early awakening. 2. a condition marked by too early waking. • Among the frequent sleep disorders of the elderly is *dysphylaxia*. [dys-, q.v., + < G *phylaxis* watching]. See **sleep & wakefulness**.

dyspnea (disp'nee-ə or disp-nee'ə) n. shortness of breath; subjective difficulty or distress in breathing; frequently rapid breathing, usually associated with serious disease of the heart or lungs. adj. = **dyspneic**. [dys-, q.v., + < G < *pnoe* breathing]. See **breathing**.

dysponderal (dis-pon'dər-əl) adj. pertaining to a disorder of weight, either overweight, obese, or underweight, **leptosomatic**, q.v. (dys-, q.v., + < L *pondus* weight]. See **physique, appearance**.

dyspragia (dis-pray'jhə, -pray'jee-ə) n. painful performance of any function. [G *dyspragia* ill success < *prasso* to do]. Cf. **dyspraxia**, q.v. See **pain**.

dyspraxia (dis-praks'si-ə) n. impaired or painful functioning in any organ. [dys-, q.v., + < G *praxis* doing]. syn. **dyspragia**, q.v. See **pain**.

dysprosody (dis-prōs'sō-dee) n. disturbance of stress, pitch, and rhythm of speech. [dys-, q.v., + < G *prosoidia* < *pros* to, towards, in addition + *oidia* ode]. See **talk**.

dysrhythmia (dis-rith'mi-ə) n. defective rhythm, generally of the heart or brain. [dys-, q.v., + < G *rhythmos* rhythm]. See **heart & rhythm**.

dyssomnia (dis-som'ni-ə) n. any disorder of sleep. • About 50% of **oldsters**, q.v., have sleep problems, especially that of falling asleep and remaining asleep: **insomnia**, q.v. [dys-, q.v., + < L *somnus* sleep]. See **sleep & wakefulness**.

dysstasia (dis-stay'zhə, zee-ə) n. difficulty in standing. [dys-, q.v., + < G *stasis* standing]. adj. = **dysstatic**. See **standing, walking, wandering**.

dyssyllabia (dis"sil-ab'bi-ə) n. syllable-stumbling. [dys-, q.v., + < G *syllabe* syllable]. See **talk**.

dyssynergia (dys"sin-ur'ji-ə) n. **ataxia**, q.v. See **standing, walking, wandering**. See **nerve, muscle, movement, touch**.

dystaxia (dys-taks'si-ə) n. mild **ataxia**, q.v. [dys-, q.v., + < G *taxis* order]. See **standing, walking, wandering**.

dysteleology (dis-tee'lee-ol'lə-jee) n. 1. lack of purposefulness or of contribution to the final result. (2. the study of apparently useless organs or parts.) [dys-, q.v., + < G *tele* far away + -*logia* < *logsos* word, study, reason & < -*logos* speaking]. See **mentality, mentation, behavior.**

dysthymia (dis-thī'mi-ə) n. any mental disorder or disease; chronically sad or depressed; a mental state of anxiety, depression, and obsession. [dys-, q.v., + < G *thymos* mind, emotion]. adj. = **dysthymic**. See **emotion**.

dystimbria (dis-tim'bri-ə) n. defect in quality or resonance of the voice. [dys-, q.v., + < F *timbre* a musical quality in a tone or sound < G *tympanon* drum.]. See **talk**.

dystonia (dis-tōn'ni- ə) n. a state of abnormal, either hyper- or hypo-, tonicity in any of the tissues; involuntary muscle contraction, as found in Parkinson's disease. [dys- + < G *tonos* tension]. adj. **dystonic**. See **standing, walking, wandering**. See **nerve, muscle, movement, touch**.

dystopia (dis-tōp'pi-ə) n. a place, imaginary or real, where everything goes wrong; malposition. [dys-, q.v.,+ < G *topos* place]. adj. **dystopic**. adj. **dystopian**. n. **dystopianism**. syn. **dystopy** (dis'tō-pee). ant. **utopia**. See **mentality, mentation, behavior**.

dystrophy (dis'trō-fee) n. defective nutrition. [dys-, q.v., + G *trophe* nutrition, nourishment]. adj. **dystrophic** (dis-trōf'fik). syn. **dystropia**

(-trō'pee-ə), q.v., **dystrophia** (-trō'fee-ə). Cf. **dystropy**, q.v. See **gastrointestinal**. See **health, illness**.

dystropia (dis-trōp'pi-ə) n. See **dystropy**. [dys-, q.v., + *tropos* a turning]. See **gastrointestinal**. See **health, illness**.

dystropy (dis'trō-pee)/**dystropia**, n. abnormal or eccentric behavior. [dys-, q.v., + < G *tropos* a turning]. adj. **dystropic**. Cf. **dystrophy**, q.v. See **mentality, mentation, behavior**.

dysuria (dis-yoor'ri-ə) n. difficult or painful urination. [dys-, q.v., + *ouron* urine + -ia, suff., a state or condition.]. alt. = **dysury** (dis'yoo-ri). syn. **dysuresia** (dis-yoor-ee'zhə, -eez'zee-ə). See **genitourinary**.

dysuriac (dis-yoor'ree-ak) n. an individual exhibiting dysuria. [dys-, q.v., + < G *ouron* urine + -ac, suff., used in forming adjs. that are often, if not always, used as nouns < -*akos*]. See **genitourinary**. See **role**.

E

Post jucundam juventutem (After youthful pastime had),/
Post molestam senectutem (After old age hard and sad). [L].

ear, hearing: anacusis, auricular, cerumen, dysacusis, dyseneia, dysphemia, logokophosis, macrotous, neurotrophins, otacoustic, otalgia, otiatrus, otology, otic, otocleisis, otology, otorhinolaryngologist, otosclerosis, otosis, ototoxic, paracusis, pinna, presbyacusis/presbyacousia/presbycusis, surdity, telepresence robots, tinnitus.

ear, hearing: Subcategories

I. Articulation (speech) loss due to deafness: **dyseneia**
II. Ear:
    1. Doctor: **otiatrus, otorhinolaryngologist**
    2. External ear: **pinna**
       a. having large ears: **macrotous**
    3. Noises, ringing: **tinnitus**
    4. Pain: **otalgia**
    5. Study: **otology**
    6. Wax: **cerumen**

III. Hearing aid: **otacoustic, telepresence robots**
IV. Hearing loss:
    1. Causing hearing loss: **ototoxic**
    2. Deafness, no hearing: **anacusis, surdity**
    3. Impaired hearing: **paracusis**
    4. Impaired hearing due to:
       a. aging: **presbyacusis/presbyacousia/pres-bycusis**
       b. ankylosis of inner-ear bones: **otosclerosis**
       c. closure of the eustachian tube: **otocleisis**
       d. closure of the external ear canal by: **cerumen**
       e. emotional or intellectual deficits: **dysphemia**
       f. misunderstanding of spoken sounds: **otosis**
       g. word deafness: **logokophosis**
V. Impaired sound discrimination: **dysacusis**
VI. Inner ear proteins: **neurotrophins**
VII. Relating to the ear: **auricular, otic**
VIII. Spoken in the ear: **auricular**

éboulement (ebulmã) nm. the crumbling or falling of a wall, especially a fortification. Fig., a crumbling of physical strength, resistance, prowess. [F]. See **tiredness, weakness**. See **physique, appearance**.

ebriection (ee-bri-ek'shən) n. mental breakdown from too much boozing. [< L *ebrius* drunk]. See **nerve, muscle, movement, touch**. See **drink, food**. See **mentality, mentation, behavior**. See **intelligence**.

ebrious (eeb'bri-əs) adj. tending to over imbibe; slightly drunk, tipsy. [< L *ebrius* drunk]. See **drink, food**.

ecchymosis (ek-i-mōs'siss), pl. **ecchymoses** (ck-i-mōs'seess) n. a purplish patch caused by extravasation of blood into the skin— ecchymoses differ from **petechiae**, q.v., only in larger size and extent. Due to decreased skin thickness atrophy with age, the skin is more subject to ecchymosis. [< G *ekchymosis* ecchymosis < *ek* out + *chymos* juice]. See **skin**. See **blood, circulation, glands**.

ecdemomania (ek"dee-mō-may'ni-ə) n. compulsive wandering. [< G *ek-*, pref., out of + *demos* people + *mania* loss of reason]. adj.

ecdemomaniacal (-mə-nī'ə-kəl). n. **ecdemomaniac**. See **manias**. See **standing, walking, wandering**.

ecdysiast (ek-dee'zi-əst) n. (1. a stripper.) 2. one unbalanced mentally who divests oneself of clothing. 3. one who sheds skin. • The long-term effect of the sun's rays on her skin had caused such **furfuration**, q.v., that the term *ecdysiast* came to mind. [an H. L. Menckenism < G *ecdysis* the zoological term for shedding skin or other outer covering]. See **skin**.

ecesis (e-sees'siss or i-sees'siss) n. the acclimation of a plant to a new environment; the successful establishment of a plant or animal species in a new environment (lit.); (fig.) refers to an old person adjusting to new living arrangements, situations. • Her *ecesis* in the nursing home was difficult. [early 20ᵗʰ C. < G *oikesis* an inhabiting < *oikos* house]. See **innovation, misoneism**. See **retirement.**

echolalia (ek"kō-lay'li-ə) n. repeating another's words. [< G *ekho* echo + *lalia* a form of speech]. See **talk**.

ecmnesia (ek-nee'zhə, -neez'zee-ə) n. loss of recent memory, with return of earlier memories. [ec-, pref, out of, away from < G prep. *ec* + *mneme* memory]. Cf. **anomia, lethonomia, senior moment, paleomnesia**, q.v. See **memory**.

ecomania (eek"kō-may'ni-ə) n. 1. any neurotic disorder supposed to result from something unpleasant or dreadful in one's home environment. 2. abnormal desire to be at home. [eco-, pref., denoting relationship to environment < G *oikos* house, household, habitation + *mania* frenzy]. adj. **ecomaniacal** (-ma-nī'ə-kəl.), q.v. **ecomaniac**, q.v. syn. **oikomania**, q.v. Cf. **philopatridomania**, q.v. See **manias**.

ectropion (ek-trōp'pi-on) (also **ectropium** {-əm}) n. (1. a turning outward of a part.) 2. a turning or rolling outward of a lower eyelid. (This leads to an inability of the punctum {tear-duct opening on the lower lid} to drain tears properly from the conjunctival sac into the lacrimal sac, which in turns leads the patient to complain of excess tearing, a not infrequent complaint in the elderly, and of tears draining onto the face.) [< G *ek* out + *trope* turning]. ant. **entropion**. q.v. See **eye**.

edacious (i-day'shəss) adj. of eating; eats a lot; voracious, greedy. [< L *edax, -acis* < *edere* to eat]. n. **edacity** (-das'ə-tee). See **drink & food**.

edea (ee-dee'ə) n.pl. the external genitalia. • The word "edea" is a useful euphemism most likely to be employed by the elderly. It's been suggested that the ancient Greek name, Medea, because of its close relation to the word, edea, is a derivative. [< G *aidoia*, genitals]. See **genitourinary**.

edema (e-deem'mə) n. the presence of abnormally large amounts of fluid in the intercellular tissue spaces of the body; usually applied to demonstrable accumulation of excessive fluid in the subcutaneous tissues. Pitting edema = edema that yields to pressure, as by a finger, by forming a depression. [< G *oidema* swelling]. adj. edematous. See **physique, appearance**.

edentate (ee-den'tayt) adj. 1. toothless. (2. pertaining to an order of mammals {*edenta*} whose members may be toothless.) [< L *edentulus* toothless < *e* without + *dens* tooth]. n. **edentia** (-ti-ə). syns. **edentulous, edentulate, agomphious**, q.v. See **mouth, gums, & teeth**.

edentulous/edentulate (ee-den'tyoo-lus, -chə-lus, -ləs/ -layt) adj. toothless; without teeth. [< L *endntulus* toothless < *e* without + *dens* tooth]. See **mouth, gums, & teeth**.

edeomania /(aidoi(o)mania) (ee-dee" ō-may'ni-ə/ aī-doy"yō-mayn'ni-ə) n. strong and, or, abnormal sexual interest or desire. [ede(o)-/ eide(o)-, pref. (alt. aidoi(o)-), < G *aidoia* genitals + *mania* frenzy]. adj. **edeomaniacal** (-mə-nī'ə-kəl). n. **edeomaniac**. syn. **aidoi(o)mania, concupiscence**, q.v. Cf. **erotomania**, q.v. See **manias**. See **sex, love**.

edipol (ed'di-pōl) n. (obs. & rare) a mild oath; any common asseveration. [< miswritten L *edepol* by Pollux, and erroneously connected with *ædis* temple]. See **talk**.

effete (i-feet'/e-feet') adj. 1. characterized by decadence, over refinement, or overindulgence. 2. no longer able to reproduce; sterile. 3. lacking in vitality, worn out, spent. [< L *effetus* effete; worn out by bearing young; spent; vain; delusive < *fetus* breeding; offspring;

growth]. adv. **effetely**. n. **effeteness**. See **tiredness, weakness**. See **sex, love**.

effleurage (ef-flur-ozh') n. a gentle rubbing with the palm of the hand; a stroking movement in massage. [< F *effleurer* to touch lightly]. See **nerve, muscle, movement, touch**. See **skin**. See **therapy**.

egad (i-gad') int. (archaic) used as an exclamation, generally to express surprise. [Late 17th C. < alteration of AH + gad, a euphemism for God. (AH {or A.H.} is an adv. indicating the number of years from the Hegira {A.D. 622}, a key date in the Islamic calendar—full form = {L} *anno Hegirae*—the Hegira {Hejira} is the withdrawal of the Prophet Muhammad from Mecca to Medina to escape punishment; uncapitalized, the word indicates flight or withdrawal from somewhere, especially to escape danger. Hegira {capitalized} can also indicate the Muslim era, which dates from the first day of the lunar year in which Muhammad's withdrawal to Medina occurred.)] See **emotion**.

egersis (ee-gur'siss) n. abnormal, extremely alert wakefulness. [G, a waking]. ants. **hypersomnia**, **sopor**; **hypnodia**, q.v. See **sleep & wakefulness**.

egotheism (ee'gō-thee"iz-əm) n. self-deification. [L, I + < G *theos* god + -ism, suff.]. See **mentality, mentation, behavior**.

eidetic (ī-det'tik) adj. 1. recalled or reproduced with startling accuracy, clarity, and vividness. 2. pertaining to the ability of visualizing something previously seen with startling accuracy, clarity, and vividness, e.g. an eidetic memory. [< G *edetikos* < *eidos* form + -ic, suff., of or relating to, having the nature of, < G *-ikos*]. See **memory**.

eidetic image (ī-det'tik im'aj) n.phr. a memory that is as intense and fresh as the actual experience. [< G *eidos* form + image]. See **memory**.

eigne (ayn) adj. first born, eldest; heir apparent (based on primogeniture). [< corrupt spelling of **ayne**, q.v., < OF *aîné* elder, eldest, first born (< earlier *aîsné, aînsné* < *aîns*) + *né* born]. See **old**.

elastosis (ee-las-tōs'siss) n. 1. degeneration of elastic tissue. 2. degenerative changes in the skin's connective tissue. [< G *elastreo*, epic form of *elauno* drive, push]. The n.phr. **actinic elastosis** = colloid degeneration of the skin that takes place in the elastic tissue of the dermis in persons who are repeatedly or almost constantly exposed to sunlight over a period of many years. [< G *aktis* a ray]. See **senile elastosis**. See **actinic keratosis**. See **skin**.

elder-care hostel (l'dər kayr hos'təl) n.phr. a relative inexpensive place for old people to stay overnight, spend leisure, vacation time. [a retronym based on the term "youth hostel" < 13 C OF *(h)ostel* < L *hospitale* guesthouse, inn < L *hospit-* host, guest]. See **old age**.

elderliness (el'də-li-ness) n. the state of being elderly, i.e., past middle age, old; having the characteristics of old age; being old-fashioned. [< OE (i)eldra < Gmc]. adj. **elderly**. See **old age**.

elder rap n.phr. slang. the general talk, language of old persons that engages, engrosses them. [< O.E. *(i)eldra* < Ger. & < L *raptus* seized, pp. of *rapere* to seize. (Elder rap is a derivative of "rap session", an informal discussion, especially of people in the same line of work, or with shared concerns.)]. syn. **elder gab**, **elder speak**. See **talk**.

eleemosynary (el"ə-mos'sə-ner"ee, -el"ee-) adj. pertaining to charity; dependent on alms; charitable; gratuitous. • One hopes that the public will have an *eleemosynary* attitude regarding the need of retirement homes for exogenous financial support. [< G *eleemosyne* pity, charity < *eleemon* pitiful < *eleos* pity]. See **mentality, mentation, behavior**.

elflock (elf'lok) n. tangled hair, tangled coil of hair (tangled as if by elves) (often plural). [< OE *elf* (MHG *elbe*) & *ælf* < Gmc. *albh-*]. See **hair**. See **physique, appearance**.

Elli (el'lee) n. an old woman; a personification of old age. (In Norse mythology Elli defeated Thor in a wrestling match.) [Icelandic *elli*, lit. old age. Cf. eld n. archaic old age < OE *eldo* < *(e)ald*, old.]. See **old woman**.

elumbated (ee-lum'bay"təd) adj. weak in the loins (that part of the body on both sides of the spine between the rib cage and the pelvic bones). • In the pornogenarian's *elumbated* state his performance was as neither he nor she expected. [< G *e-*, pref., < *ex* out of, from, away from + < L *lumbus* loin, pl. = loins, including genital organs (as in "fruit of one's loins", "child of one's loins", "sprung from one's loins","loin cloth", "gird one's loins"; **edea**, q.v.)]. adj. **loined**. See **genitourinary**. See **sex, love**. See **tiredness, weakness**.

Elysium (i-liz'hee-əm, ə-liz'-hee-) n. 1. in Greek mythology, the home of the blessed after death. 2. any ideally delightful or blissful place or condition. [< G Elysium]. n.pl. **Elysian fields** = **Elysium**. adj. **Elysian** (i-lizh'ən). See **end of life, death**.

embo(lo)lalia (em-bō{lō}-lay'li-ə) n. hesitation forms inserted frequently in speech, e.g., *ah's, uh's, um's, you know, like*, extra *o.k.'s*. [< G *embolus* something thrown in < *embollo* to throw in (< em- {= en- often before *b, p*, or *m*}, pref., in < L *in* in + < OE *beall* < Ger. ball) + < G *lalia* talk]. adj. **embolalic**. See **talk**.

embrocation (em-brō-kay'shən) n. 1. lubricating or rubbing the body with liniment, oil, etc., to relieve muscular pain, etc. 2. the liquid used for this. [< L *embrocatio* a fomentation: poultice, warm application]. Cf. **effleurage**, q.v. See **skin**. See **therapy**.

emeritus (i-mer'ri-təss), m.adj., **emerita** (-taa), f.adj., retired from active service, usually for age, but retaining rank or title; honorably discharged from service. [< L pp. of *emerere* serve out, earn deserve < *merere* to serve, earn]. nm. **emeritus**, nf. **emerita**, pl.nm. **emeritii** (-tee), pl.nf. **emeritae** (-tī) = one (or more) who has (have) retired but retains (retain) former rank or title, especially in re: professor(s). See **retirement**. See **role**.

emollient (i-mol'yənt, ee-mol'lee-ent). adj. softening or soothing. [< L *emolliens* softening < *e*-out + *mollis* soft]. n. **emollient** an agent that softens or soothes the skin, or soothes an internal surface. syn. **malactic**, q.v. Cf. **embrocation**, q.v. [< G *malaktikos* softening]. syn. n. **malagma**. [< G, a poultice]). See **skin**. See **therapy**.

emotion: acescent, acherontic, anautarchia, anhedonia, antithalian, anxiolytic, ataraxia, atrabilarian, atrabilious, autognosis, autophobia, cathect, cathexis, choleric, congruence, cyclothyme, dacryagogue, dacrygelosis, daphnean, dudgeon, dysphemia, dysthymia, egad, epicedian, erubescence, eudaemonia/eudemonia, eumoirous, euthymia, evancalous, gadzooks, horsefeathers, hypothymia, impassible, importunate, importune, importunity, impotentia, iracund, irascible, languish, larmoyant, lowering, lugubrious, lypemania, lypemanic, lypophrenia, lypothymia, mawkish, megrims, morose, nosothymia, phatic, rectopathic, saturnine, Schadenfreude, serotonin, sough, zounds.

emotion: Subcategories

negative

I. Against enjoyment: **antithalian**
II. Anger: angry, displeased, upset; angry: **iracund, irascible, lowering; dudgeon, choleric**
III. Anxiousness: **dysthymia**
IV. Bashful, shy: **daphnean**
V. Cheerless, depressing, sad, gloomy: **acherontic, atrabilious, epicedian, lowering, lugubrious, morose, saturnine**
VI. Depression: depression, sadness:
    1. general: **dysthymia**
    2. due to illness: **nosothymia**
    3. without cause: **lypophrenia**
    4. one who is depressed: **atrabilarian**
VII. Easily hurt: **rectopathic**
VIII. Emotionally-caused disordered phonation: **dysphemia**
IX. Fear of oneself: **autophobia**
X. One with mood swings: **cyclothyme**
XI. Overly sentimental: **mawkish**
XII. Pleasure in another's suffering: **Schadenfreude**
XIII. Sadness: melancholy, melancholic: **hypothymia, megrims, lypemania; larmoyant, lypemanic, lypothymia**
XIV. Sour: **acescent**
XV. Undergo hardship: **languish**
XVI. Unfeeling: **impassible**
XVII. Unhappiness: **anautarchia, anhedonia**
XVIII. Weakness: *impotentia*, **languish**

neutral

I. A blush: **erubescence**
II. Emotional: **phatic**
III. Interjections: **egad, gadzooks, horsefeathers, zounds**
IV. Insistent; insist; insistence: **importunate; importune; importunity**

V. Invest emotional or mental activity in something or someone: **cathect**
VI. Investment of emotional or mental activity in something or someone: **cathexis**
VII. Promoting the secretion of tears: **dacrygenic**
VIII. Self awareness: **autognosis**
IX. Sigh: **sough**
X. That which induces a flow of tears: **dacryagogue**
XI. The condition of alternately crying and laughing: **dacrygelosis**

positive

I. Calmness: **ataraxia**
II. Embraceable: **evancalous**
III. Happiness:
  1. general happiness: **eudaemonia/eudemonia, euthymia, congruence**
  2. happiness from being good: **eumoirous**
IV. Lessens inertness and depression: **serotonin**
V. Reducing anxiety: **anxiolytic**

emphysema (em-fi-see'mə) n. (1. the presence of air in the interstices of the connective tissue of a part.) 2. increase in the size of air spaces distal to the terminal bronchioles (of the lung), either from dilation or from destruction of their walls. • COPD, chronic obstructive pulmonary disease, affects mainly the elderly; a major component of this is *emphysema*. [< G *en* in + *physema* a blowing < *physa* bellows]. See **breathing**.

emphysematous (em-fi-sem'mə-təs) adj. 1. bloated, swollen. 2. pertaining to **emphysema**, q.v.

empressement (ãprɛsmã) nm. attentiveness, extreme politeness, display of cordiality; eagerness, zeal, enthusiasm; in a hurry. [F < *empresser* to hasten, to be eager, to hurry]. See **mentality, mentation, behavior**.

empyrean (em"pī-ree'ən, -pir'ree-) n. (literary) the sky or celestial sphere. The firmament (considered as an arch). 2. the highest, i.e., the fifth, part of heaven, which was codified by the Alexandrian mathematician and astronomer, Ptolemy (fl.127-151 A.D.), and thought by the ancient Greeks and Romans to consist of pure fire. By

Christian doctrine the empyrean was the seat of deity and the angels. [< G *empyrios* fiery]. adj. **empyrean.** adj. **empyreal** (em"pī-ree'əl) = heavenly, celestial. syn. **supernal,** q.v. See **religion, theology, morality**.

emunctory (ee-munk'tə-ree, -mungk') adj. excretory or depurant, i.e., cleansing or purifying. • The old dear was unaware of the *emunctory* noises she made in clearing simultaneously both her nose and her intestinal gas. [< L *emunct-*, pref., < *emungere* to cleanse + -ory]. n. **emunctory** = any excretory organ or duct. See **gastrointestinal**. See **genitourinary**. See: **nose, smell**.

enchiridion (en-kir-id'di-ən) n. a manual, handbook. [G < *en* in + *kheir* hand]. Arrian, the best-known pupil of the famous Greek stoic philosopher, Epictetus (AD 55-135), compiled Epictetus's sayings outlining his philosophy and entitled it "Enchiridion". • The antiquarian would be lost without his *enchiridion*. Cf. *vade mecum*, q.v. See **memory**.

encraty (en'krə-tee) n. abstinence, self-restraint. [G]. See **mentality, mentation, behavior**.

encephalopathy (en-sef"fə-lop'pə-thee) n. any disease of the brain, cerebropathy. [encephal(o)-, pref., indicating the brain or some relationship thereto < G *enkephalos* brain + *pathos* disease]. syn. **cerebropathy**. See **brain**.

encephalophonic (en-sef"fə-lō-fon'nik) adj. refers to hearing noises, talk, voices in one's head. [encephal(o)-, pref., < G *enkephalos* brain + *phone* voice]. See **talk**. See **mentality, mentation, behavior**.

encopresis (en-kō-pree'siss) n. incontinence of feces not due to organic illness or defect. Due to a decrease in contractile strength of the pelvic floor muscles—particularly the external and internal puborectal muscles—with age, sphinctal pressure may decrease, and smaller distention volume can inhibit anal sphincter tone, thus facilitating fecal incontinence. • *Encopresis* is much more frequent in the aged. [G < *en* in + *kopros* dung + -*esis* a suff. denoting action, process, or condition; see also -sis] See **gastrointestinal**.

end-of-life, death: acrotism, advesperate, biometry, *alieni juris*, apopemptic, apoptosis, *apud se*, athanasia, brumal, cenotaph, Cerberus, cerements, chthonic, cinerarium, cinerary, cinereous, coimetromania, coimetrophilia, coimetrophobia, columbarium, commorant, cremains, desinence, dormition, Elysium, epicedian/epicedium/epicede, epitaph, eschatology, escheat, eulogy, evening of life, exequies, exheredate, Extreme Unction, feuillemorte, fey, finifugal, funest, gloming, Gompertz Law, great assize, Hadephobia, Hayflick's limit, hibernacle, hiemal, *immortel*, immure, intestate, inhumation, latibulize, lethe, lethiferous, moirologist, moribund, necrologist, necromania, necromimesis, necromorphous, *non compos mentis*, *nunc dimittis*, nuncupate, obituary, obsequies, *à outrance*, pareschatology, patrimony, preagonal, QALYS, quietus, relic, relics, relict, rhytidosis, senicide, September, sepulcher, sepulture, *shpilkes*, sough, Struldbrug, Stygian, Styx, *sui juris*, sunset clause, supernal, taisch, taphephobia, taphophilia, Tartarus, testate, thanatoid, thanatology, thanatomania, thanatophobia, thanatopsis, tilmus, Valhalla, viaticum, welkin, wraith.

end-of-life, death: Subcategories

I. Approaching or near death:
1. Anointed and prayed over for salvation: **Extreme Unction**
2. Approaching death, at or toward life's end: **advesperate, brumal, evening of life, gloming, hibernacle, hiemal, moribund, preagonal, quietus, rhytidosis, September, tilmus**
3. Calculation of life expectancy: **biometry**
4. Cell-division limit controlling aging: **Hayflick's limit**
5. Color of death: **feuillemorte**
6. Crossing the river from life to death: **Stygian**
7. Difficulties governmental and social planners have with prolonging life in those who are decrepit: **Struldbrug**
8. Farewell: **apopemptic**
9. Fated to die: **fey**
10. Forgotten past: **lethe**. harbinger of death: **funest**
11. Hibernate: **latibulize**
12. Last rites, Eucharist: **viaticum**

13. Prolonging life via fidgeting, inability to sit quietly: *shpilkes*
14. Something surviving from an earlier age: **relic, relict**
15. Willingness to die: *nunc dimittis*
16. A formula for deciding the worthiness of treatment: **QALYS**

II. Signs of death:
 1. Breathe one's last: **sough**
 2. Chance of continuing to live: **Gompertz Law**
 3. Corneal wrinkling (a sign of death): **rhytidosis**
 3. Death like: **thanatoid**
 5. Pulseless: **acrotism**

III. Death:
 1. Causing death, deadly: **lethiferous**
 2. Cell death: **apoptosis**
 3. Contemplation of death: **thanatopsis**
 4. Corpse: **relics**
 5. Death: **dormition**
 6. Death delusion: **necromimesis**
 7. Deathlessness, immortality: **athanasia**
 8. Death phantom: **taisch, wraith**
 9. Death preoccupation: **thanatomania**
 10. Death pun: *à outrance*
 11. Death words: **epitaph, eulogy, obituary**
 12. Death writer: **necrologist**
 13. Death feign: **necromimesis, necromorphous**
 14. Dying together: **commorant**
 15. End: **desinence**
 16. Fear of cemeteries: **coimetrophobia**
 17. Fear of death: **thanatophobia**
 18. Fear of Hades: **Hadephobia**
 19. Killing old men: **senicide**
 20. Peaceful, painless death: **dormition**
 21. Preoccupation with dead bodies: **necromania**
 22. Shunning, avoiding death: **finifugal**.
 23. Study of death: **eschatology, thanatology**
 24. To the death, to the extreme: *à outrance*

IV. Burial, funeral:
 1. Ashes: **cinerary, cinereous, cremains**
 2. Burial clothes: **cerements**
 3. Burial vault, tomb: **columbarium, sepulcher, sepulture**

4. Bury in a wall: **immure**
5. Container for storing ashes of a corpse: **cinerarium**
6. Corpse: **relics**
7. Fear of being buried alive: **taphephobia**
8. Funeral: **exequies, obsequies**
9. Funeral ode: **epicedium/ epicede**
10. Interring, burying: **sepulture, inhumation**
11. Love of cemeteries, graveyards: **coimetrophilia**
12. Love of funerals: **taphophilia**
13. Paid mourner: **moirologist**
14. Re: a funeral ode: **epicedian**

V. After death, burial, heaven & hell:
   1. A widow: **relict**
   2. Artistic image after death: *immottel*
   3. Dog who guards the gates of hell: **Cerberus**
   4. Heaven, heaven-like: **welkin, Valhalla, Elysium**
   5. Heavenly: **supernal**
   6. Hades, hell: **Tartarus**
   7. Last judgment, judgment day: **great assize**
   8. Love of collecting tombstone epitaphs: **coimetrophilia**
   9. Life after death: **pareschatology**
   10. Memorial erected to a dead person(s) buried elsewhere: **cenotaph**
   11. Morbid attraction, compulsion to visit cemeteries: **coimetromania**
   12. Relating to the underworld: **chthonic, Stygian**
   13. River in Hades: **Styx, Lethe** (river of forgetfulness, oblivion)

VI. Will, inheritance:
   1. Future date when a will's specifications end: **sunset clause**
   2. In one's senses: *apud se*
   3. Inheritance: **patrimony**
   4. Mentally competent to manage one's affairs: *sui juris*
   5. Mentally incompetent to manage one's affairs; not sound of mind, insane: *alieni juris*; *non compos mentis*
   6. Reversion of property in absence of legal heirs: **escheat**
   7. To disinherit: **exheredate**
   8. Will: **intestate, nuncupate, testate**

endogamy (en-dog'gə-mee) n. The practice of marriage within a specific social group. ● *Endogamy* within this assisted-living facility is surprisingly frequent. [endo-, pref., within, inside < G *endo* in + < G *gamos* marriage]. See **marriage**.

enervate (en'ner-vayt) vt. to weaken or take energy away from; weaken. (Enervate is a phantonym, i.e., a word the meaning of which is different from what it would seem.) [< L *enervate-*, pp. of *enervare* extract the sinews of, weaken < *nervus* sinew]. adj. **enervate** (en-er'vayt) wanting in (physical, moral, literary, artistic) vigor. n. **enervation** (-vay'shən). Cf. **denervate** = to remove or destroy the nerve(s), and **innervation** = the distribution of nerves to an organ or body part, or the activation of a muscle or other body part. See **tiredness, weakness**.

enfin (ãfɛ̃) adv. finally; at last; in short, in a word; that's to say. [F]. int. *enfin!* at last! well! See **talk**.

enissophobia (en-is"sō-fōb'bi-ə) n. morbid fear of being reproached. [? + *phobos* fear]. adj. **enissophobic**. n. **enissophobe**. See **phobias**.

enophthalmos/enophthalmus (en-of-thal'məs, -mos/-mus) n. displacement of the eye(s) backward into the orbit. It is caused by loss of orbital fat in the elderly. [< G *en* in + *ophthalmos* eye]. See **eye**. See **physique, appearance**.

enosimania (en-ōs"si-may'ni-ə) n. belief that one has committed an unpardonable sin. [< G *enosis* a quaking + *mania* frenzy]. adj. **enosimaniacal** (-mə-nī'ə-kal). n. **enosimaniac**. Cf. **enosiphobia**, **hamartomania**, q.v. See **manias**. See **religion, theology, morality**.

enosi(o)phobia (en-ōs"si-(ō)-fōb'bi-ə) n. morbid fear of having committed an unpardonable sin. [< G *enosis* a quaking + *phobos* fear]. adj. **enosiphobic**. n. **enosiphobe** (en-ōs'si-fōb). Cf. **enissophobia**, **hamartophobia, peccatiphobia; enosimania**, q.v. See **phobias**. See **religion, theology, morality**.

ensorcell (en-sor'səl) vt. to bewitch, enchant, fascinate. [< OF *ensorceler* < *en-* put into or on something + *sorceler* < *sorcier* sorcerer < Roman *sortiarius* caster of lots < *sors sortis* lots, casting of lots].

ensynopticity (en"sin-op-tis'si-tee) n. the ability to take a general view of something. adv. **ensynoptically** (en"sin-op'ti-kəl-ee). [< G *en-*, pref., in < prep. *en* in + *synopsis* seeing, a general view < *syn* with, together, or alike + *opsis* sight < *ops* eye]. See **mentality, mentation, behavior**.

entelechy (en-tel' lə-kee) n. (1. the real existence of a thing, not merely its theoretical existence.) 2. in some philosophies, a life-giving force believed to be responsible for the development of all living things—that vital force directing an organism toward full realization of its potential. [early 17th C. via late L < G *entelekheia* having completeness < *enteles* complete < *telos* end]. See **religion, theology, morality**.

entheal/enthean (en'thee-əl/ -ən) adj. (obs.) divinely inspired. [< G *entheos* divinely inspired < *en* in + *theos* god]. See **religion**.

entheomania (en"thee-ō-may'ni-ə) n. an abnormal state in which one thinks one is divinely inspired. [< G *enthetos* implanted < *en*, a preposition meaning "in", + *thesis* a placing + *mania* frenzy]. adj. **entheomaniacal** (en-thee"ō-mə-nī'ə-kəl). n. **entheomaniac** (-may'ni-ak). See **manias**. See **religion**.

entropion/entropium (en-trō'pi-ən, -on/-əm) n. (1. inversion or turning inward of a part.) 2. infolding of the margin of an eyelid (especially a lower one) such that the eyelashes touch the conjunctiva giving the false sensation of a foreign body in the eye. This is not uncommon in the elderly. [< G *en* in + *trope* a turning]. syn. **enstrophe**. ant. **ectropion**, q.v. See **eye**.

enuresis (en-yoo-rees'siss) n. bed-wetting, involuntary discharge of urine while asleep. [< G *enourein* urinate in < *ouron* urine]. See **genitourinary**.

epicaricacy (ep"pi-kər-ik'kə-see) n. taking pleasure in others' misfortune. [?]. Cf. **Schadenfreude**, q.v. See **mentality, mentation, behavior**.

epicedian (ep"pi-seed'di-ən) adj. sad, mournful, elegiac. [< L *epicedium* < G *epikedeion* a dirge, neuter of *epikedeios* of or for a funeral < *epi-* upon + *kedos* care]. n. **epicedium** or **epicede** (ep'i-seed) (pl. **epicedia** {ep-i-seed'di-ə, -aa}/**epicedes** {-see'deess})

= a funeral ode, dirge. adj. **epicedial**. See **emotion**. See **end-of-life, death**.

epicene (ep'pi-seen") adj. having characteristics of: 1. both sexes; 2. of neither sex; 3. of a man having typically female characteristics. 4. weak, lacking physical vigor or strength. (5. having only one grammatical form for both masculine and feminine in languages the nouns of which have gender.) [< G *epikoinos* in common < *koinos* common]. **epicene** n. 1. someone or something epicene. (2. a noun having the same masculine and feminine form.) n. **epicenism**. See **sex, love**. See **tiredness, weakness**. See **role**.

epigone (ep'pi-gōn) n. a follower; of a later—and presumably inferior—generation; used especially literarily or artistically; a mediocre imitator or follower of an important person. [< G *epigonoi*, pl. of *epigonos* offspring < *gignesthai* be born. *Epigonoi* was a term applied to the sons of the seven conquerors of Thebes in ancient Greece]. See **youth, younger generation**. See **role**.

epigonous (ee-pig'ə-nəs) adj. of a later generation; pertaining to an imitative school of art or science. [See **epigone**]. See **youth, younger generation**.

epilegomenon (ep"pi-lee-gom'mi-non) n. an added remark [epi-, pref., after, in addition < G *epi*, on, upon + *legos* word + pres.p. form of the verb *legein* to speak]. See **talk**.

epiolatry (ep"pi-ol'lə-tree) n. the worship of words. ● One is more inclined to *epiolatry* in old age. [< G *epos* word + -*latry*, suff., worship—first citation: Oliver Wendell Holmes in his 1860 book "Professor at the Breakfast Table" (< A.Word.A.Day)]. See **talk**. **religion, theology, morality**.

epiphora (ee-pif'fawr-aa, -ə) n. watery eye; an overflow of tears upon the cheek—a frequent complaint in the elderly. Epiphora may be due, paradoxically, to dryness of the eye, which results in tearing that dilutes the oil in normal tears. That oil keeps tears adherent to the eyeball and directed into the tear duct. Another cause is **ectropion**, q.v., an eversion of the lower eyelid that displaces the tear duct entrance away from the eye so tears aren't drained normally. A blocked tear duct is also a possible cause of epiphora. [G, a sudden flow, burst < *epi* on + *phero* to bear]. See **eye**.

epistaxis (ep"pis-taks'siss) n. nosebleed, which is relatively common in the elderly. Old-age-related atrophy of the nasal mucosa (mucous membrane) causes thinning of the mucosal blood vessels rendering them more subject to minor injury, the effect of drugs (aspirin), hypertension, etc. [< G *epistazo* to bleed at the nose < *epi* on + *stazo* to fall in drops]. See **nose & smell**. See **blood, circulation, glands**.

epitaph (ep'pi-taf) n. words written in memory of a dead person, esp. as a tomb inscription. [< G *epitaphion* funeral oration < *epi* upon + *taphos* tomb]. See **end-of-life, death**.

epizeuxis (ep-i-zooks'siss) n. emphatic verbal repetition (rhetoric). • The old professor seemed unaware of his recurrent *epizeuxis*. [G, *epizeuxis* a fastening upon < *epizeugnunai* < *epi* upon + *zeugnunai* to yoke]. See **talk**.

epulotic (ep-yoo-lot'tik) adj. having healing power. n. 1. cicatrizing (scaring). 2. an agent that promotes cicatrization. 3. a medicine that heals. [< G *epoulosis* a scarring over]. See **therapy**.

equipoise (ek'kwi-poyz", eek'kwə-) n. 1. equilibrium (often fig.); balance; a condition in which weights are in balance, or there is a balance between different social, emotional, intellectual, etc., influences. 2. something that creates a balanced state, usually by counterbalancing some other force or thing. • In addition to aerobics and muscle- strengthening exercises, *equipoise*, i.e., balance training, is a needful practice for seniors. [equi-, pref., equal < L *aequus* equal + < Fr. *pois* weight, balance < *penser* to weigh < L *pensare* to keep on weighing < *pendere* weigh]. vt. to counterbalance a weight or influence (formal); hold (mind) in suspense. See **health, illness**.

equivoque (ek'kwi-vōk, -kwə-) an amusing use of an ambiguous word, expression; a pun; a double meaning. [F *équivoke* < L *aequivocuus* ambiguous < *vox* voice]. Cf. **dittology**, *double entendre*, q.v. See **talk**.

erem(i)ophobia (er"ree-m(i-)ō-fōb'bi-ə) n. a morbid fear of loneliness, of being alone. [< G *eremia* solitude + *phobos* fear]. adj. **eremophobic**. n. **eremophobe**. syns. **autophobia**, **isolophobia**, **monophobia**, **solophobia**, q.v. See **loneliness, solitude, silence**. See **phobias**.

eremomania (er-eem"mō-may'ni-ə) n. abnormal interest in stillness. [< G *eremia* solitude + *mania* frenzy]. adj. **eremomaniacal** (er-eem"mō-mə-nī'ə-kəl). n. **eremomaniac**. Cf. **erem(i)ophobia**, q.v. See **manias**. See **loneliness, solitude, silence**.

erethism (er'rə-thiz"əm) n. excessive irritability or excitability; an abnormal sensitivity to stimulation, either generalized or restricted to a body part. Cf. **erythrism**. See **sleep & wakefulness**. See **mentality, mentation, behavior**.

ergasiomania (ur-gas"si-ō-may'ni-ə) n. 1. overeagerness to be at work, working. • His *ergasiomania* prevents any enjoyment of retirement. (2. undue eagerness to perform surgery.) [< G *ergon* work + *mania* frenzy]. **ergasiomaniacal** (-ma-nī'ə-kal). n. **ergasiomaniac**. See **manias**.

ergomania (ur"gō-may'ni-ə) n. compulsion to be constantly at work. [< G *ergon* work + **mania** frenzy]. adj. **ergomaniacal** (-mə-nī'ə-kl, -nī-i-kl). n. **ergomaniac**. Cf. **ergasiomania**, q.v. See **manias**.

ergophile (ur'gō-fīl) n. someone who loves work. [< G *ergon* work + *philos* loving]. adj. **ergophilic** (ur"gō-fil'ik). See **role**.

eristic (er-is'tik)/**eristical** (-ti-kəl) adj. controversial; disputatious, contentious, argumentative. [< G *eristikos* < *eris* strife]. n. **eristic** 1. disputation; art of disputing, debating. 2. a disputant, debater. n. **eristic** one who is argumentative, contentious; syn. **philopolemist**, q.v. adv. **eristically**. See **talk**. See **role**.

ermitophobia (er-mit"tō-fōb'bi-ə) n. morbid fear of solitude. [< OF *hermite* hermit < L *eremita* < G *eremites* < *eremia* desert < *eremos* solitary + *phobos* fear]. adj. **ermitophobic**. n. **ermitophobe**. syns. **autophobia**, **erem(i)ophobia**, **isolophobia**, **monophobia**, **solophobia**, q.v. See **phobias**.

erotomania/eroticomania (er"rō-tō-may'ni-ə)/(er"rot'ti-kō-) n. excessive or morbid inclination to erotic thoughts and behavior; preoccupation with sexuality. [< G *eros* love + *mania* frenzy]. adj. **erotomaniacal** (-mə-nī'ə-kəl). n. **erotomaniac**. Cf. **aidoimania**, **edeomania**, q.v. See **manias**. See **sex, love**.

errabund (er're-bund) adj. 1. (rare) erratic; random. 2. wandering to and fro or about. [< L *errabund* wandering to and fro, wandering about < *errare* to wander, lose one's way, stray, roam; to waver; to err, make a mistake, be mistaken]. See **mentality, mental, behavior**. See **standing, walking, wandering**. See **talk**.

erstwhile (urst'wīl) adj. who in the past was something, e.g., a friend or supporter, but now no longer is. [O.E. *ærest* first < Ger.]. adv. **erstwhile** = (arch.) at a time in the past. syn. **whilom**, q.v. See **past, time**.

erubescence (air-yoo-bes'sənz) n. a reddening, flushing of the skin; a blush. [< L *erubescere* to redden]. adj. erubescent (-sənt). See **skin**. See **color**. See **emotion**.

eructation (er"ruk-tay'shən) n. 1. belching or something produced by belching: the raising of gas or a small quantity of acid fluid from the stomach. 2. any violent expulsion, e.g., intestinal gas from the rectum via the anus. [< L *eructo*, pp. of *eructatus* to belch]. syns. **crepitus**, **flatus**, q.v. See **gastrointestinal**.

erugate (er'roŏ-gayt) adj. freed from wrinkles, smoothed, smooth. [e- < ex-, q.v., + < L *ruga*, pl. *rugae*, wrinkle]. See **skin**.

eschatology (es"kə-tol'lə-jee) n. the study of last things; the body of religious doctrines concerning the human soul in its relation to death, resurrection, judgment, immortality, heaven, and hell. adj. **eschatological** (-ka"tō-loj'ji-kal). adv. **eschatologically** (-loj'ji-kəl-lee). [< G *eskhatos* last + -logy, suff., speech, expression; science, study < -*logia* < *logos* word, study, speaking, reason]. n. **eschatologist** (-tol'). See **religion, theology, morality**. See **end-of-life, death**. See **role**.

eschaton (es'kə-tawn) n. the end of the world, the end of time. [< G *eskhatos* last]. See **religion, theology, morality**. See **end-of-life, death**.

escheat (es-cheet') n. 1. reversion of a deceased person's property—in the U.S. to the state—when there are no legal heirs. 2. the property that reverts by escheat. (3. reversion of property to a feudal lord in medieval England.) [13th C. OF *eschete* < assumed vulgar L *excadere* fall away < L *cadere* to fall]. adj. **escheatable** (-ə-bəl). See **finance**. See **end-of-life, death**.

esclandre (es-klaan'drə) n. notoriety; disturbance; a disgraceful occurrence or scene, an unpleasant public scene: *faire un esclandre* (fɛr œ~ ɛsklɑ~dr) = to make a scene. [F]. See **mentality, mentation, behavior**.

ethnophaulism (eth-nŏ-fawl'liz"zəm) n. any racial pejorative, slur. [< G *ethnos* nation +?]. See **talk**.

etiolate (eet'tee-ə-layt", -ō-layt") vt. to make pale, whiten, esp. to whiten a plant by excluding light; to give sickly hue to (a person). [< F *étioler* to become sick, emaciated; to blanch]. n. **etiolation** (eet"tee-ə-lay'shən). adj. **etiolated** (eet"tee-ə-lay'təd). • Her *etiolated* visage attests to her age and **dyscrasia**, q.v. See **color**. See **skin**. See **health, illness**.

eu - (yoo) a particle used as a pref. meaning good, well, true, easily. [via L < G *eus* well].

euania (yoo-ay'ni-ə) n. ease of awakening in the morning. [eu-, pref., q.v., +?]. ant. **dysania**, q.v. See **sleep & wakefulness**.

eucrasy (yoo'krə-see) n. a normal state of good health. • Such *eucrasy* at the age of 100 years is rare. [< eu-, pref., q.v., + *krasis* a mixing]. syn. **eucrasia**. [< G *eukrasia* good temperament]. ant. = **dyscrasy**, q.v. See **health, illness**.

eudaemonia/eudemonia (yoo-dee-mōn'ni-ə, -də-mon') n. a feeling of well-being or happiness; true happiness, well-being (which, according to Aristotle, results from a life of reason). • One hopes fervently that one's old age is blessed by *eudaemonia*. [eu-, pref., q.v. + < G *daimon* guardian genius, spirit—therefore, happy]. n. **eudaemonism**. adj. **eudaemonic** (-mon'ik). See **emotion**. See **health, illness**.

eugeria (yoo-jer'ri-ə) n. a normal and happy old age. [< G *eu-*, pref., well + *geras* old age]. See **old age**. See **health, illness**.

eulogy (yoo'lə-jee), pl. **–ies**, n. 1. a speech or piece of writing that praises somebody or something very highly, especially a tribute to somebody who has recently died. 2. great praise (formal). [< G *eulogia* < *eu-*, pref., well + -*logia* speaking]. n. **eulogist**. adj. **eulogistic** (-jis'-). adv. **eulogistically** (-jis'ti-kal-lee, -jis'tik-lee). vi.&vt. **eulogize**. n.

eulogizer. syn. **eulogium** [L]. See **talk**. See **death, end-of-life**. See **role**.

euneirophrenia (yoo-nī"rō-freen'ni-ə) n. peace of mind after a pleasant dream. [eu-, pref., q.v., + < G *neiron* dream + *phren* mind (intellect), heart (the seat of emotions), diaphragm (partition)]. See **sleep, wakefulness**.

eumoirous (yoo-moy'rus, -rəs) adj. lucky or happy as a result of being good. [eu-, pref., good, well < G *eus* good, well +?]. See **emotion**. See **religion, theology, morality**.

eupatrid (yoo-pat'trid), pls. **eupatridae** (-dī) or **eupatrids** (-tridss), n. (1. any hereditary aristocrat of ancient Athens or of other Greek city-states; eupatrids were usually lawmakers and administrators.) 2. by extension, fig., someone who is upper class, of higher rank. • His condescension would suggest that **grognard**, q.v., thinks he is a *eupatrid* in this retirement community. [G *eupatrides* < *eu-*, pref. well, + *pater*, father]. See **role**.

euphelicia (yoo-fə-lis'si-ə) n. healthiness resulting from having all one's wishes granted. [eu-, pref., q.v., + < L *felicitatem* < *felix* happy]. See **health, illness**.

euthermic (yoo-thur'mik) adj. inducing warmth. [eu-, pref., q.v., + < G *thermos* warm]. n. **euthermia**. See **therapy**.

euthymia (yoo-thī'mi-ə) n. mental tranquility; joyfulness. [eu-, pref., q.v., + <G *thymos*

mind]. See **emotion**. See **mentality, mentation, behavior**.

evagation (ee-va-gay'shən) n. mental wandering, straying, digression. [e- < G & L ex-, pref., out, away from + < L *vagari* to wander, range, roam]. See **mentality, mentation, behavior**.

evancalous (ee-van"kə-ləss) adj. pleasant to embrace. [? < OF *evangile* < G *euaggelion* good news < *euaggelos* bringing good news < *eu* good + *aggelein* to announce + *kalos* beautiful]. See **sex, love**. See **mentality, mentation, behavior**.

evening of (one's) life n.phr. (fig.) the end of life. • On a 1927 trip to Stalin's Soviet Union, Lincoln Steffans, a man of the left, offered this ironic compliment, "I would like to spend the *evening of my life* watching the morning of a new world." syn. (fig.) **September**, q.v. See **old age**. See **end of life, death**.

Ewig-Weibliche (ay"vik-vīp'li-kə) n. according to Goethe, "eternal-feminine characteristics". [Ger., *ewig* eternal, everlasting, forever + *weiblich* female, feminine]. See **sex, love**.

ex- (eks), **exo-** (eks-ō {used before vowels}), **ef-** (used before f), or **e-** (ee) a particle used as a pref. denoting out of, from, away from; not without; former. [via L < G *ex, ek* (before vowels) out].

exallotriote (eks-al-ō'tri-ōt) adj. foreign. [ex-, pref., q.v., + < G *allotrios* foreign < *allos* other]. See **innovation, misoneism**.

exaugurate (eks-aug'gyoor-ayt) vt. to secularize; to desecrate. [ex-, pref., q.v., + < L *augur* priest, prophet, seer]. See **talk**. See **religion, theology, morality**.

ex capite (eks kaap'pee-tay) adv. (collocation) from memory. [L, (lit.) out of the head]. See **memory**.

excerebrose (ek-ser're-brōs) adj. having no brains, no intelligence, brainless. [ex-, pref., q.v., + < L *cerebrum* brain]. See **intelligence**.

excoriate (eks-kor'ree-ayt) vt. (1. a. to remove part of the skin of a person, etc., by abrasion. b. strip or peel off skin; skin.) 2. censure severely; berate severely. [< L *excoriare* < ex-, pref., q.v., + *corium* hide]. n. **excoriation**. See **talk**. See **skin**.

exeat (eks'ee-ət) n. a permit for temporary leave, e.g., from college or university, usually, or, perhaps, from a residence for the elderly. • His assisted-living center has granted him an *exeat* of three days while his daughter is visiting. [< L *exire* to go out, to go forth; to go away, depart, retire].

execrate (eks'ə-krayt) vt. detest greatly, feel loathing for; denounce, declare someone or something loathsome. vi. curse, utter curses upon. • In her confused state of mind she was prone *to execrate* without cause attendants at her nursing home. [< L *execrari* undo consecration < *sacrare* < *sacr-*, stem of *sacer* holy, sacred]. n. **execration** (eks'sə-kray'shən). n. **execrator**. adj. **execrative** & **execratory** (eks'sə-krə-tawr"ree). See **talk**.

Exelon®Patch (eks'ə-lon) n.phr. a drug (revastigmine transdermal system made by Novartis Pharmaceuticals) used to treat mild-to-moderate Alzheimer's disease) and mild-to-moderate dementia of Parkinson's disease. The drug is applied once a day as a patch. It is said to improve cognition. See **Aricept**. See **therapy**.

exequies (eks'ə-kweez) n.pl. (n.s. **exequy**) 1. funeral rites; obsequies. 2. funeral procession(s). [< L *exequiae* those following out to the grave < *exsequi* follow out < *sequi* follow]. See **end-of-life, death**.

exheredate (eks-her'rə-dayt) vt. to disinherit. [ex-, pref., q.v., + < L *hereditas* inheritance]. syn. **forisfamiliate**, q.v. See **finance**. See **end-of-life, death**.

exility (eks-il'li-tee) n. 1. thinness. 2. (pedant.) subtlety. • Such extreme *exility* in old age may be an indication of serious disease. [< L *exilitas* < *exilis* thin]. See **physique, appearance**.

eximious (eks-im'mi-əss) adj. excellent, distinguished, or eminent. [< L *eximius* taken out, exempted; exempt, excepted; select, choice, special, exceptional < *emere eximere* to take out; exempt; make an exception].

exinanition (eks-in"nə-nish'ən) n. (obs.) extreme fatigue. [ex-, pref., q.v., + *initio* < *inanire* to make empty]. See **tiredness, weakness**.

exosculate (eks-os'kyoo-layt) vt. to kiss, especially to do so heartily. [ex-, pref., q.v. + < L *osculari* to kiss, make a fuss over]. See **sex, love**.

exostosis (eks'os-tōs'siss) n. a benign bony growth projecting outward from the surface of a bone and characteristically capped by cartilage. [ex-, pref., q.v., + < G *osteon* bone]. adj. **exostotic** (-tot'tik). See **joint, extremities, back**.

expatiate (eks-pay'shee-ayt) vi. 1. speak or write about a subject at great length or in detail. 2. (arch.) to wander or roam at will. [< L *exspatiari* to go off course, walk out; to digress < *spatiari* to walk <

spatium space]. n. **expatiation** (-spay"shee-ay'shən). n. **expatiator**. See **talk**. See **standing, walking, wandering**. See **role**.

explaterate (eks-plat'tər-ayt) vi. (slang) to talk a lot. [? ex-, pref., q.v. +? < G *platus* flat + -ate, suff.]. See **talk**.

expostulate (eks-pos'chə-layt, -choo-layt) vi. 1. make a friendly protest; express disapproval, disagreement. 2. reason or argue with a person; attempt to dissuade. [< L *expostulate-*, pp. of *expostulare* demand from < *postulare* to demand]. n. **expostulation**. n. **expostulator** (-lay'tawr). adj. **expostulatory** (-lə-tawr"ree). See **talk**. See **role**.

expuition (eks"pyoo-ish'ən) n. a spitting. [ex-, pref., q.v., + < L *sputare*, *spuere* to spit]. See **mouth, gums teeth**.

exsuccous (eks-suk'kəss) adj. dry, sapless, dried up, without moisture. • The **supercentenarian**, q.v., not surprisingly, had an *exsuccous* appearance. [ex-, pref., q.v., + < L *succus* sap, juice; taste, flavor]. See **physique, appearance**. See **skin**.

exsufflicate (eks-suf'lə-kayt) n. (obs.) forcible breathing or blowing out. • The old gentleman's *exsufflicate* immediately attracted his doctor's attention. [ex-, pref., q.v., + < L *sufflatio* a blowing up]. See **breathing**.

Extreme Unction (eks'treem unk'shən, eks'tree-munk'shən) n.phr. (dated) a rite practiced by a Roman Catholic priest in which a very sick, injured, or dying person is anointed with oil and prayed over for salvation. (In 1972 the term was changed to "Anointing of the Sick".) [< L *extremus* farthest, last + *extremus* farthest, last < *ex* out & < *unction-* < *unguere* to smear, anoint]. See **end-of-of-life, death**.

exungulate (eks-ung'gyoo-layt, -ung'gyə-layt) vi. to trim, cut, or cut off the nails or hooves. [ex-, pref., q.v., + < L *ungula* hoof, claw < *unguis* fingernail, toenail, claw, hoof, talon]. See **therapy**. See **joint, extremities, back**.

eye [L *oculis*, G *ophthalmos*]: **ablepsia, amaurosis**, *amaurosis fugax*, **AMD, anaphalantiasis**, *arcus corneae/arcus cornealis*, *arcus senilis*, **bleareye, blepharitis, cataract, cecity, cecutiency,**

chalazion, collyrium, dacryagogue, dacryocystitis, dacryogenic, dacrygelosis, dysopia, dysopsia, ectropion,

enophthalmos/enophthalmus, entropion, epiphora, gerontopia, gerontoxon, glusk, hemeralopia, hordeolum, hyperope, hyperopia, idiopsia, idiopt, lippitude, luscition, lutein/luteine, macular degeneration, maculopathy, madarosis, meibomian cyst, miosis, mydriatic, myopia, nyctalopia, obnubilate, occecation, orthoscopy, pinguecula, presbyope, presbyopia, presbytia, presbytism, pseudophakic eye, pterygium, purblind, retinitis, retinopathy, retinosis, rheum, senopia, squintifego, telepresence robots, typhlology, uveitis. xanthelasma, xanthoma xerophthalmia.

eye: subcategories

I. Conjunctiva:
    1. Conjunctival thickened area; patch: **pinguecula**; **pterygium**
II. Decreased vision & blindness:
    1. Blindness: **ablepsia, amaurosis, cecity, occecation, purblind**
    2. Clouded vision: **obnubilate**
    3. Day blindness: **hemeralopia**
    4. Deteriorative changes in the macula retinae: **macular degeneration**
    5. Knowledge of blindness: **typhlology**
    6. Night blindness: **nyctalopia**
    7. Partial blindness: **cecutiency, luscition, purblind**
    8. Transient blindness: *Amaurosis fugax*
III. Eye:
    1. Backward displacement of the eyeball: **enophthalmos/enophthalmus**
    2. Examination of the eye by looking through a layer of water: **orthoscopy**
    3. Treatment: eye salve or eyewash: **collyrium**
IV. Eyebrow:
    1. Falling out of the eyebrows; &/or eyelashes: **anaphalantiasis; madarosis**
V. Eyelid:
    1. Inflammation: **bleareye, blepharitis, lippitude**, (See No. 5., Stye.)

2. Turning in: **entropion**
3. Turning out: **ectropion**
4. Skin deposit: **xanthelasma, xanthoma**
5. Stye: **chalazion, hordeolum, meibomian cyst**
6. Watery discharge from the eye(s): **rheum**

VI. Iris, cornea, pupil, uvea:
    1. Corneal-inserted telescope: **AMD**
    2. Pupil size:
        a. **miosis**
        b. **mydriatic**
    3. Uveal tract inflammation: **uveitis**
    4. White or gray ring at the corneal margin: *arcus corneae/arcus cornealis, arcus senilis*, gerontoxon

VII. Lens:
    1. Lens-implanted eye: **pseudophakic eye**
    2. Lens opacity: **cataract**

VIII. Retina, macula:
    1. General, non-inflammatory retinal disease: **retinosis**
    2. Inflammation of the retina: **retinitis**
    3. Macular degeneration: **maculopathy**
    4. Protects the macula: **lutein/luteine**
    5. Retinal disease: **retinopathy**

XI. Sight:
    1. Far sighted:
        a. generally: **hyperope, hyperopia**
        b. due to aging: **presbyope, presbyopia, presbytia, presbytism**
    2. Impaired sight: **dysopia, dysopsia, idiopt, idiopsia**
    3. Near (short) sighted: **myopia**
    4. Robotic vision: **telepresence robots**
    5. Second sight: **gerontopia, senopia**

XI. Squinting; squinter: **glusk; squintifego**

XII. Tears:
    1. Alternately laughing & tearing (crying): **dacrygelosis**
    2. Producing: **dacryagogue, dacryogenic**
    3. Overflow: **epiphora**
    4. Not enough tears: **xerophthalmia**
    5. Sac inflammation: **dacryocystitis**

F

*"One likes to sit back and let the world turn
by itself without trying to push it."*
—Sean O'Casey, who wrote in his eighties.

fabulist (fab'yoo-list) n. a composer of fables or apologues (moral fables). [< F *fabuliste* < L *fabula* story, tale; talk, conversation, conversation piece; small talk; affair, matter, concern; myth; legend; drama, play < *fabulari* to say; invent; talk, chat, gossip + -ist, suff., practicing a particular skill or profession < OF *-iste*, < L *-ista*, < G *-istes*]. See **talk**. See **role**.

factious (fak'shəss) adj. 1. having factions, causing or taking part in conflict within a group. 2. creating dissension; turbulent. [< L *factiosus* < *factio*, s *faction-* act of making < *fact-* pp. of *facere* do, make]. adv. **factiously**. n. **factiousness**. See **talk**. See **mentality, mentation, behavior**.

faff (faf) vi. (obs.) 1. to dither or fumble, or **catachrestically**, q.v., to **fart about**, q.v. (2. to blow in sudden gusts.) [dialectal; of echoic origin.]. n. **faff** = a puff of wind. Cf. a related word, **faffle** vi., a. to stutter or stammer, or utter incoherent sounds. b. to saunter; to fumble. c. (of a sail) to flap idly in the wind. See **mentality, mentation, behavior**. See **talk**.

fag-ma-fuff (fag'mə-fuf) n. a garrulous old woman. [?]. See **old woman**.

fainéant, -e (fɛneã, ãt) adj. lazy; doing nothing, idle; sluggish, slothful. [F]. nm., nf. **fainéant, -e** = an idler, sluggard, slacker. See **work, activity**. See **role**.

famulus (fam'yoo-ləs) n. a private secretary or factotum; an attendant, especially one assisting a magician or scholar. [L, a servant]. See **role**.

fanfaronade (fawn-far-rən-naad') n. arrogant bluster, boastful, ostentatious talk or behavior, bragging, bravado. [< F *fanfaronade* < Sp. *fanfarronada* < Arabic *farfar* garrulous + the suff. -ade, an action via OF < L *-ata* f. of *-atus*, pp. of v(s). ending in *-are*]. nm.&f.

fanfaron (fɑ~farɔ~, ɔn) a braggart (or fanfare)]. syns. **braggadocio**, **gasconade, rodomontade; thrasonical,** q.v. See <u>talk</u>. See <u>role</u>.

fart around/about (faart) vi. (slang) an offensive, indecent term— literally, to fart, i.e., to expel rectal gas—meaning to waste time by behaving foolishly. [OE *feortan* < I-E (Aryan); Cf. G *perdomai*]. syn. **faff.**, q.v. See <u>mentality, mentation, behavior</u>.

feckless (fek'less) adj. 1. unable or unwilling to do anything useful. 2. lacking the thought or organization necessary to succeed. • Attempts to organize her life were rendered *feckless* by advancing age. [late 16ᵗʰ C. < obs. *feck* value, efficiency; shortening of effect]. adv. **fecklessly.** n. **fecklessness.** See <u>mentality, mentation, behavior</u>. See <u>work, activity</u>.

feculent (fek'yə-lənt) adj. very dirty, foul, stinking, fetid, full of dregs, esp. if polluted by excrement, feces. [< L *faeculentus* < *faeces*, pl. of *faex* sediment, dregs]. n. **feculence.** See <u>nose, smell</u>.

feisty (fïs'tee) adj. 1. Characterized by spirited, sometimes aggressive behavior. 2. likely to respond in an irritable or touchy way. [informal, regional < late 18ᵗʰ C., a variant of *fist*, shortening of *fisting cur* < obsolete *fisten* to break wind < Gmc.]. adv. **fesitily.** n. **feistiness.** See <u>mentality, mentation, behavior</u>.

feuillemorte (fœjmɔrt) adj. having the color of a faded or dead leaf; yellow, yellow-brown, brown. • Chronic illness, liver disease, and advanced age gave her a distinctly *feuillemorte* appearance. [F *feuille* leaf + *mort* dead]. See <u>color</u>. See <u>end-of-life, death</u>. See <u>physique, appearance</u>.

fey (fay) adj. 1. behaving in an irrational, unusual, uninhibited way suggestive of a possible psychiatric disorder. (2. supernatural or clairvoyant.) 3. (Sc) fated to die; believed to be doomed or destined to die, especially as indicated by peculiar, especially elated, behavior. [< OE *fæge* doomed, fated to die < Ger.]. See <u>mentality, mentation, behavior</u>. See <u>end-of-life, death</u>.

fibrillation (fi-bril-lay'shən) n. 1. ventricular (lower heart chambers) twitching, usually slow, of individual muscle fibers, commonly occurring in the atria (upper heart chambers) or ventricles of the heart—auricular or ventricular fibrillation—(as well as in recently denervated skeletal muscle fibers) in which the regular forceful, coordinated contractions of atrial or ventricular cardiac walls are replaced by irregular twitching. Cardiac output suffers. (2. the condition of being fibrillated.) (3. the formation of fibrils.) 4. exceedingly rapid contractions or twitching of muscular fibrils, but not of the muscle as a whole.) [< L *fibrilla*, diminutive of *fibra* fiber + -tion, suff.]. See **heart, rhythm**.

fideism (feed'day-iz"əm) n. depending upon faith rather than reason; belief that religious knowledge and access to heaven depend upon faith and revelation. [< L *fides* faith + -ism, suff.]. n. **fideist**. adj. **fideistic**. See **religion, theology, morality**. See **role**.

filiopietistic (fil'lee-ō-pī"ə-tis'tik) adj. 1. having great reverence for ancestors. 2. excessive reverence for tradition, or great men in history. [< L *filius* son, *filia*, daughter + via Ger. *pietismus* < L *pietas* < *pius* devout]. syn. **old-fashioned**. See **past, time**. See **mentality, mentation, behavior**.

finance: *alieni juris*, *apud se*, COLA, *compos mentis*, coacervate, coparcener, dotation, escheat, exheredate, forisfamiliate, frugalista, health-care REIT, intestate, locust years, Morton's fork, *non compos mentis*, nuncupate, parcener, parsimony, patrimony, *rente*, subvention, succursal, *sui juris*, sunset clause, testate, testator, testatrix, usufruct, usufructuary. See **end of life, death**.

finance: Sub-categories

I. Pertaining to inheritance, a will, making a will:
    1. A coheir or joint heir: **coparcener, parcener**
    2. A date certain when a will's provision(s) will no longer prevail: **sunset clause**
    3. Endowment: **dotation**
    4. Having made a legally valid will: **testate**
    5. Inheritance: **patrimony**
    6. Mentally competent to handle one's affairs: *sui juris*, *apud se*
    7. Mentally incompetent to handle one's affairs; not of sound mind: *alieni juris*; *non compos mentis* (See FHW&P.)

8. One who can legally use—as through inheritance—another's property: **usufructuary**
9. One who jointly inherits undivided property: **coparcener**
10. One who makes a legally valid will: **testator, testatrix**
11. Property, etc., not having been assigned in a valid will: **intestate**
12. Property unassigned to someone in a legally valid will: **intestate**
13. Someone not having made a valid will: **intestate**
14. The legal right to use another's property: **usufruct**
15. To declare orally or make an oral will: **nuncupate**
16. To disinherit: **exheredate, forisfamiliate**

II. Other:

1. Annual adjustments in Social Security and Medicare payments: **COLA.**
2. Annual income, annuity: *rente*
3. A period of economic hardship: **locust years**
4. Carefulness or economy in the use of money or things: **parsimony**
5. Exchange-traded health-care investment fund: **health-care REIT**
6. Mentally competent to handle one's affairs: *apud se, compos mentis, sui juris* (See FW&PD.)
7. Mentally incompetent to handle one's affairs; not of sound mind: *alieni juris; non compos mentis* (See FW&PD.)
8. One who can legally use another's property: **usufructuary**
9. One who lives frugally: **frugalista**
10. Property of an intestate reverting to the state: **escheat**
11. Re: Subsidiary help, support, especially of a chapel: **succursal**
12. The giving of financial aid, support: **subvention**
13 Someone having no legally valid will: **intestate**
14. Sound of mind: *compos mentis* (See FW&PD.)
15. Tax levied regardless of one's economic situation: **Morton's fork**
16. The legal right to use another's property: **usufruct**
17. To amass, accumulate: **coacervate**

18. To dedicate or inscribe: **nuncupate**
19. To shed parental authority: **forisfamiliate**

finifugal (fi-nif'fyoo-gəl) adj. shunning the end (of anything, e.g., life itself). [L *finis* end + *fugere* flee]. See **end-of-life, death**. See **mentality, mentation, behavior**.

flannel (flan'nəl) n. nonsense, evasive talk; flattery. (The fabric, washcloth, trousers, and undergarment definitions are not considered). [< Welsh *gwlanen* (woolen article) or < OF *flaine* a kind of coarse wool, blanket. Flannel's metaphysical sense is probably derivative of the material's soft and smooth texture]. See **talk**.

flatulent (fla'chə-lənt) adj. 1. causing excessive gas to be created in the stomach and intestines. 2. having excessive gas in the digestive system. 3. (fig.) having or showing excessive self-importance. [< L *flatuentus* < *flatus* blowing, blast < *flare* to blow]. n. **flatulence** (-lənz). n. **flatulency** (-len-see). n. **flatulosity** (-los"si-tee). adv. **flatulently**. Cf. **ventose**, q.v. See **gastrointestinal**.

flatulopetic (fla'chə-lō-pet'tik) adj. 1. pertaining to gas production in the bowels. 2. pretentious, pompous, inflated. • Seniors, generally, are more *flatulopetic* than younger age groups; he was *flatulopetic* in both senses of the word. [< L *flatus* a blowing, breathing, a breath; wind; snoring; arrogance +? < G *poiein* to make]. See **gastrointestinal**. See **mentality, mentation, behavior**.

flatus (flay'təs) n. 1. gas or air in the gastrointestinal tract: flatulence. 2. (indecent) emission, of gas, wind, or air through the anus. [L *flatus* a blowing, breathing, a breath; wind; snoring; arrogance]. (*flatus vaginalis* [L] = noisy expulsion of gas from the vagina.) syn. **crepitus**, q.v. Cf. **eructation**, q.v. See **gastrointestinal**. See **genitourinary**.

flavescent (flaa-ves'sənt) adj. yellowish. Cf. **luteolus**, q.v. [< L *flavescere* to become gold colored < *flavus* yellow]. See **color**. See **skin**.

floccilation (flok-sil-lay'shən) n. an aimless plucking at the bedclothes, as if one were picking off threads, or tufts of cotton, occurring in the delirium of a fever; it is a sign that a person is approaching death. [L *floccus*, a tuft of wool; *flocculus* a little tuft].

syns. **carphology/carphologia**, **crocidismus**, **floccilegium**, **flocculation**, **tilmus**, q.v. See **mentality, mentation, behavior**.

floccilegium (flok-si-lej'ji-əm) n. See **flocculation**. [< L *floccillus*, dim. of *floccus* flock, a tuft of wool, or cotton, a lock of hair, or a material consisting of coarse wool or cotton tufts + *lego* to gather together]. See: **mentality, mentation, behavior**.

flocculation (flok-yoo-lay'shən) n. an aimless, delirious picking, plucking motion at the bedding, as happens in certain prolonged illnesses often with delirium and fever, or as a sign of impending demise. [< L *floccillus*, dim. of *floccus* flock, a tuft of wool, or cotton, a lock of hair, or a material consisting of coarse wool or cotton tufts + -ation, suff.]. syns. **carphology**, **crocidismus**, **floccilegium**, **tilmus**, vs. See **mentality, mentation, behavior**.

floruit (flaw-roo'it) vi. flourished—(lit.) he flourished—a (formal) term that is placed before a name or numeric designation of a previous period to indicate when a specific person or movement was most active. • The octogenarian's paintings *floruit* in the 19th C. when in his forties. [L, he flourished < *florare* to flourish]. See **work, activity**.

flounder (flown'dər) vi. 1. make uncontrolled movements, struggle and plunge, as in mud, wading. 2. make mistakes, blunder; act confused or without purpose; manage business badly, or with difficulty. (Note: possible confusion with **founder** (vi.) meaning: 1. sink or cause to sink, 2. break down, 3. crumple, 4. be bogged down, 5. stumble, or 6.{vi.&vt.} make or become ill by overfeeding.) [imitative, perhaps, and associated with founder (be wrecked and to sink), or blunder]. n. **flounder**, **floundering** = an act or piece of blundering, struggling attempts to get on. See **mentality, mentation, behavior**.

fogram/fogrum (fō'grəm)/(fō'grəm) n. an old-fashioned or conservative person who resists change or novelty. [unk.]. adj. **fogram** = old-fashioned, passé. (Cf. **filiopietistic**). syn. **fogy**. See **old man**, **old woman**. See **old**.

fogy, fogey (fōg'gee) pl. **–ies**. n. usually old fogy; old, or old-fashioned, fellow; old man behind the times. [late 18th C. Sc, abbr. of **fogram**, q.v.]. n. **fog(e)ydom**. n. **fog(e)yism**. adj. **fog(e)yish**. n. (old) **fogyism** (See under **old age**). syns. **buffer**, **duffer**, **fogram**, q.v. See **old man**. See **old age**.

footle (foo'təl) vi. to wile away time; trifle, play the fool, hence **footling**: to speak or act foolishly. [unk.]. n. **footle** = twaddle, folly. See **mentality, mentation, behavior**.

forfoughen (fawr'fōk'ən, -fooch'ən', -faak'en) adj. a Sc term meaning tired out, exhausted. [?]. syn. **forjesket**, q.v. See **tiredness, weakness**.

forisfamiliate (fawr"ris-fə-mil'li-ayt) vt. to disinherit; to shed parental authority. [< L *foris*, door, (fig.) door; gate + *familia* family, family estate]. syn. **exheredate**. See **finance**.

forjesket/forjeskit (fawr-jes'ket, -kit) adj. a Sc term meaning worn out, extremely tired. [?]. syn., **farfoughen**, q.v. See **tiredness, weakness**.

fossil (fos'səl) n. (1. the remains of an animal or plant preserved from an earlier era inside a rock or other geological deposit, often as an impression or in a petrified state.) 2. (fig.) a very old person belonging to the past, hopelessly out of date, unwilling to change, set in his/her ways (informal insult). Often **fossil** is preceded by *old* for emphasis, even though tautological. (3. Something that is old, outdated, having outlived its usefulness.) (4. a word or part thereof that was once used generally but now survives only in a few contexts, e.g., *couth* in *uncouth*, *apron* in *napron* {rhetorically = aphaeresis}.) [< F *fossile* < L *fossilis* dug up < *fodere* to dig]. See **old man, woman**.

FOX03A n. the name of a gene with a single biochemical misprint in DNA typography. The gene appears to double or triple one's chance of living to be 100 years or more, i.e., to be a **supercentenarian**, q.v., one of the **wellderly**, q.v. Inheriting two copies of this gene, one from each parent, results in unusual **longevity**, q.v., (Pacific Health Research Institute, Hawaii). The Los Angeles Research Group reported a few years ago that ". . . there are only 79 men and women alive today aged 110 years or more . . ." However, recent evaluation of reputed Japanese longevity indicates a number of unsubstantiated instances. Recently reported, after a genetic analysis of 108 centenarians, is the finding of 150 genes associated with longevity. Some control the response to famine and drought; others have a role in preventing or postponing certain diseases. There are some 3 billion DNA characters of the human genome; 150 markers among millions distinguish centenarians from those less long lived. Using these 150 markers, there is a 77% prediction rate re: one's longevity. There are economic implications: It is said that the medical expenses during the last two years before death are three times greater for someone dying at age 80 than for someone dying at age 100. See **old age**.

fractious (frak'shəss) adj. irritable, whiny, quarrelsome, rebellious, and likely to complain or misbehave. [< L *fraction*- < *fract*-, pp. of *frangere* to break]. n. **fractiousness**. adv. **fractiously**. See **mentality, mentation, behavior**.

frampold (fram'pōld) adj. (obs. except dialectical) peevish, touchy, quarrelsome, irritable, sour-tempered. [of obscure origin]. See **mentality, mentation, behavior**.

franion (fran'yən) n. the perennial hedonist, reveler; a gay reckless fellow; a dirty old man; a paramour. [of obscure origin]. • The role of a *franion* was difficult for him to relinquish despite his superannuation. See **mentality, mentation, behavior**. See **role**.

fremescent (frəm-es'sənt) adj. (rare) growling, muttering. [< L *fremere* to growl]. n. **fremescence**. See **talk**.

froward (frō'wərd) adj. perverse, willfully contrary; obstinately disobedient; refractory. [fro, adv. < ON *frá*, prep., = OE *fram*, from; OS, OHG, & Goth. *fram* < Gmc *fra*-, pref., forward + -ward, suff., < OE –*weard*, primarily forming adjs. with a sense of having a specified direction]. adv. **frowardly**. n. **frowardness**. See **mentality, mentation, behavior**.

frowsty (frow'stee) adj. (UK) musty, having a stale smell. [origin uncertain, possibly a var. of **frowzy**, q.v. Earliest documented use: 1865 (Anu Garg)]. syn. **frowzy**, q.v. Cf. **fusty**, q.v. See **nose, smell**.

frowzy (frow'zee) adj. 1. dirty and untidy, unkempt; slovenly; slatternly; blowzy. 2. ill-smelling or musty or **fusty**, q.v., environment. [17th C. of unk. origin]. n.**frowziness/frowstiness**. syn. **frowsty**, q.v. See **nose, smell**. See **physique, appearance**.

frugalista (froog"-gə-lees'tə) n. a neologism indicating a person who lives a frugal life-style, but stays fashionable and healthy by swapping clothes, buying secondhand, growing his/her own produce, etc.—the *nom de guerre* of the "recession warrior" of late 2008 and beyond. • The 2008 Great Recession, which has so devastated savings and pensions, has made old skinflints and *frugalistas* of us oldsters. [< L *fructus* fruit + < E –ist, suff., following a specific belief or school of thought < Sp & L -*ista* < G -*istes*. The word *frugal* was first applied to the careful apportioning of food, but Shakespeare in his *Merry Wives of Windsor* (1598) applied it metaphorically to mean "sparingly supplied, thrifty of anything."—William Safire, *On Language* article, New York Times, Oct. 23, 2008]. Cf. **skinflint**, q.v. See **role**. See **finance**.

fubsy (fub'see) adj. fat or squat. [E, < obs. *fubs* a small, fat person]. Cf. **adipose**, **lardy**, **pinguid**, **pursy**; **abdominous**, **ventricous**, q.v. See **physique, appearance**.

fuddle (fud'dəl) vt. to confuse, perplex, e.g., by inebriation, give confused instruction. vi. (arch.) to drink too much alcohol regularly. [late 16th C. <?]. n. **fuddled state** = a state of confusion due to drunkenness. syn. **befuddle**, q.v. See **mentality, mentation, behavior**. See **drink, food**. See **talk**.

fuddy-duddy (fud'dee dud"dee) n.pl. –ies, n. an old-fashioned or dull person, especially an elderly one; it's often preceded by *old*: "old fuddy-duddy" (informal; sometimes offensive). [early 20th C.,? origin]. See **old man**. See **old woman**.

fuliginous (fyoo-lij'ji-nəss) adj. smoky, sooty, dusky, dingy, of the color of soot, dark gray, dull brown, black; fig., darkly mysterious. • His *fuliginous* appearance bespoke his advanced age. [< L *fuliginosus* < *fuligo* soot]. See **color**. See **physique, appearance**.

fumacious (fyoo-may'shəss) adj. fond of smoking. [< L *fumus* smoke + -acious, suff.- forming adjs. meaning "inclined to", "abounding in", < -*axacis*, suff., added to verb stems to form adjs. + -ous]. See **mentality, mentation, behavior**.

funest (fyoo-nest') adj. harbinger of evil or death; dire. [< L *funer-*, stem of *funus* death ritual]. See **end-of-life, death**.

furfuraceous (fur-fyoo-ray'shəss) adj. fine and loose; said of scales resembling bran or dandruff; pertaining to skin falling off in small flakes. [< L *furfur* bran]. n. **furfur** (fur'fur) = dandruff, scurf. n. **furfuration** = a flaking off, such as dandruff. See **skin**.

fustigate (fus'ti-gayt) vt. (1. to cudgel, bludgeon with a stick.) 2. to criticize severely. [< L *fustigare* < *fustis* cudgel, wood club + *agere* to do]. n. **fustigation** (-gay'shən). See **talk**.

fustilugs (fus'tee-lugss) n. (obs. except dialectal) a fat, unkempt, frowsy woman—often preceded by *old*. • "Come on, you old fustilugs," he called, for she wheezed and blew and mounted with difficulty."— Julian Rathbone; Joseph, Little Brown; 2001. [uncertain, perhaps < **fusty**, q.v., in the sense of stale, smelly, musty + lug, in the sense of something heavy, or slow]. See **physique, appearance**. See **old woman**.

fusty (fus'tee) adj. 1. smelling of damp dust, mildew, or age. 2. old-fashioned and conservative in style, appearance, habits, or attitudes; clinging unyieldingly to the past. • "I passed up a side street, one of those deserted ways . . . dim places, *fusty* with **hesternal** {q.v.} excitements and thrills of yesteryear."—Rupert Brooke (Anu Garg; my emphasis). [< obsolete *fust* wine cask, via OF < L *fustis* wood, club]. n. **fusty/fustiness**. adv. **fustily**. Cf. **frowsty**, **frowzy**, q.v. See **physique, appearance**. See **mentality, mentation, behavior**. See **nose, smell**.

G

"One should never make one's debut with a scandal; one
should reserve that to give interest to one's old age."
—Oscar Wilde.

gadzookary (gad-zook'kə-ree) n. the use of archaic words or expressions, e.g., wight (brave), prithee (I pray), ye (you, the). [< gadzooks, int., arch., an expression of surprise, etc., < gad, God + zooks, unk., + -ary, suff., forming nouns < F –*aire* or L –*arius* connected with]. See **talk**.

gadzooks (gad-zooks') int. (archaic or humorous) used to express surprise or a mild oath. [Late 17th C. < gad, God + zooks, unk.]. See **emotion**.

gaffer (gaf'fer) n. 1. an elderly rustic old fellow; also used as a pref. to a name, e.g., gaffer-John. (2. non-U.S.: foreman of a gang.) [< a contraction of "godfather"; ga- of **gaffer** is, alternatively, associated with "grandfather"; Cf. **gammer** & gossip]. See **old man**.

gait speed n.phr. refers to a simple emerging measure of geriatric frailty: the length of time taken to walk five meters, i.e., about 16 feet (J. Am. Coll. of Cardiol., Nov. 2, 2010). A gait speed longer than six seconds is considered abnormal. Those having such are about three times as likely to die of or suffer such complications as a stroke or kidney failure, and twice as likely to have a prolonged hospital stay, or be discharged to a nursing home after open heart surgery as those whose speed was six seconds or less. Gait speed allows more accurate estimation of surgical risk, or may suggest to physicians that less invasive measures are indicated, or to patients that they opt for less aggressive treatment strategies. Gait speed or velocity can be predicted by **double stance/double support**, q.v. (Other simple measures of gauging health in the elderly are useful: a sudden weight gain of two pounds or more, or a waist measurement of > 40" in men and > 35" in women; they both are indicators of increased risk for medical problems, e.g., diabetes, kidney failure, and heart disease. Other tests for frailty in the aged are such simple things as how easily an elder gets out of a chair or onto an examination table, or the strength of a man's handshake.) syn. **walking speed**, q.v. See <u>health and illness</u>.

galimatias (gal"li-may'shee-əss, -mat'tee-əss) n. gibberish; confused, meaningless, unintelligible talk or jargon that is possibly pompous as well. [F, *galimatias*, a word of unknown origin first found in the 16th C. Cf. *galimafrée*, gallimaufry (any preposterous mixture), a jumble, mishmash, farrago, but with the suff., *-atias*, which is? < G *amathia* ignorance]. Cf. **glossolalia**, etc. See <u>talk</u>.

gammer (gam'mər) n. an old wife; an old woman; a rustic old woman, the counterpart of a **gaffer**, q.v. [< contraction of godmother, ga- by association with grandmother; Cf. **gaffer**, **gossip**]. vi. **gammer** = to idle. See <u>old woman</u>.

garrulous (gar'rə-ləs) adj. talkative, inclined to chatter, babble, ramble; loquacious, wordy. [< L *garrulous* < *garrire* to chatter]. n. **garrulity** (-roo'lə-tee). n. **garrulousness**. adv. **garrulously**. See <u>talk</u>.

gasconade (gas-kə-nayd') n. is inordinate boasting, extravagant bragging. [< Gascony, in France *Gascoigne*, once a province in southwestern France, the natives of which, the *Gascons*, traditionally poor, were noted for their boastful ways]. vi. to brag, boast outrageously. nm., nf. **gascon**, **gasonne** (lower case "g") (gas'kən,

-kon-ə; gaskɔ~, ɔn) = a braggart—an upper-case G is used for one from Gascony. syns. **braggadocio, fanfaronade, rodomontade, thrasonical**, q.v. See **talk**. See **role**.

gastrointestinal: anorectic, aperient, aperitive, apositic, asitia, borborygmus, cachexia, carminative, clyster, clysterize, coprolite, coprostasia, coprotasophobia, costive, crepitus, devorative, dyschezia, dysgeusia, dyshepatia, dysmasesis, dysmetabolism, dysorexia, dyspepsia, dysphagia, dystrophy, dystropia, emunctory, encopresis, eructation, flatulence, flatulent, flatulopetic, flatus, incontinence, inccontinentia alvi, lapactic, laparoscopy, mephitic, mulligrubs, obstipation, peritoneoscopy, physagogue, procidentia, ventoseness, ventricous, void, wamble.

gastrointestinal (g.i.): Subcategories

I. Abdomen:
   1. Big-bellied: **ventricous**
   2. Examination of the abdomen's interior by means of a scope: **laparoscopy**
   3. Percutaneous examination of the peritoneum (membrane lining the internal abdomen): **peritoneoscopy**
   4. Stomach-ache: **mulligrubs**

II. Appetite, eating, digestion:
   1. Abnormal digestion: **dyspepsia**
   2. Capable of being swallowed whole: **devorative**
   3. Defective metabolism: **dysmetabolism**
   4. Defective nutrition: **dystrophy, dystropia**
   5. Difficult mastication: **dysmasesis**
   6. Diminished/perverted appetite: **dysorexia**
   7. Food loathing: **asitia**
   8. Impaired swallowing: **dysphagia**
   9. Impaired taste: **dysgeusia**
   10. Having no appetite: **anorectic**
   11. Severe undernourishment: **apositic, cachexia**
   12. Stimulates the appetite: **aperitive**

III. Constipation, defecation, fecal incontinence, feces:
   1. Difficult/painful defecation: **dyschezia**.
   2. Difficult/painful/severe constipation: **coprostasia, costive; obstipation**

3. Enema: **clyster, clysterize**
4. Evacuate fecal matter: **void**
5. Excretory: **emunctory**
6. Fear of constipation: **coprotasophobia**
7. Fecal incontinence: **encopresis**
8. Fossilized feces, turd: **coprolite**
9. Laxative: **aperient, lapactic**
10. Passing feces involuntarily: **incontinence, incontinentia alvi**
11. Rectal prolapse: **procidentia**

IV. Gas, abdominal pain:
1. Anti-flatulent: **carminative**
2. Belching, perhaps violently: **eructation**
3. Colic: **mulligrubs**
3. Epigastric discomfort: **dyspepsia**
4. Excessive gas: **flatulence, flatulent, ventoseness**
5. Excretory: **emunctory**
6. Fart: **crepitus, eructation, flatus**
7. Fart-producing: **carminative, physagogue**
8. G.I. gas: **flatus**
9. Gas producing: **flatulopetic**
10. Noxious emanation, odor: **mephitic**
11. Sound of flatulence: **borborygmus**
12. Stomach rumble, nausea: **wamble**

V. Liver (hepar):
1. Abnormal liver (hepatic) function: **dyshepatia**

gawkocracy (gaw-kok'krə-see) n. persons who watch television frequently or for long periods, often interminably. [a neologism of the 20th C. & a portmanteau word < 18th C. gawk, vi., (origin unk.) = stare stupidly + -cracy, suff., added to G stems, & as -ocracy to E words, meaning rule of, ruling body of, class influential by]. See role. See work, activity.

geezer (gee'zər) n. a man—often preceded by *old*. [late 19th C., representing dialectical pronunciation of guiser < guise < F < Gmc. deceptive or changed form or appearance]. See wheezy, as in the collation **wheezy geezer**. See old man.

geezerhood (gee'zər hoŏd") n. a slang neologism referring to old people in general. [< geezer, q.v. + hood < OE *hod* < I-E to cover]. syn. = **geezersphere**, q.v. See old age.

geezersphere (gee'zər- sfeer") n. a neologism and slang expression referring to the whole group of old people in general—used by Wm. Safire in his "On Language" column, NYTimes Magazine, 7/19/09. Grandparents were not long ago considered geezerhood members, but a 2009 study from Grandparents.com finds the median ages when men and women first become U.S. grandparents are 54 and 50 years of age, respectively. In 2010 there were 69.9 million grandparents in the U.S.: 3 of every 10 adults. [< geezer, q.v., + sphere < G *sphaira* ball—the sphere ending is probably analogous to that in blogosphere, i.e., blogs, i.e., logs, being sent on the Web]. syn. = **geezerhood**, q.v. See **old age**.

gelotripsy (jel'lō-trip'see) n. nerve-point massage; rubbing away an indurated swelling or tender point in neuralgia and myalgia. [gelosis < G *gelo* to freeze, congeal + *tripsis* a rubbing]. See **nerve, muscle, movement, touch**. See **therapy**.

geniophobia (jeen'ni-ō-fōb'bi-ə) n. morbid fear of chins, e.g. double ones. [geni(o)-, pref., denoting relationship to the chin, < G *geneion* chin, + *phobos* fear]. adj. **geniophobic**. n. **geniophobe**. See **phobias**.

genitourinary: aconuresis, ADAM syndrome, atrophic vaginitis, benign prostatic hypertrophy (BPH), colporrhaphy, DIAPPERS, dyspareunia, dysuria, dysuriac, edea, elumbated, emunctory, enuresis, flatus vaginalis, incontinence, impotentia, improcreant, Kegel's exercises, laparoscopy, medomalacophobia, micturition, nocturia, pediculosis, pelvic support disorders, piddle, piss-proud, procidentia, prostatism, prostatomegaly, urethremphraxis, urination, uropathy, void, voiding, vulvar dystrophies, vulvitis, vulvovaginitis, xeronisus.

genitourinary: Subcategories

I. Male:
    1. Erection, ejaculation:
        a. fear of losing an erection during sexual intercourse: **medomalacophobia**
        b. having a false erection: **piss-proud**
        c. inability to have an erection, or to copulate, or to ejaculate: **impotentia**
        d. inability to reach orgasm: **xeronisus**

2. Hormonal:
   a. low testosterone level: **ADAM syndrome**
3. Loins:
   a. weak in the loins: **elumbated**
4. Prostate:
   a. benign prostatic enlargement: **benign prostatic hypertrophy (BPH)**
   b. enlargement of the prostate: **prostatomegaly**
   c. symptoms of prostate enlargement: **prostatism**
   d. pelvic-floor exercises for urinary incontinence, e.g., after radical prostatectomy: **Kegel's exercises**

II. Female:
   1. Pelvic support:
      a. herniation of various pelvic organs in various directions: **pelvic support disorders**
      b. treatment of pelvic support disorder; urinary incontinence: **colporrhaphy**; **Kegel's exercises.**
   4. Vagina, vulva, & uterus:
      a. inflammation of the vulva and vagina, or of the vulvovaginal glands: **vulvovaginitis**
      b. inflammation of the external genital organs of the female: **vulvitis**
      c. noisy expulsion of gas from the vagina: **flatus vaginalis**
      d. prolapse of the uterus and vagina: **procidentia**
      e. vaginal changes of old age: **atrophic vaginitis**
      f. vulvar non-neoplastic epithelial disorders: **vulvar dystrophies**

III Both genders:
   1. Abdominal:
      a. examination of the abdomen's interior by means of a scope: **laparoscopy**
   2. Genitalia:
      a. the external genitalia: **edea**
   Infection:
      a. lousiness: **pediculosis**

4. Procreation:
   a. inability to procreate: **improcreant** (*impotentia generandi.* See **impotentia**.)
5. Sexual intercourse:
   a. painful sexual intercourse: **dyspareunia**
6. Urination:
   a. Any affection of the urinary tract: **uropathy**
   b. difficult or painful urination: **dysuria**
   c. excretory: **emunctory**
   d. involuntary urinary or fecal discharge: **incontinence**
   e. involuntary discharge of urine while sleeping: **enuresis**
   f. one with difficult or painful urination: **dysuriac**
   g. passage of urine, pissing: **urination, voiding**
   h. urethral obstruction: **urethremphraxis**
   i. urinary incontinence: **aconuresis, DIAPPERS, incontinence**.
   j. urinary-incontinence treatment: **Kegel's exercises**
   k. urinate: **micturition, piddle, void**
   l. urinate (act or work) triflingly: **piddle**
   m. urinating at night: **nocturia**

gerascophobia (jer-as"kō-fōb'bi-ə) n. the morbid fear, dread of growing old, or of old age. [< G *geras* old age + *phobos* fear]. adj. **gerascophobic**. n. **gerascophobe** (-as'kō-). syn. **gerontophobia**, q.v. See **phobias**. See **old age**.

geriatric care manager/geriatric case manager n.phr. one who looks after an elderly person, but much more comprehensively, managerially than a home-health aide. A care manager can arrange doctor visits, accompany elders on such visits and others, administer medication, follow patients' progress in hospital, help with financial paperwork, vet nursing homes and assisted living facilities, provide companionship, etc. Such a role and concept is relatively new, and such managers usually have nursing and/or social work degrees. They are hired after an initial assessment charge, and at a substantial hourly rate. There's a National Association of Professional Geriatric

Care Managers: www.caremanager.org. See **health, illness**, **therapy**. See **role**. See **work, activity**.

geriatric center (jer-ree-at'rik) n.phr. a place for care of the aged. [G < *geras* old age + *iatrike* surgery, medicine]. Cf. **assisted-living residence** or **facility, convalescent home, hospice, nursing home, rest home, retirement home**. Cf. **CCRC, elder-care hostel**, geriatric center, **gerontocomium, hibernacle**, q.v. See **old age**. See **therapy**.

geriatrics (jer-ree-at'trikss) n. the branch of medicine that deals with the illnesses and medical care of the aged, senior citizens—the word, geriatrics, takes a singular verb. [G < *geras* old age + *iatrike* surgery, medicine]. n. **geriatrician** (-ə-tri'-shən) = a practitioner of geriatrics (Jerry Atrics!). adj. **geriatric** 1. relating to the diagnosis, prevention, and treatment of illness in the aged, seniors. 2. an offensive term meaning showing the effects of age. n. **geriatric** a senior citizen in a medical context. syn. = **presbyatrics** & **presbytiatrics**, q.v. See **old age**. See **role**.

gero-, geron-, geront-, geronto- prefs. relating to aging, old age. [< G *geras* old age & *geron*, old man].

gerocomical (jer"ō-kom'i-kəl) adj. (obs.) pertaining to the treatment of the aged. • *Gerocomical* attempts are sometimes comical. [G *gerokomikos* < *gerokomia* < *gero-*, pref., q.v., < *geras* old age + *-komia* tending]. See **old**. See **therapy**.

geroderma (jer-ō-der'mə) n. 1. the atrophic skin of the aged. 2. any condition in which the skin is thinned and wrinkled, resembling the integument of old age. [gero-, pref., q.v., + < G *derma* skin]. See **skin**.

gerodontics/gerodontology (jer-ō-don'tiks/jer"ō-don-tol'ō-jee, -ə-jee) n. the branch of dentistry focusing on the needs of the aged, senior citizens; dental geriatrics (takes singular v.). [< gero-, pref., q.v., + < G *odous* tooth + *logos* study]. adj. **gerodontic**. n. **gerodontist** = a practitioner of gerodontics. n. **gerodontologist** (jer"ō-don-tol'lə-jist) = a practitioner of, or one who specializes in, gerodontics. syns. **dental geriatrics, gerodontia**. See **mouth, gums, teeth**. See **old age**. See **role**.

geromarasmus (jer"rō-ma-ras'məs) n. senile atrophy or wasting. [gero-, pref., q.v., + < G *marasmos* a wasting]. See **physique, appearance**.

geromorphism (jer"rō-mor'fis-səm) n. the condition of appearing older than one's age or of being prematurely senile. [gero-, pref., q.v., + < G *morphe* form]. adj. **geromorphic**. ants. **paedomorphism, neanimorphism**, q.v. See **physique, appearance**. See **old age**. See **intelligence**.

gerontal (jer-on'təl)/**gerontic** (-tik) adj. 1. pertaining to old age; senile. 2. pertaining to an old man. [geron-, pref., q.v., + -al, suff., relating to or characterized by < L –*alis*]. See **old**. See **old man**.

gerontarchical (jer"rən-taar'ki-kəl) adj. pertaining to, or of the nature of, government by old men. [< G *geront-*, *geron* old man + *archos* ruling + -ic, suff., + -al, suff.]. n. = **gerontarchy** (jer'rən-taar"kee) = a government by old men. See **old man**. *See* **work, activity.**

gerontic (jer-on'tik) adj. of or pertaining to old age, senile. ("geronic" is an erroneous form.) [geron-, pref., q.v., + -ic, suff.]. See **old age**.

gerontiloquence (jer"ron-til'lō-kwənss) n. 1. speaking among the aged. 2. speaking about the aged. [< geront-, pref., q.v. + < L *loqui* speak + E -ence, suff., forming nouns of quality or action < L pres.p(s). in -*ent*- & earlier -*entia*]. See **talk**.

gerontocomium (jer-ən"tō-kōm'mi-əm) n. (obs.) an institution for care of the aged, a nursing home; old-age residence. [geronto-, q.v., + -*komia* tending]. Cf. **assisted-living residence** or **facility, convalescent home, hospice, nursing home, rest home, retirement home**. Cf. **geriatric center, gerontocomium, hibernacle**, q.v. See **old age**. See **therapy**.

gerontocracy (jer"rən-tok'krə-see) n. government by the elderly or aged, perhaps in the form of a council. [geronto-, q.v., + < G *kratos* power]. adj. **gerontocratic** (jer-ron"tō-kra'tik). See **old age**.

gerontogenes (jer-on'tō-jeenss) n. genes that govern antiaging effects. The gerontogene TOR (target of rapamycin) is a compound controlling the production of cell protein and other actions.) Rapamycin, in drug form, in small doses, appears to activate TOR's benefits. Rapamycin was recently found to extend the lifespan of mice by 14%. Another gerontogene is SIRT-1, which instructs the body to make certain enzymes that extend the lives of worms, flies, and mice. **Resveratrol**, q.v., activates SIRT-1, and Resveratrol-like compounds, called "sirtuin drugs"—probably named for the company, Sirtris, a pioneer in investigating gerontogenes, and acquired by GlaxoSmithKlein in 2008—that are popularly known as "The Youth" or "Fountain-of-Youth" pills. [-geronto-, pref., q.v., + gene, early 20th C. via Ger. *Gen* < G *genos* birth, race]. See **therapy**.

gerontolagnia (jer-ən"tō-lag'ni-ə) n. strong sexual desire in an older man. [geronto-, pref., q.v., + < G *lagneia* lust; coition]. See **sex, love**.

gerontology (jer"ən-tol'lō-gee, -lə-gee) n. the scientific study, process of aging and its effects, problems. [geronto-, pref., q.v., + -logy, suff., study, science < G *logos* word, reason]. adj. **gerontologic** (-ron"tō-log'ik), **gerontological** (-ron"tō-loj'ji-kəl). n. **gerontologist** (ger"rən-tol'lə-jist) = 1. one who studies and researches aging. 2. one who diagnoses and treats the aged. syns. **geroscience**, **nostology**, q.v. Cf. **geriatrics**, q.v. See **old age**. See **role**. See **Therapy**.

gerontophilia (jer"rən-tō-fil'li-ə) n. morbid love of old persons. [geronto-, pref., q.v., + < –philia, suff., intense or abnormal attraction to, or tendency toward < G *philia* < *philos* loving, fond]. n. **gerontophile/gerontophilist** (ger"rən-tof'fil-ist). See **sex, love**. See **old age**. See **role**.

gerontophobia (jer"rən-tō-fō'bi-ə) n. 1. the dread, or morbid fear, of growing old. 2. morbid fear of old persons. [geronto-, pref., q.v., + < G *phobos* fear]. adj.

gerontophobic. n. **gerontophobe** (ger-on'tō-fōb). syn. **gerascophobia**, q.v. See **phobias**. See **old age**.

gerontopia (jer"ron-tōp'pee-ə) n. second sight: an apparent decrease in **presbyopia**, q.v., in the elderly, which is related to the development of nuclear (lens) sclerosis (hardening and thickening) with resultant myopia (inability to see distant objects). [geront-, pref., q.v., + < G *ops* eye]. syn. **senopia**, q.v. See **eye**.

gerontotherapeutics (jer-on'tō-thair"rə-pyoo'tikss) n. the science dealing with treatment of the aged. [geronto-, pref., q.v., + < G *therapeutike* medical practice]. n. **gerontotherapy** (-thair'-ə-pee). n. **gerontotherapist** (-thair'ə-pist) = **gerontologist**, q.v. See **therapy**.

gerontoxon (jer-on-tok'son) n. an opaque, grayish ring at the periphery of the cornea, just within the sclerocorneal junction, of frequent occurrence in the aged, and a mark of old age. [geron-, pref., q.v., + G *toxon* bow]. syns. *arcus corneae/arcus cornealis, arcus senilis*, q.v. See eye.

geroscience (jer'ō sī'əns) n. the science of old age, aging. [geronto-, pref., q.v., + < L *scientia* < *scire* to know]. syns. **gerontology, nostology**, q.v. See old age.

Gerousia (jer-roo'si-ə) n. ancient Sparta's legislative body; it was composed of 28 aristocrats and two kings (the *archabetai*). Five *ephors* from the Gerousia ranked higher governmentally then the remainder of the Gerousia, and the kings had to answer to the *ephors*—a system of checks and balances. Gerousia members, who had to be over 60 years of age, served for life. Upon a Gerousia member's death, male citizens, constituting the *Apella*, elected a new member. Parallels with the U.S. government are apparent. [G]. See old men (men).

glabrous (glayb'brəs) adj. smooth; hairless; a term applied to areas of the body where hair does not normally grow. • At age 79 the playwright Aeschylus was so bald that his pate was mistaken by an eagle flying overhead to be a stone. The eagle dropped the turtle carried in its beak in order to break it on the "stone". The turtle struck Aeschylus's *glabrous* dome and killed him (456 B.C.). [< L *glibber* smooth]. syns. glabrate, baldpated. See **physique, appearance**. See **hair**.

gleet (gleet) n. a viscous, transparent discharge from a mucous surface. [OF *glette, glecte*, a flux]. vt. to discharge gleet. adj. **gleety**. See **physique, appearance**.

gloming (glō'ming) n. twilight; dusk. Used fig., gloming = toward the end of life: in life's gloming. [< ME *gloming* < OE *glomung* < *glom* dusk < I-E stem *ghel-* to shine]. syn. **September, evening of life, gloming, golden years**, q.v. See **end-of-life, death**.

glossolalia (glos"sō-lay'li-ə) n. 1. nonsense talk; gibberish. 2. "speaking in tongues" (Chistian religion). [< G *glossa* tongue, language + -lalia, suff., speech, speech disorder < G *lalia* talk <

lalein to talk]. adj. **glossolalic**. Cf. **balderdash, galimatia, idiolalia, jabberwocky, prate, prattle,** q.v. See **talk**.

glusk (glusk) vi. (obs.) to squint. [derivation obscure]. n. **glusker** = squinter. vbl.n. **glusking** = squinting. See **eye**. See **role**.

gnarled (naarld) adj. (of a tree, hands, etc.) knobby; twisted; rugged. • Her old, gnarled hands were busily knitting an afghan. [var. of knarled < knurl, a small projecting knob, ridge, etc., < knur, a hard excrescence on a tree trunk; a hard concretion < ME *knorre* var. of *knar*, a knot or protuberance in a tree trunk, root, etc., rel. to MLG, MDu, MHG *knorre* knobbed protuberance]. adv. **gnarly**. See **physique, appearance**.

gnoff (noff)/**gnof/gnoffe/gnooffe/gnuffe/knuffe** n. (obs.) a curmudgeon, churl, boor, lout. It is preceded frequently by *old*. [uncertain origin. Cf. East Frisian *knufe* lump, *gnuffig* thick, rough, coarse, ill-mannered]. syn. **curmudgeon**, q.v. See **old man**. See **old woman**. See **old person(s), people**.

gnome[1] (nōm) n. one of the legendary small, hunchbacked, shriveled, ugly old men of folklore who had long white beards, lived in the interior of the earth, were chthonic or chthonian characters guarding treasure, and were known also as a trolls, goblins, and dwarfs. Figuratively and insultingly, someone supposedly fitting this description was a gnome. [< L *gnomus* (Paracelsus), perhaps irregular or erroneous for G. *genomos* < *ge* earth & *-nomos* dwelling]. See **old man**.

gnome[2] (nōm) n. a terse expression of general truth, a maxim, aphorism, or proverb. [< G *gnome* opinion, judgement < *gignoskein* to know]. adj. **gnomic**, q.v. See **talk**.

gnomic (nom'mik, nōm'mik) adj. 1. sententious, full of aphorisms or maxims. 2. wise and pithy. (3. {grammar} **gnomic aorist** = a verb tense that is indefinite, usually in a past form, but used without a past sense to express sententiously a general truth, e.g., ". . . men were deceivers ever."; the aorist is used frequently in G drama.) [< G *gnomikos* < *gnome* < *gignoskein* to know]. See **talk**.

golden ager (gōl-den ayg'gur) n.phr. an old person; someone over retirement age. [golden, as in golden years, i.e., old age + ager, i.e., old person (slang)]. See **old man, old woman**.

golden years n.phr. the years toward the end of life; a metaphor for old age. syn. **September, gloming,** q.v., **hiemal,** q.v., years, winter of life—neologistically: **goldentopia.** See **old age.**

Gompertz Law (gom'pertz) pr.n.phr. the chance of continuing to live doubles roughly every nine-and-one-quarter years. It applies roughly until age 70-75, then mortality rates increase, but more gradually. Although the law's validity has been questioned, recently there is some support for it. [< E 19th C. mathematician, Benjamin Gompertz]. See **end of life, death.**

gormless (gawrm'less) adj. dull or stupid; lacking in intelligence, sense, or discernment [< E dial. *gaum* attention or understanding < ME *gome* < ON *gaumr*]. See **intelligence.**

grandam(e) (graN'daam") n. grandmother or a woman no longer young; (but only without a terminal "e") an animal's dam's dam; ancestress; old woman. [ME < AF *graund dame* < L *grandis* full grown + < ME *dam,* alt. *dame,* mother < L *domina* mistress]. See **old woman.**

granocracy (gran-nok'rə-see) n. rule by old women. [< L *grandis* full grown + < G *kratos* power]. See **old woman.** See **old age.**

graybeard (gray'beerd) n. 1. (dated) a man of advanced years. (2. an earthenware container for alcohol.) [OE *græg* < Gmc. *græwaz* gray + beard < OE < I-E]. adj. **graybearded.** See **old man.** See **hair.**

gray power (gray pow'ər) n.phr. the collective political and consumer influence of old people that has come about and increased with their increasing number. (Note: In England "gray" is spelled "grey".) See **old age.**

gray rights (gray rīts) n.phr. a collocation referring to a U.S. movement of the 1990s asserting entitlements due the aged, e.g., not to be fired from a job without cause except age. [< gray, the hair color of many of the elderly & thus a surrogate for the aged, < OE *græg* < Gmc., & probably based on the concurrent women's rights movement]. See **old age.**

gray tech n.phr. a collocation referring to technology directed at and devoted to the problems, health, and care of the aged. The

Oregon Health and Science University has Oratech, an acronym for the school's Oregon Center for Aging & Technology. A study aid for technological development is an "age empathy suit" named AGNES (age-gain-now empathy system), developed by the M.I.T. Age Lab. The suit, with its instant add-on decades, can be donned by a young adult and calibrated to simulate the impaired dexterity, mobility, strength, and balance of, e.g., a 74-year-old. See **therapy**.

great assize (as-sīz) n.phr. last judgement, judgement day. [ME < OF *asise*, F *asseoir* sit at < L *assidere* to sit down beside]. syns. **doomsday**, **final reckoning**. See **end-of-life, death**.

grimalkin (grim-awl'kin) n. (1. an old female cat.) 2. an old frumpy spiteful woman. [< E grey < OE *gr-aeg* < Gmc. + E Malkin (Matilda), (obs.) a cat, + -kin, suff., little, dear, probably < MDu -*ki(j)n*]. See **old woman**.

grinch (grinch) n. someone who ruins others' enjoyment. • He was both an octogenarian and a grinch. [< the Grinch, a character in "How the Grinch Stole Christmas", a 1957 story by Dr. Seuss, nom de plume of Theodore Seuss Geisel (1904-1991)]. See **mentality, mentation, behavior**.

grisard/grizard (griz'ərd) n. a grey-haired person. [< F *gris* gray (*gris* can also mean "dismal" or "tipsy".) + -ard, suff., forming nouns, sometimes of censure, ME & OF < Gmc.]. syns. **canities**, **graybeard** (man only), q.v. See **old man**. See **old woman**. See **old person(s)**. See **physique, appearance**.

grognard (grɔɲar) nm. an old soldier, seasoned veteran. [F. The term was first applied to men of Napoleon's Old Guard]. See **old man**.

grouse (growss) vi. to complain in a grumbling, often self-serving, way. [early 19th C.?]. n. **grouse**. n. **grouser**. See **talk**. See **role**.

gudgeon (guj'jən) n. 1. a credulous person. 2. a dupe. (3. a small freshwater fish that is often used for bait. 4. a socket into which a pin fits.) [via OF *goujon* < L *gogionem* < *gobius* a fish (with ventral fins joined into a sucker) < G *kobios* gudgeon: a socket (in which a rudder works)]. See **mentality, mentation, behavior**. See **role**.

gynecomania (gī"neek-kō-mayn'ni-ə) n. morbid or excessive sexual desire in a male. [gyn(o)-, gyne(o)-, prefs., relating to women < G gyne woman + *mania* frenzy, madness]. adj. **gynecomaniacal** (-mə-nī'ə-kəl). n. **gynecomaniac**. syns. **cretomania, satyromania**, q.v. See **manias**. See **sex, love**.

H

"That happy age when a man can be idle with impunity."
—Washington Irving.

habitué, -e (f.) (abitye) n. a person who frequents a particular place; a regular visitor or resident. • The owner of the country store considered them *habitués*, old **cronies**, q.v., who gathered there daily. [F, pp. of *hjabituer* < L *habituare* < *habitare* inhabit]. See **mentality, mentation, behavior**.

Hadephobia (hay"dee-fōb'bi-ə) n. morbid fear of hell. [< OE *hel(l)* Gmc *hel-, hal-* to hide < I-E *conceal* + -phobia, suff., fearing < G -*phobia* < *phobos* fear]. n. **hadephobe** (hay'dee-fōb). adj. **Hadephobic**. syn. **stygiophobia**, q.v. See **phobias**. See **end-of-life, death**.

hair: acomia, alopecia, alopeciaphobia, atrichia, calvities, canescent, canities, combover, depilous, dyschromia, elflock, glabrous, graybearded, hirsutulous, madarosis, pediculosis, peladophobia, phalacrophobia, phalacrosis, pilgarlic, plica polonica, poliosis, psilosis.

hair: Subcategories

I. Color:
    1. Abnormal color: **dyschromia**
    2. Premature graying/loss of hair color: **poliosis**
    3. White/gray hair: **canescent, canities, graybearded**
II. Scalp hair:
    1. Baldness, hairless: **acomia, alopecia, atrichia, calvities, depilous, glabrous, phalacrosis, pilgarlic**
    2. Fear of baldness/becoming bald: **alopeciaphobia, peladophobia, phalacrophobia**

      3. Fear of bald people: **peladophobia**
      4. Hair loss: **psilosis**
      5. Louse infestation: **pediculosis**
      6. Partial baldness cover-up: **combover**
      7. Tangled hair: **elflock**
      8. Various other hair conditions: matted, tangled, crusted, dirty, neglected hair: **plica polonica**
  III. Eyebrows/eyelashes:
      1. Loss: **madarosis**
  IV. Hairiness:
      1. Minutely hirsute: **hirsutulous**

hakam (haak'kaam) n. 1. a sage. (2. a rabbinical commentator, especially one during the first two centuries, A.D.) [< Hebrew *hakham* wise]. Cf. **polymath**, q.v. See role.

halcyon (hal'see-ən) adj. 1. peaceful; tranquil. 2. carefree; joyful. 3. golden; prosperous. [via L and M E < G *halkyon* kingfisher. The halcyon was a mythical bird, identified with the kingfisher, that was said to breed around the winter solstice. It nested at sea and had the power to charm the wind and waves so that they became calm. In Greek mythology, *Alcyone* was the daughter of Aeolus and wife of Ceyx. When Ceyx drowned in a shipwreck, *Alcyone* threw herself into the sea. Out of compassion, the gods transformed them into a pair of kingfishers. To protect their nest, the winds were forbidden to blow for a week before and after the winter solstice—Anu Garg.] (n. **halcyon** any of various kingfishers of the genus Halcyon.) See **mentality, mentation, behavior**.

hamartithia (ham"maar-tith'hi-ə) n. mistake prone. [< G *hamartion* a bodily defect < *hamartanein* miss the mark, make a mistake]. See **mentality, mentation, behavior**.

hamartomania (ha-mawr"tō-may'ni-ə) n. Abnormal interest in sin. [< G *hamartion* a bodily defect + *mania* frenzy]. adj. **hamartomaniacal** (-mə-nī'ə-kəl). n. **hamartomaniac.** Cf. **hamartophobia**, q.v. See **manias**. See **religion, theology, morality**.

hamartophobia (ha-maar"tō-fōb'bi-ə) n. morbid fear of error, sin, or sinning. [< G *hamartion* a bodily defect + *phobos* fear]. adj. **hamartophobic.** n. **hamartophobe** (-maar'tō-fōb. syn.

peccatiphobia, q.v. Cf. enosiophobia or enissophobia, q.v. See phobias. See religion, theology, morality.

harpaxophobia (haar-paks"sō-fōb'bi-ə) n. morbid fear of thieves (or of becoming a thief). ● As she grew old *harpaxophobia* became an increasing concern. [< G *harpax* robber + *phobos* fear]. adj. harpaxophobic. n. harpaxophobe (-paks'so-). syn. kleptophobia/cleptophobia, q.v. See phobias.

harpy (haar'pee) n. 1. a predatory person. 2. a bad-tempered woman (often used with *old*). [< G *harpuiai* (pl.) harpies, rapacious monsters in Greek mythology who had a woman's head, face, and body, but a bird's wings and claws < *harpazein* to snatch. They were ordered by the gods to snatch King Phineus's food as punishment for his revealing secrets]. See old woman. See role.

harridan (har'ri-dən) n. a bad-tempered old woman; a hag, a shrew, a vixen; she deliberately insults her age and temperament. [?, perhaps < F *haridelle* old jade]. See old woman.

hartshorn (haarts'hawrn) n. ammonia water, or any volatile ammonium salt, e.g., the carbonate. It is used as a stimulant, e.g., to revive one who has fainted: smelling salts. [< OE *her(o)t*, < OS *herut*, < OHG *hir(u)z*, < ON *hjqrtr* < Gmc. *herutaz* stag (male {especially red} deer + the horn of the hart, *cornu cervi* (*cerva, -ae* f. hind, deer). Hartshorn was formerly the chief source of ammonia]. See therapy.

Hayflick's limit (hay'flikss lim'it) n.phr. the limit to cellular replicative capacity. When human cells reach this biologic limit, after about 50 cell divisions, the cells die. Fibroblast cells removed from elderly persons divide fewer times. (One explanation for why a cell-division limit is reached is that the end pieces, telomeres, of cell chromosomes get shorter with each cell division until they become so short that the cell can no longer divide.) [< the laboratory work of Dr. Leonard Hayflick at the Wistar Institute]. See end-of-life, death.

health-care REIT (reet) n.phr. an investment vehicle, i.e., an exchange-traded fund (ETF) that invest in health care, often, if not predominantly, in senior health-and-retirement facilities: assisted-living units, skilled nursing, Alzheimer's facilities, medical office buildings, hospitals, senior housing, independent-living facilities, long-term-care facilities, senior housing, nursing homes, senior apartments, rehabilitation hospitals, specialty-care units, etc. Examples of such REITS, with their stock-exchange symbols are: Health Care REIT (HCN), Senior Housing Properties (SNH), LTC Properties (LTC), Ventas (VTR), Cogdell Spencer (CSA), etc. [REIT is an initialism: real-estate-investment trust]. See **finance**.

health, illness: agnosia, anosognosia, CCRC, comorbidity, detumescence, dyscrasia, dyscrasy, dyscrinism, dystrophy, dystropia, entelechy, equipoise, etiolate, eucrasy, eudaemonia/ eudemonia, eugeria, euphelicia, gait speed, geriatric care manager/geriatric case manager, herpes zoster, *hors de combat*, hygieolatry/hygeiolatry, hysteresis, iatrophobia, idiopathic, idiosyncrasy, immune senescence, inanition, inappetence, ingravescence, insanable, invalescence, invaletudinary, klotho, lectual, lentor, longevity, longevous, macrobian, marasmus, marcescent, marcescible, megrim, megrims, miosis, molys(o) mophobia, nocebo, nosocomephrenia, nosomania, nosophobia, obstruent, oligotrophia/oligotrophy, orthocrasia, paralysis agitans, patharmosis, pathocryptia, pathomimesis/pathomimicry, pathomimetic, pathomiosis, pathoneurosis, pathophobia, patroiophobia, reable, recrudescence, reddition, redintegrate, redivivous, redux, refocillation, refractory, regimen, repullulate, resipiscent, revalescent, salubrious, sarcopenia, serotonin, succorance, tabefaction, tabescence, tabefy, tendsome, tophaceous, tophus, trypanophobia, tutelage, tutelary, uratic arthritis, valetudinarianism, virtual visit, walking speed, wan, wanze, wellderly, xeniatrophobia, zoster.

health, illness: Subcategories

I. Doctors, caregivers, medical treatment tests:
    1. Acting in the role of guardian, caregiver: **tutelary**
    2. Care, guidance, and supervision: **tutelage**
    3. Continuing care in a retirement community: **CCRC**
    4. Geriatric care giver: **geriatric care manager/ geriatric case manager**
    5. How fast an elder can walk: **gait speed**
    6. Morbid fear of doctors: **iatrophobia**
    7. Morbid fear of going to a foreign doctor: **xeniatrophobia**
    8. Morbid fear of injections or inoculations: **trypanophobia**

9. Physical fitness and longevity test: **walking speed**
10. Requiring much attendance: **tendsome**
11. Visiting doctors: **virtual visit**

II. Bad health:

1. Altered (decreased) immunity: **immune senescence**
2. An invalid state: **invalescence**
3. Bedridden: **lectual**
4. Defective nutrition: **dystrophy**, **dystropia**
5. Disabled, out of action: *hors de combat*
6. Emaciation due to disease: **tabefaction**
7. Illness based on awareness of side effects: **nocebo**
8. Loss of the ability to recognize the input of sensory stimuli: **agnosia**
9. Pale, sickly looking: **wan**
10. Producing and obstruction: **obstruent**
11. Reactivation of disease: **recrudescence**
12. Sluggishness: **lentor**
13. Stubborn, refractory, unyielding: **refractory**
14. Tending to wither or fade: **marcescible**
15. The state of needing assistance from another: **succorance**
16. The state of progressive wasting, withering away, decay; becoming emaciated: **tabescence**
17. To sprout again; to recur, as might a disease: **repullulate**
18. To waste away gradually: **tabefy**
19. Two diseases present simultaneously: **comorbidity**
20. Unable to be cured: **insanable**
21. Unhealthy: **invaletudinary**
22. Waste away, wither, become emaciated: **wanze**
23. Wasted away, withered: **marasmus**
24. Withering, wasting away, becoming emaciated: **marcescent**
25. Weak, sickly, or convalescent state; thinking only of one's illness; tendency to hypochondria: **valetudinarianism**
26. Worsening in disease severity: **ingravescence**

III. Good health:

1. Equilibrium (often fig.); a balance between different social, emotional, mental, and physical influences; something creating a balanced state, usually by counterbalancing some other force or thing: **equipoise**
2. Healthful state:
   a. a feeling of well being, happiness: **eudaemonia/eudemonia**
   b. a life-giving, vital force productive of full realization of potential: **entelechy**
   c. normal state of good health: **eucrasy**.
   d. wholesome, healthy, and beneficial: **salubrious**
3. Healthiness/wishes granted: **euphelicia**
4. Longevity gene: **klotho**
   a. long-lived: **longevous, macrobian**
   b. neologism indicating collectively those elderly who live the longest, 100 years or more: **wellderly**
5. Normal, happy old age: **eugeria**
6. Renewed, restored health: **redux**
   a. recovering from illness or injury: **revalescent**
   b. restoration of previous condition: **reddition, refocillation**c. restoration program of exercise, diet, etc., intended to improve health: **regimen**
   d. restore health completely: **redintegrate**
   e. restore self or condition: **reable**
   f. restored to life: **redivivous**
   g. restored to sanity; learned from experience; to come to one's senses; having returned to a saner mind: **resipiscent**
7. Stimulant neurotransmitter: **serotonin**
8. The quality or condition of being long lived: **longevity**
9. When symptoms diminish: **miosis, detumescence**

IV. <u>Organ systems, disease</u>:
1. Blood abnormality: **dyscrasia, dyscrasy**
2. Endocrine glands:
   a. endocrine gland abnormality: **dyscrinism**
3. Eyes: contracted pupils: **miosis**
4 Drugs:
   a. reaction to drugs, etc.: **orthocrasia**

5. Gastrointestnal, nutrition:
   a. deficient nutrition: **oligotrophia/ oligotrophy**
   b. lack of appetite: **inappetence**
   c. severe malnutrition, exhaustion due to disease: **inanition**
6. Immunity:
   a. **immune senescence**
7. Infection: **herpes zoster**, **zoster**
8. Joints:
   a. gouty arthritis: **uratic arthritis**
9. Metabolic:
   a. characteristic of hard or gritty gouty nodules: **tophaceous**
   b. the nodule(s) of gout: **tophus (tophi)**
10. Muscle:
   a. loss of muscle—both the number and size of muscle fibers—associated with disuse, old age: **sarcopenia**
11. Neuro-psychiatric, emotional, mental, neurologic:
   a. depression from a long hospital stay: **nosocomephrenia**
   b. fear of disease, illness: **nosophobia**, **pathophobia**
   c. fear of hereditary disease: **patroiophobia**
   d. fear of infection: **molys(o)mophobia**
   e. fear of the doctors: **iatrophobia**
   f. feigning disease: **pathomimesis/patho-mimicry**
   g. health fanaticism: **hygieolatry/ hygeiolatry**
   h. irrational belief that one has a disease: **nosomania**
   i. loss of the ability to recognize the input of sensory stimuli: **agnosia**
   j. low spirits: **megrims**
   k. mental adjustment to disease: **patharmosis**
   l. migraine headache: **megrim**
   m. minimizing disease: **pathomiosis**.
   n. neurotic preoccupation with true disease: **pathoneurosis**
   o. Parkinsonism (type of): **paralysis agitans**
   p. one feigning disease: **pathomimetic**

      q. time lag in the elderly between stimulus & response: **hysteresis**

      r. unawareness or denial of disease, illness: **anosognosia**

      s. unusual way of thinking, behaving, feeling: **idiosyncrasy**

      t. unwillingness to discuss or to believe in one's disease: **pathocryptia**

12. Penis: **detumescence**
13. Skin:
    a. To give a sickly hue to someone: **etiolate**
    b. Vesicular rash along a body segment (s): **herpes zoster, zoster**
14. Unknown organ system:
    a. disease cause unknown: **idiopathic**

<u>**heart, heart rhythm**</u>: **angina, angina pectoris, atrial fibrillation, bradycardia, bruit, calcium CT cardiac scan, CIMT, coronary angiography, dysrhythmia, tachyarrhythmia, tachycardia, ventricular fibrillation**.

<u>**heart, heart rhythm**</u> Sub-categories

I.   <u>Cardiac chest pain</u>: **angina, angina pectoris**
II. Coronary-artery thickness prediction: **CIMT**
III. <u>Coronary artery visualization</u>:
    1. Heart scan: **calcium CT cardiac scan**
    2. Radiographic visualization of the coronary arteries by contrast media injected into them: **coronary angiography**
IV. <u>Heart rate</u>:
    1. Abnormal heart rate:
        a. fast heart rate: **tachycardia, tachyarrhythmia**
        b. slow heart rate: **bradycardia**
    2. Dysfunctional slow, fast, or irregular heart beat: **atrial fibrillation**
V. <u>Heart rhythm</u>:
    1. Abnormal rhythm: **dysrhythmia**
    2. Ineffective, irregular heart beat: **ventricular fibrillation**
VI. <u>Heart sound</u>: **bruit**

Heberden's nodes (heb'bur-denss) n.phr. hard nodosities, nodules (**exostoses**, q.v.) occurring on the terminal phalanges (digit-end bones) of the fingers in **osteoarthritis**, q.v., a common disease of the elderly. These nodes are found in some elderly who are genetically predisposed and consist of enlargements of the tubercles at the articular extremities (knuckle joints) of the distal phalanges. Similar nodes found at the proximal interphalangeal joints are called **Bouchard's nodules**. [< Dr. William Heberden, an 18th C. London physician]. See **joint, extremities, back**.

hebetude (heb'bə-tood) n. slow in perceiving, dullness; mental lethargy, obtuseness, stupidity. [< L *hebetudo* < *hebetare* to be blunt, dull, dim]. vi.&vt. **hebetate** = make, become dull. adj. **hebetudinous** (-tood'di-nəss). See **intelligence**.

heliophobia (heel"li-ō-fōb'bi-ə) n. morbid fear of sunlight. • Her *heliophobia*, based on preventing **actinic keratosis**, q.v., kept her indoors. [helio-, pref., relating to the sun, < G *helios* sun + *phobos* fear]. adj. **heliophobic**. n. **heliophobe**. syn. **phengophobia**, q.v. See **phobias**.

hellhag (hel'hag) n. an evil old woman; a hellcat. [O.E. *hel(l)* hell < I-E hide, conceal + hag, 14th C. <?]. See **old woman**.

heloma (hee-lō'mə) n. a corn, a **clavus**, q.v. [< G *helos* nail + *-oma*, suff., tumor]. See **skin**. See **joint, extremities, back**.

heloma durum (hel-lō'mə dur'rəm) n.phr. a hard corn, which occurs over joints of the toes. [< G *helos* nail + *-oma*, suff., tumor, and L, *durum* hard, tough; callous]. See: **joint, extremities, back**. See **skin**.

heloma molle (hel-lō'mə mol'lee) n.phr. a corn, which is usually found between the toes, and due to pressure from adjacent toes. See: **joint, extremities, back**. See **skin**.

hemartia (hem-aar'shə) n. 1. a single defect of character in an otherwise decent person; the classic tragic character flaw, but which could actually, and more likely, have been just an instance of bad judgment. (2. a localized defect in tissue combination or arrangement as a result of deranged fetal development.) [G, defect]. See **religion, theology, morality**.

hematoma (hee-ma-tōm'mə, hee-mə-, pl. -tō-məs, -tōm-ma-tə) n. a localized mass of extravasated blood that is relatively or completely confined within an organ, a tissue, a space, or a potential space; the blood is usually clotted, or partly so, and, depending on how long it has been there, may manifest various degrees of organization and decolorization. ● The skin of the elderly is fragile and particularly susceptible to *hematoma* from even rather minor trauma (injury). [hemato- pref., meaning blood, < G *haima* (*haimat-*) blood, + *-oma*, suff., tumor]. See **blood, circulation & glands**. See: **skin**.

hemeralopia (hem"mər-al-ōp'pi-ə) n. day blindness; inability to see as distinctly in bright light as in dim light. [< G *hemera* day + *alaos* obscure + *ops* eye]. n. **hemeralope**. syn. **hemiablepsia**, q.v. Cf. **ablepsia**. See **eye**. See **role**.

heresiarch (hə-reez'zee-aark) n. a leader or founder of a heretical religious sect, or of a group or movement. [mid 16th C. ecclesiastical L < ecclesiastical G *hairesiarkhes* < G *hairesis* choice, group < *haireisthai* to choose + *-arkhes*, suff., ruler]. See **role**. See **religion, theology, morality**.

heresyphobia (her"ri-see-fō'bi-ə) n. morbid fear of heresy. [< G *hairesis* choice, group < *haireisthai* to choose + *phobos* fear]. adj. **heresyphobic**. n. **heresyphobe** (her'-ri-see-fōb). See **phobias**. See **religion, theology, morality**.

herpes zoster (hur'pees zoss'ter, -zoss'-tə) n.phr. an acute, vesicular (blistered) eruption, along a dermatome, caused by reactivation of latent varicella (chickenpox) virus in the dorsal root ganglia, in the context of a patient's naturally waning, or absent, cellular immunity, or immunosuppressed immunity. Herpes zoster's peak incidence is between 50 and 70 years of age. Other predisposing factors include use of immunosuppressants or corticosteroids, malignancy, local irradiation, trauma, and surgery. Zoster is associated with acute neuralgic pain. Postherpetic (after the eruption has healed) neuralgia (nerve pain) occurs particularly in the elderly, and the duration and severity increase with age. syn. **zoster**, q.v. See **skin**. See **nerve, muscle, movement, touch**. See **health, illness**.

hesternal (hes-tur'nəl) adj. of yesterday. ● "I passed up a side street, one of those deserted ways . . . dim places, **fusty** {q.v.} with *hesternal* excitements and thrills of yesteryear."—Rupert Brooke (Anu Garg) (my emphasis). [< L *hesternus* of yesterday]. See **past, time**.

hesternopathic/hesternopothic (hes-tur"nō-pa'thik/ -pō'thik) n. one who pathologically yearns for the good old days. adj. pertaining to pathologic yearning for the good old days. [< L *hesternus* yesterday + -pathy, a suff., disorder, disease; remedial treatment; feeling, perception < G -*ptheia* < *pathos* feelings of, or what makes people feel, pity]. n. **hesternopathia/hesternopothia** = pathologic yearning for the good old days. See **mentality, mentation, behavior**. See **role**.

heteroclitic (het"tər-ō-klit'tik) adj. 1. eccentric, unconventional. (2. of a word that is formed in an unusual or irregular way.) • The older, the more *heteroclitic*, he became. [< G *heteroclitos* < *heteros* other + *klinein* to lean]. n. **heteroclite** (-klīt) = an eccentric, a maverick. Cf. **idiosyncratic, heteromorphic**. See **mentality, mentation, behavior**. **role**.

heteromorphic (het"tər-ō-mor'fik)/**heteromorphous** (-mor'əs) adj. 1. (fig.) having different forms at different stages of its life cycle. 2. differing in size or shape. 3. differing in shape, size, or structure from the normal form of the organism. 4. (fig.) characterized by an abnormal form or forms. [< hetero-, pref., different, other < G *heteros* other + -morph, suff., something having a particular form, shape, or structure < G *morphe* form]. n. **heteromorphism, heteromorphy**. Cf. **heteroclite, idiosyncrasy**, q.v. See **physique, appearance**.

hibernacle (hīb'bur-nak-əl) n. a winter retreat—can be used figuratively: old-age residence—the winter home of a hibernating animal. [< L *hibernacula* winter bivouac; winter residence < *hiems* or *hiemps* winter, cold, storm]. adj. **hibernal** (-bur'nəl) relating to winter (as one of the six divisions of the year: *pre-spring* (adj. prevernal) and *late summer* (adj. seritonal) as distinct seasons, along with the traditional four spring, summer, winter, and fall.) [< L *hibernus*, adj., winter, in winter, wintry]. adj. **hiemal**, q.v. Cf. **assisted-living residence** or **facility, convalescent home, hospice, nursing home, rest home, retirement home**. Cf. **geriatric center, gerontocomium, hibernacle**, q.v. See **end-of-life, death**. See **old age**.

hiemal (hī'ə-məl, -ee-mal) adj. of winter; wintry; hibernal, used fig.: pertaining to winter, the end of life. [< L *hiems* or *hiemps* winter, cold, storm]. See **end-of-life, death**.

hieromania (hī"ər-rō-may'ni-ə) n. religious insanity. [< G *hieros* holy + *mania* insanity]. See **manias**. See **religion**.

hierophobia (hī"ər-rō-fōb'bi-ə) n. morbid fear of religious or sacred objects. [< G *hieros* holy + *phobos* fear]. See **phobias**. See **religion**.

hippocampus n. (hip"pō-kam'pəss) a complex area of the temporal lobe of the brain: the seat of memory; it is crucial to the formation of new memories, which function tends to become impaired with age. The hippocampus typically shrinks after one's mid-50s resulting in memory loss, but sustained regular exercise in older adults can result in hippocampal growth. New research indicates memories are repeatedly recast and with some alteration. [< G *hippokampos* sea horse]. adj. **hippocampal**. See **memory**.

hirsutulous (hir-soo'chə-ləss) adj. minutely hirsute, i.e., hairy. [< L *hirsutus* rough, hairy]. See **physique, appearance**. See **hair**.

hoarhead (hawr'hed) n. an old grey-haired or white-haired man. [< OE *har*, OHG *her*, ON, *harr* < I-E *shine* + head]. See **old man**. See **color**.

hoary (hawr'ree) adj. (of hair) gray, grayish-white, white with age; having hair of such color; venerable. [< OE *har*, OHG *her*, < Gmc *hairaz*]. n. **hoariness**. See **physique, appearance**. See **color**.

hobble (hob'bəl) vi. to walk haltingly, unsteadily, limp along. vt. **hobble** = to restrict someone (or thing) to slow or prevent progress. [13th C., probably < LG]. See **nerve, muscle, movement, touch**. See **standing, walking, wandering**.

holagogue (hōl'lə-gog) n. a medication that removes all trace of a disease (or, formerly, to get rid of all four morbid humors); a panacea. • The aged, suffering serially from physical ailments, hope in their despair for a *holagogue*. [holo-, or hol- before a vowel, < G *holos* whole, entire, complete + *agogos* drawing forth]. See **therapy**.

homophobia (hō"mō-fō'bi-ə) n. 1. morbid fear of monotony, sameness. • *Homophobia* is not unexpected in nursing homes absent such diversions as special activities, occupational therapy, and extracurricular activities. 2. fear, disapproval, or hatred of homosexuals, lesbians, or of homosexuality and its culture. [homo-, pref., meaning the same or alike, < G *homos* the same + *phobos* fear.

(< L *homo* human being)]. adj. **homophobic**. n. **homophobe**. See **phobias**.

horaphthia (haar-af'thi-ə) n. a neurotic preoccupation with one's youth. [?]. See **youth, younger generation**.

horbgorgling (hawrb-gawrg'ling) n. the act of puttering around aimlessly. [?]. See **mentality, mentation, behavior**.

hordeolum (hor-dee-ōl'ləm) n. a sty. [L *hordeolus* sty]. See **meibomian cyst**. See **eye**.

hors de combat ('ɔr də kōba) adv.phr./adj.phr. disabled; out of action.
• As the **grognard**, q.v., became increasingly decrepit, it was obvious he was *hors de combat*. [F, out of the fight]. See: **work, activity**. See **health, illness**.

hors de concours ('ɔr də kōkur) adv.phr./adj.phr. beyond competition. [F, out of competition, contest]. See: **work, activity**.

horsefeathers (hawrs' feth"ərss) int., n. (humorous slang) nonsense. (used with a sing. v.) [< Early 20th C. euphemistic alteration of the scurrilous "horseshit"]. See **emotion**.

huggermugger/hugger-mugger (hug'gər-mug'gər) n. (1. a disorderly mess or muddle {syn. **imbroglio**}). 2. secretive behavior or concealment, chaotic or obsessive secrecy. [early 16th C.? origin (a ricochet word like higgledy-piggledy {a partial syn.}, or willy-nilly. Cf. hubbub)]. adj. 1. confused or jumbled. 2. clandestine or secret. **huggermugger/hugger-mugger** vt. = to keep something secret. **huggermugger/hugger-mugger** vi. = to behave in a secretive, clandestine manner. See **mentality, mentation, behavior**.

hunkerousness (hunk'kər-us-ness") n. opposition to progress; **old-fogyism**, q.v. [< *hunker* (U.S.) as used familiarly, initially in the New York region, to designate a surly, crusty, or stingy old fellow, a curmudgeon, but also to designate one who sticks to his post or home: hunkers down. In U.S. politics: applied as a nickname to a conservative, one opposed to innovation or change + suffixes]. n. **hunker** = an old fogy who opposes progress. See **old age**. See **old man**. See **role**. See **innovation, misoneism**.

hunks (hungkss)/**hunx** (hungk) s.n. a term of obloquy for a surly, cross-grained, crusty, bad-tempered old man; a close-fisted, stingy man, a miser; generally used with *close, covetous, niggardly,* or other uncomplimentary epithet—certainly not a "hunk" as understood currently, i.e., "beefcake": a very muscular, handsome, young, male-model type of guy. [appeared soon after 1600; origin unknown]. See **old man**.

hygieolatry/hygeiolatry (hī-gee-ol'lə-tree) n. an extreme observance of the laws of health; health fanaticism. [< G *hygieia* health + the suff. -latry, worship < G *latreia* worship]. See **health, illness**.

hypaesthesia/hypesthesia (hip-es-thee'zhə) n. diminished power of sensation or sensitiveness to stimuli; hypoesthesia; diminished sensibility. [< G *hypo* under + *aesthesis* feeling]. See **nerve, muscle, movement, touch**.

hypegiaphobia (hip"pə-jee"ə-fō'bi-ə) n. morbid fear of responsibility. [probably a variant of **hypengiaphobia**, q.v.]. adj. **hypegiaphobic**. n. **hypegiaphobe** (hip"pə-jee'ə-phob). syn. **hypengyophobia**, q.v. See **phobias**.

hypengyophobia (hī-pen"ji-ō-fō'bi-ə) n. morbid fear of responsibility. [< G *hypengyos* responsible + *phobos* fear]. adj. **hypengyofobic**. n. **hypengyiophobesy** (-fō'bə-see). n. **hypengiaphobe** (-pen'-). syn. **hypegiaphobia, paralipophobia**, q.v. See **phobias**.

hyper - pref. above, more than normal, beyond, over. [< G *hyper* above, over].

hypercholesterolemia (hī"per-kō-les"ter-ōl-eem'mee-ə) n. excess of cholesterol in the blood. [< hyper-, pref., q.v., + chole- (chol{o}-), pref., denoting relationship to the bile. < G *chole* bile + *stereos* solid + *haima* blood + -ia, suff.]. adj. **hypercholesterolemic**. n. syns. **hypercholesteremia, hypercholesterinemia**. adj. syns. **hypercholesteremic; hypercholesterinemic**. See **blood, circulation, glands**.

hyperglycemia (hī'per-glī-seem'mi-ə) n. abnormally increased content of sugar in the blood, especially with reference to a fasting level, and typical of diabetes. [< hyper-, pref., q.v., + < G *haima* blood]. adj. **hyperglycemic**. See: **blood, circulation & glands**.

hyperkeratosis (hī"per-ker-ə-tōs'siss) n. hypertrophy of the horny layer of the epidermis. This is common in the feet of the elderly, especially in those with bony changes resulting from **arthritides**, q.v. [< hyper-, pref., q.v., + kerat(o)- (also cerato-), pref., < G kerat(o), pref., denoting (1. the cornea) or 2. horny tissue or cells < G *keras*, gen. *keratos* horn + -osis, suff.]. adj. **hyperkeratotic**. syns. **keratosis**, q.v., **keratoderma, hyperkeratinization**. See **skin**.

hyperlipidemia (hī"per-lip"i-deem'mee-ə) n. a general term for elevated concentrations of any or all of the lipids in the plasma, including **hyperlipoproteinemia, hypercholesterolemia**, q.v., etc. [< hyper-, pref., q.v., + < G *lipos* fat + *haima* blood]. syn. **hyperlipemia**. See **blood, circulation, glands**.

hyperlipoproteinemia (hī"per-līp"pō-prōt"teen-eem'mi-ə) n. an excess of lipoproteins in the blood, due to a disorder of lipoprotein metabolism, and occurring as an acquired or familial condition. [< hyper-, pref., q.v., + < G *lipos* fat + *protos* first + *haima* blood]. See **blood, circulation, glands**.

hypermnesia (hī"perm-neez'zhə, -neez'zee-ə) n. unusually sharp memory; a vivid memory of impressions that seemed long forgotten. [< hyper-, pref., q.v., + < G *mneme* memory]. See **memory**.

hyperope (hī'per-ōp) n. one who is visually far sighted, i.e., can see distant things better than those nearby—a condition apt to develop with age. [< hyper-, pref., q.v., + < G *ops* eye]. n. **hyperopia** (hi"per-op'i-ə). syn. **presbyope**, q.v. See **eye**. See **role**.

hyperprosexia (hī"per-prō-seks'si-ə) n. 1. excessive sexuality. [< hyper-, q.v., + pro-, pref., in favor of < L *pro* for + *sexus* sex + -ia, suff.]. syn. **paraprosexia**, q.v. See **mentality, mentation, behavior**. See **sex, love**. 2. excessive, abnormal concentration on one thing (a phantonym). [< hyper-, pref., q.v., + < G *prosexis* attention < *pros-echo* to hold to]. See **mentality, mentation, behavior**. **intelligence**.

hypersomnia (hī"per-som'ni-ə) n. a condition, probably toxic, in which one sleeps for an excessively long time, but is normal when awake; it is distinguished from **somnolence**, q.v., in which one is always inclined to sleep. [< hyper-, pref., q.v., + < G *somnos* sleep]. See **sleep, wakefulness**.

hypersteatosis (hī"per-stee'ə-tō'sis) n. increased or excessive sebaceous secretion, as in **seborrhea**, q.v. Hypersteatosis of the face and chest is most common in the elderly. [< hyper-, pref., q.v., + steato-, pref., < G *stear* (*stear-)* tallow + -osis, suff.]. See **skin**.

hyperthermalgesia (hī"per-therm-al-jeez'zee-ə, -jeez'zhə) n. abnormally increased sensitivity to heat. [< hyper-, pref., q.v., + < G *therme* heat + < *algesis* pain]. See **nerve, muscle, movement, touch**.

hypesthesia (hip"es-thee'zee.ə, -thee'zhə): See **hypaesthesia**.

hypn(o)- pref., relating to sleep or hypnosis. [< G *hypnos* sleep].

hypnodia (hīp-nōd'di-ə) n. somnolence (constant unnatural sleepiness). [< hypn(o)-, pref., q.v., < ME *nodden* to bend the head forward, then raise it again; to be drowsy; very sleepy + -ia, suff., denoting condition < -ia, suff. denoting diseases or medical conditions < G -*ia* denoting action or an abstract]. See **sleep, wakefulness**.

hypnolepsy (hip'nō-leps'see) n. **narcolepsy**, q.v. [< hypn(o)-, pref., q.v., + < G *lepsis* a seizing]. See **sleep, wakefulness**.

hypnomogia (hip'nō-mōj'jee-ə) n. insomnia. [< hypno-, pref., q.v., + < G *mogis* with difficulty]. See **sleep, wakefulness**.

hypnopathy (hip-nop'pə-thee) n. sleep abnormality, disorder, or disease. • The aged are unusually subject to *hypnopathy*. [< hypn(o)-, pref., q.v., + -pathy, suff., meaning disease < G *pathos* suffering, disease]. adj. **hypnopathic** (hip-nō-paht'ik). See **sleep, wakefulness**.

hypnophobia (hip'nō-fōb'bi-ə) n. morbid fear of sleep (and not waking). [< hypn(o)-, pref., q.v., + < G *phobos* fear]. adj. **hypnophobic**. n. **hypnophobe**. See **phobias**. See **sleep, wakefulness**.

hypnophrenosis (hip'nō-fre-nōs'siss) n. a general term for any sleep disturbance. [< hypn(o)-, pref., q.v., + phren-, pref., meaning mind < G *phren* mind + -osis, suff.]. Cf. **hypnopathy**, q.v. See **sleep, wakefulness**.

hypnopompic (hip-nō-pom'pik) adj. pertaining to the fuzzy, semi-conscious state between sleep and wakefulness. [< hypn(o)-, pref., q.v., + < G *pompe* a sending away, sending home]. Cf. **semisomnous**, q.v. See **sleep, wakefulness**.

hypnosia (hip-nōs'si-ə) n. uncontrolled drowsiness. [< hypno-, pref., q.v., + -ia, suff., denoting condition < G -ia, suff., denoting action or an abstract]. See **sleep, wakefulness**.

hypnosophy (hip-nos'sō-fee) n. the study of sleep and its phenomena. [< hypn(o)-, pref., q.v., + < G *sophia* wisdom]. adj. **hypnophystic** (-nos"sō-fis'-tik). See **sleep, wakefulness**.

hypo-, pref. under; diminution or deficiency; the lower or least. [< G *hypo* under].

hypobulia (hī"pō-byool'li-ə) n. difficulty in acting, making decisions. [< hypo-, pref., q.v., + < G *boule* will]. adj. **hypobulic**. Cf. **abulia**. See **mentality, mentation, behavior**.

hypogonadism (hī"pō-gōn'nad-iz"əm) n. inadequate gonadal function as manifested by deficiencies in gametogenesis and/or the secretion of gonadal hormones, gonadotropin, testosterone. Celibacy may result. (In men, about 70% of those 70 years of age are hypogonadal. This results in a symptom complex of reduced muscle mass, strength, and cognitive function. Failure of the hypothalamic-pituitary axis to secrete gonadotropin results in decreased testosterone levels). [hypo-, pref., q.v., + < G *gone* seed]. adj. **hypogonadic**. syns. **ADAM syndrome**, q.v., (obs.) **hypogonadia** (-nad'di-ə), **hypogenitalism**. See **sex, love**.

hyposmia (hī-poz'mi-ə) n. a diminished sense of smell. Due to neural degeneration, the sense of smell starts to diminish gradually at about 50 years of age, but hyposmia can be due to a variety of causes, e.g., smoking, viral infection, head trauma. Gustatory (taste) function consists of fine taste, such as the ability to distinguish one type of meat from another, an **olfactory**, q.v., (nasal) function, and crude taste, e.g., sweet vs. sour, which is a lingual (tongue) function. adj. **hyposmic**. [hypo-, pref., q.v., + < G *osme* smell]. See **anosmia**, **dysosmia**. See **nose, smell**.

hyposomnia (hī"pō-som'ni-ə) n. lack of sleep; sleep for shorter periods than normal. [hypo-, pref., q.v., + < G *somnos* sleep + -ia, suff., denoting condition < -*ia*, suff., denoting action or an abstract]. See **sleep, wakefulness**.

hypothermalgesia (hī"pō-therm-al-jeez'zi-ə) n. abnormally increased sensitivity to cold. [hypo-, pref., q.v., + < G *therme* heat + *algesis* pain]. See **nerve, muscle, movement, touch**.

hypothymia (hī-pō-thī'mi-ə) n. profound melancholy or mental prostration. [hypo-, pref., q.v., + < G *thymos* mind + -ia, suff., denoting condition < -*ia* denoting action or an abstract]. See **emotion**.

hysteresis (his-tər-ees'siss) n. 1. the lag between cause and effect, e.g., the increasing lag time in the elderly between stimulus and response, i.e., reaction time or human latency, < L *latere* to lie concealed. • There is a *hysteresis* associated with retirement: The longer one is retired, the more working or professional skills are lost. (2. In physics, the lagging behind of an effect when its cause varies in amount, etc., especially of magnetic induction behind the magnetizing force.) [< G *hysterein* to come late, to be behind < *husteros* late, coming after]. See **health, illness**.

I

"I'm too young to retire and too old to go back to work"
—Barry Goldwater.

"I have measured out my life with coffee spoons."
—T.S. Eliot: "The Love of J. Alfred Prufrock".

iatrophobia (ī-at"trō-fōb'bi-ə) n. morbid fear of (going to) the doctor. [iatro-, pref., denoting relation to physicians or to medicine < G *iatros* physician + -phobia, suff., fearing < G -*phobia* < *phobos* fear]. adj. **iatrophobic**. n. **iatrophobe** (-at'trō-). Cf. **xeniatrophobia**, q.v. See **phobias**. See **health, illness**.

icterical (ik-tair'ri-kəl) adj. tinged with yellow. [< L *ictericus* jaundiced]. n **icterus** (ik'tair-əs) = jaundice. adj. **icteric** = jaundiced. Cf. **luteolous**, q.v. See **color**. See **skin**.

idée fixe (ide fiks) pl. *idées fixes* (ide fiks) n.phr. an idea that dominates the mind, monomania. • The dear old **fossil**, q.v., has an *idée fixe* that she is still a performing ballerina. [F, lit., fixed idea]. See **mentality, mentation, behavior**.

idio- (id'dee-ō) pref. denoting private, individual, proper, or distinctive. [< G *idios* one's own, private].

idiolalia (id"dee-ō-lay'li-ə) n. a mental state characterized by use of invented language. [idio-, pref., q.v., + < G *lalia* talk < *lalein* to talk]. adj. **idiolalic**. Cf. **glossolalia**, etc. See **talk**.

idiopathic (id"ee-ō-path'ik) adj. pertaining to a disease, medical condition of unknown cause: a state peculiar to the patient or which a physician can't diagnose. [< G *idiopatheia* subjective feeling peculiar to oneself < *idios* own, peculiar + *pathos* suffering]. n. **idiopathy** (id"dee-op'pə-thee). syn. = **essential**, not in the sense of necessary or indispensable, but "what it is by its very nature". See **health, illness**.

idiopt (id'di-opt) n. (rare) someone whose vision is less than perfect. [idio-, pref., q.v., + < G *ops* eye]. n. **idiopsia** (id"di-op'si-ə). Cf. **cecutient**, q.v., (if not cecutient). See **eye**. See **role**.

idiosyncrasy (id'dee-ō-sink'kra-see), pl. **–sies**, n. a way of behaving, thinking, or feeling that is peculiar to an individual or group, especially an odd or unusual one. 2. an unusual or exaggerated reaction to a drug or food that is not caused by allergy. • One's *idiosyncrasy* often becomes more prominent with old age. [< G *idiosugkrasia* personal mixing together < idio-, pref., q.v., + *krasis* mixing]. adj. **idiosyncratic** (-sink-kra'tik). adv. **idiosyncratically** (-kra'ti-kal-lee). Cf. **heteroclitic**, q.v. See **health, illness**. See **mentality, mentation, behavior**.

idioticon (id-dee-ōt'ti-kon) n. a dialect dictionary, i.e., one of words used in one region only. [< idio-, pref., q.v., + *lexicon*, a form of *lexicos* of words < *lexis* word < *legein* speak]. See **talk**.

ignavy (ig-nay'vee) adj. sluggish, lethargic, slothful. [L *ignave* listlessly, lazily]. See **sleep, wakefulness**. See **work, activity**.

illinition (il-li-nish'ən) n. 1. rubbing with liniment. (2. treatment of metals with corrosives; the crust produced by so doing.). [< L *illinere* to cover; to smear; to smear or spread something in + -tion, suff., an action or process, or the result of it < L –*tion*-]. See **therapy**. See **skin**.

im-, pref. = **in-** before b, m, and p. [in-, pref., privative < L *in*, a privative, i.e., that which expresses negation].

immorigerous (im"mawr-ij'jer-əss) adj. (obs.) unyielding, inflexible, set in one's ways. [im-, pref., q.v., + < L *morigerus* < *mor-*, *mos* custom, humor + *gerere* to bear, carry (after the L phrase *morem gerere* to humor, to comply with the wishes of a person) + -ous, suff.]. See **mentality, mentation, behavior**.

immortel (imɔrtɛl) n.m. immortality. 1. (fig.) an artistic image of remembrance after death. (2. a. a member of the French Academy. b. {pl.} the immortals, the gods.) 3. n.f., *immortelle* (imɔrtɛllə), everlasting: a shortening of *fleur immortelle* (flœr imɔrtɛllə), or E, immortelle (im-mawr"tel'), an undying plant, flower. [F, *im-*, pref., q.v., + *mortalis* < *mors, -rtis* death]. See **end of life, death**.

immune senescence (im-myoon' sə-nes'sənz) n.phr. the progressive dysfunction of the immune system with age. Clinically this results in an increasing and important number of age-related disorders: allergic reactivity, reactivation of infectious diseases, response to immunization, impaired recognition of cancer cells, dysglobulinemia and T-lymphocyte dysfunction, increased autoantibody production, age-related degenerative disease, etc. [< L *senescent-*, pres.p. of *senescere* to grow old; decline, become feeble, lose strength; to wane, draw to a close < *senex* advanced in age, aged, old; n. = old man; old woman]. See **old age**. **Blood, circulation, glands**.

immure (im-myoor') vt. 1. to lock up, to confine, to imprison. 2. to build into or entomb within a wall. ● She was convinced her family immured her in that nursing home. [< L *immurare* to wall in < im-, pref., q.v., + *murus* wall]. See **end-of-life, death**.

impassible (im-pas'sə-bəl) adj. 1. insusceptible to pain or suffering or injury. 2. unfeeling, incapable of feeling emotions. ● **Superannuation**, q.v., had seemingly reduced her to an *impassible* state. [< L *impassibilis* "not feeling" < im-, pref., q.v., + *passibilis* < *pass-*, pp. of *pati* suffer + -ble, suff.—passible = capable of feeling or suffering]. n. **impassibility**. n. **impassibleness**. adv. **impassibly**. See **emotion**.

importunate (im-pawr'choo-nət) adj. 1. making insistent requests, especially in a forceful, troublesome manner. 2. requiring immediate attention and action. [< L *importunari* < *importunus* inconvenient, unseasonable < *Portunus*, god of harbors]. adv. **importunately.** n. **importunateness.** See **talk**. See **emotion**.

importune (im-pawr'chən, im-pər-toon') vt. 1. to ask continually, repeatedly, or forcefully in a troublesome way. (2. to ask to have sexual relations in exchange for money.) • The **dowager**, q.v., daily *importuned* the resident-home's staff for their immediate attention to her suspect needs. [< L *importunari* < *importunus* inconvenient, unseasonable < *Portunus*, god of harbors]. adj. **importunate.** n. **importunacy** (-pawr'chən-nəs-see). adv. **importunely.** n. **importuner.** See **importunate**. See **talk**. See **emotion**. See **role**.

importunity (im''pər-toon'nə-tee) n. (pln. **-ties**) 1. the fact of being troublesomely demanding or insistent. 2. a demand made repeatedly or insistently. [See **importune**]. See **emotion**. See **talk**.

impotentia (L = im-paw-ten'tee-aa; E = im-pō-ten'shə) n. 1. impotence, i.e., weakness, lack of power. 2. in men, specifically, inability to copulate, cohabit (*impotentia coeundi* {< *coire* to come together, to combine; to mate, copulate}) due to inability to achieve penile erection (*impotentia erigendi* {< *erigere* to set up straight, to straighten out, erect}), or to achieve ejaculation, or both. This dysfunction may be due to neurological, psychological, or emotional factors, and can imply inability to reproduce (*impotentia generandi* {*genero*, -*are* to beget, procreate}). • *Impotentia* and old age are fellow travelers. [L, < *in*-, pref., q.v., + *potentia* power < *potens* (-*ent*-) powerful]. See **genitourinary**. See **nerve, muscle, movement touch**. See **emotion**. See **sex, love**.

imprecate (im'prə-kayt) vti. to call down or invoke (harm, an evil, or a curse) upon a person. [< L *imprecari* < im-, pref., q.v., + *precari* to entreat < *prec*- stem of *prex* prayer]. n. **imprecation** (im''-prə-kay'shən). n. **imprecator.** adj. **imprecatory** (-kay'tawr-ee). See **talk**. See **role.**

improcreant (im-prō-kree'ənt) adj. impotent. [im-, pref., q.v., + < L *procreare* to beget < pref. pro- before, precursor < L & G pro- before + *creare* to create]. See **genitourinary**. See **sex, love**.

in-, pref. 1. privative, not. [< L *in*- pref., expresses negation].

in-, pref.—**im-** before b, m, and p. [L *in*, 1. a privative, i.e., that which expresses negation, not. 2. in, into, toward, within].

inaniloquent (in-an-il'ə-quent) adj. full of idle talk, babbling, or nonsense. [< L *inanis* inane + *loqui* to speak]. adj. **inaniloquous**. n. **inaniloquence** or **inaniloquation** (-il"ə-kway'-). adv. **inaniloquently**. See **talk**.

inanition (im-an-ish'ən) n.1. exhaustion caused by lack of food or water as a result of disease. 2. lethargy or lack of vigor, vitality. [< L *inanition* < *inanis* empty]. Cf. **cachexia**, q.v. See **health, illness**. See **tiredness, weakness**.

inappetence (in-ap'pə-tənss) n. lack of appetite. • *Inappetence is a frequent problem in the superannuated.* [< in-, pref., q.v., + < L *appetitus* desire < *appetere* to seek after < *petere* to seek]. n. **inappetency**. adj. **inappetent**. See **health, illness**.

incontinence (in-kon'ti-nenz) n. 1. inability to prevent the discharge of any of the excretions, especially of urine or feces. This can be "active" with normal bladder size and capacity, or "passive", i.e., "overflow incontinence", e.g., with continuous over distention of the bladder, or "paradoxical" with discontinuous overflow, both with dribbling of urine. 2. Lack of restraint of the appetites, especially of the sexual appetite; Cf. **intemperance**. [< L *incontinentia* < in-, pref., q.v., + *contineo* to hold together < *con-* with + *teneo* to hold]. syn. **incontinentia**—*incontinentia alvi*, q.v. = incontinence of feces, fecal incontinence. See **genitourinary**. See **gastrointestinal**.

incontinentia alvi (in"kawn-ti-nen'ti-aa, or –nen'shə, al'vī) n.phr. fecal incontinence. [L, *incontinentia alvi* < in-, pref., q.v., + *contineo* to hold together < *con-*, pref., with + *teneo* to hold + *alvi* belly, bowels, stomach]. See **gastrointestinal**.

incruental (in-kroo-en'təl) adj. bloodless. [in- pref., q.v., + < L *cruor* blood (< G mythology, *ichor* = the fluid flowing in the veins of the gods) that flows from a wound]. See **blood, circulation, glands**.

indocible (in-dos'si-bəl) adj. unteachable. [in-, pref., q.v., + < L *docere* to teach].

n. **indocibility** (-dos"si-bil'li-tee). syn. **indocile**, q.v. See **intelligence**. See **mentality, mentation, behavior**.

indocile (in-dos'-səl, -sīl) adj. resisting discipline or instruction. [in-, pref, q.v., + < L *docere* to teach]. n. **indocility**. syn. **indocible**, q.v. See **intelligence**.

inductile (in-duk'til) adj. unyielding, inflexible, rigid, unbending. [in-, pref., q.v., + < L *ductilis* that may be led < *ducere* to lead]. See **mentality, mentation, behavior**.

ingeminate (in-jem'i-nayt) vi.&vt. to repeat; to reiterate; to emphasize by repetition. • The nurse *ingeminated* instructions to the old biddy, but she remained **indocible**, q.v. [< L *ingeminare* vt. redouble; repeat, reiterate; vi. to redouble < in-, pref., q.v, + *geminare* < *geminus* twin]. See **talk**.

ingravescence (in-grə-ves'sənz) n. a worsening or increase in severity, especially of disease, medical condition, e.g., increasing, worsening health problems of the aged. [in-, pref., q.v., + *gravare* to weigh upon < *gravis* heavy]. adj. **ingravescent** = becoming worse. See **health, illness**.

inhume (in-hyoom') vt. (literary) to bury a dead body. [< L *inhumare* < in-, pref, q.v., + *humus* earth]. n. **inhumation** (in-hyoo-may'shən) n. **inhumer**. See **end-of-life, death**. See **role**.

innovation, misoneism: androgogy, caino(to)phobia/kaino(to) phobia, centophobia, ecesis, exallotriote, hunkerousness, kilobytophobia, Luddite, misocainea, misoneism/misoneistic, moss-grown, neophobia/neophobic, obsolescent, ossify/ ossific, prosophobia/prosophobic, technophobia, tropophobia, vicissitude, wonted.

innovation, misoneism: Subcategories

  I.   Adjustment to a new environment: **ecesis**
  II Customary: **wonted**
  III. Fears:
      1. Fear of change: **tropophobia**
      2. Fear of computers: **kilobytophobia**
      3. Fear of progress: **prosophobia/prosophobic**

4. Fear of the new: **centophobia, caino(to)phobia/ kaino(to)phobia, neophobia/neophobic**
5. Fear of technology: **technophobia**

IV. Foreign: **exallotriote**
V. Hatred:
    1. Of anything new: **misocainea, misoneism/ misoneistic**
VI. Obsolescence:
    1. Becoming obsolete: **obsolescent**
VII. Old fashioned: **moss-grown**
VIII. Opposing innovation: **Luddite, hunkerousness**
IX. The science of teaching adults: **androgogy**
X. To become rigidly conventional/becoming so: **ossify/ossific**
XI. Variable, unexpected change: **vicissitude**

insanable (in-san'nə-bəl) adj. unable to be cured. [in-, pref., q.v., + < L *sanare* to heal]. See **therapy**. See **health & illness**.

insomnia (in-som'nee-ə) n. sleeplessness, lack of sleep. [< in-, pref., q.v., + L *somnus* sleep]. n. **insomniac** (–ak) = a sufferer from insomnia. adj. **insomniac** = exhibiting, tending toward, or producing insomnia. syn. **insomnolence**, q.v. Cf. **somnipathy, parahypnosis**, q.v. See **sleep & wakefulness**. See **role**.

insomnolence (in-som'nō-lənz) n. insomnia. [in-, pref., q.v., + L *somnolentus* sleepy < *somnus* sleep]. adj. **insomnolent**. adv. **insomnolently**. syn. **insomnia**, q.v. Cf. **somnipathy, parahypnosis**, q.v. See **sleep & wakefulness**.

insusurration (in-sus"sər-ray'shən) n. (obs.) whispering in the ear; insinuation. [in-, pref., q.v., + < L *susurrare* to whisper < *susurrus* whisper: onomatopoeic]. See **talk**.

intelligence: abderite, *abus de faiblesse*, addled, addlepated, **Alzheimer's disease, anencephalia, anencephalotrophia, anility, anserine, ApoE4, aprosexia,** *apud se*, **bapineuzumab, blather/ blether, blateroon, blatherskate, blatherskite, blithering, CLU, cognition, cognitive dysfunction,** *compos mentis*, **dementia, desipient, dotage, dott(e)rel, dyscalculia, dysgnosia, dyslogia, dysmentia, dysphemia, ebriection, excerebrose, geromorphism,**

gormless, hebetude, indocibility, indocility, musard, noetic, nous, oligophrenia, Parkinson's disease, percipience, phrontistery, PICALM, pixilated, pneuma, prepresbyophrenia, presbyophrenia, presenile, presenile dementia, presenilin, presenility, progeria, pump head, purblind, Rember®, resipiscent, sagacious, sapient, senior moment, TOMM4, wooly

intelligence: Subcategories

I. In one's senses:
    1. Intelligence, common sense: **nous, pneuma**
    2. Perceptiveness: **percipience**
    3. Restored to sanity: **resipiscent**
    4. To be in one's senses: *apud se, compos mentis*
    5. Wise: **sagacious, sapient**
II. Out of one's senses:
    1. Alzheimer's Disease:
        a. Alzheimer-disease antibody: **bapineuzumab**
        b. Alzheimer-disease lipid-indicator gene: **ApoE4**
        c. Alzheimer-disease: other gene indicators: **CLU, PICALM**
        d. Alzheimer-disease early onset gene variant: **TOMM4**
        e. Alzheimer-disease treatment: **Rember®**
    3. Dementia:
        a. brain atrophy: **anencephalotrophia**
        b. onset of dementia: **geromorphism, prepresbyophrenia, presenile, presenile dementia, presenility, progeria**
        c. type of dementia: **Alzheimer's disease**
    4. Brainless: **anencephalia, excerebrose**
    5. Cognitive decline post cardiac-bypass surgery: **pump head, cognitive dysfunction**
    6. Dotage in a woman: **anility**
    7. Dull or stupid: **gormless, dyslogia, dementia, dysmentia**
    8. Loss of phonation or hearing due to intellectual deficit: **dysphemia**
    9. Mental breakdown: **ebriection**

10. Senile dementia: **presbyophrenia**, **dotage**, **Parkinson's disease**, **cognitive dysfunction**
11. Simpleton, silly, gullible person: **abderite**, **dott(e)rel**
12. Stupidity: **hebetude**, **oligophrenia**
13. Talking nonsensically: **blithering**
14. Thinking disorder: **addled**, **addlepated**, **dysgnosia**, **dotage**, **cognitive dysfunction**
15. Vague, fuzzy, disorganized: **wooly**

III. Of uncertain senses, mentality:
1. Absent-minded dreamer or fool: **musard**
2. Constant talker: **blateroon**
3. Exploitation of frailty associated with age, mental incapacity: ***abus de faiblesse***
4. Inability to pay attention: **aprosexia**
5. Mathematical impairment: **dyscalculia**
6. Momentary absent mindedness, befuddlement: **senior moment**
7. One who talks nonsense: **blatherskite**, **blatherskate**
8. Pertaining to the mind: **noetic**
9. Place for thinking: **phrontistery**
10. Resisting instruction: **indocility**
11. Senility gene: **presenilin**
12. Senselessly talking: **blather/blether**
13. Slightly crazy, whimsical: **pixilated**
14. Talking silly: **desipient**
15. Talking silly like a goose: **anserine**
16. Thinking: **cognition**
17. Unteachability: **indocibility**
18. Unwilling to understand: **purblind**

intestate (in-tes'tayt) adj. 1. not having made a legally valid will. 2. property, etc., not having been assigned to somebody in a legally valid will. [< L *intestatus* not having made a will < in-, pref, q.v., + *testari* to make a will]. n. **intestate** somebody who has died without having made a legally valid will. n. **intestacy** the state of not having made a will. See **finance**. **See end-of-life, death**. See **role**.

intractable (in-trak'tə-bəl) adj. stubborn or obstinate, not flexible, refractory; not easily led. [in-, pref, q.v., + < L *tractabilis* tractable <

tractare to handle]. n. **intractability** (-bil'li-tee). n. **intractableness.**
adv. **intractably.** See **mentality mentation, behavior**.

intransigent/intransigeant (in-tran'si-jənt) adj. uncompromising,
firmly refusing even to consider changing an attitude or decision,
especially in politics. [< F *intransigeant* < Sp. *los intransigentes* a
political party of extreme republicans < in-, pref., q.v., + < L *transigere*
to drive through, do, accomplish, come to an understanding < *agree*
drive, do]. n. **intransigence.** n. **intransigent** = an irreconcilable
person, especially in politics. See **mentality, mentation, behavior**.
See **role**.

invalescence (in-val-es'ənz) n. (rare) 1. being an invalid. (2. strength,
health, force. {inceptive of *invalere*}). [< L *invalidus* not strong < in-,
pref., q.v., + *validus* strong < *valere* to be strong + suff. –escence <
L verbs ending in –*escere* expressing the beginning of action]. See
health, illness.

invaletudinary (in-val"lə-too'din-nair"ee) adj. unhealthy. [< L
invalidus not strong < in-, pref., q.v., + *valetude* health + -ary, suff.].
n. **invaletudinarian** (-too'din-air'ee-ən) = a sickly, infirm, or feeble
person; a weakling. See **health, illness**. See **role**.

inveigh (in-vay') vi. to protest or criticize angrily; attack violently or
bitterly in words; revile. • The recent resident *inveighed* against many
of the attendants and routines in the retirement home. [< L *invehere*
carry in < *vehere* to carry]. n. **inveigher.** See **role**. See **talk**.

ipsedixitism (ip-see-diks'i-tiz"zəm) n. the authoritative, dogmatic
assertion of something as if it were fact. [< L *Ipse dixit.* He himself
said (it).]. n.phr. **ipse dixit** (ip-see-diks'sit) = something asserted
dogmatically and without proof. See **talk**.

iracund (īr'rə-kund) adj. easily angered. (Thomas Jefferson in his
"Decalogue of Canons for Observation in Practical Life" states, "When
angry, count ten, before you speak, if very angry, an hundred." Mark
Twain in parody advised, "When angry count four; when very angry,
swear.") [< L *iracundus* hot-tempered, quick-tempered, irritable; angry;
resentful]. syns. **irascible, lowering; dudgeon, choleric,** q.v. See
emotion. See **mentality, mentation, behavior**.

irascible (ir-as'sə-bəl) adj. of an irritable temperament, hot-tempered; easily annoyed—often associated with cantankerous old men. [< L *irascibilis* quick to anger < *irasci* to grow angry < *ira* anger]. n. **irascibility** (-bil'-li-tee). n. **irascibleness**. adv. **irascibly**. See **emotion**. See **mentality, mentation, behavior**.

irenicist (ir-ren'nə-sist) n. a peace maker; one who promotes a compromise, finds a third way, soothes hurt feelings. [< G *eirenikos* peaceable < *eirene* peace]. adj. **irenic**, **irenical**. adv. **irenically**. Cf. **dimbox**, q.v. See **role**.

irreverent (ir-rev'vər-ənt) adj. wanting in reverence; lacking in respect. [< L ir*reverent*- < pres.p *revereri* < *vereri* to be in awe of]. n. **irreverence**. adj. **irreverential** (-ren'shəl). adv. **irreverently**. See **religion, theology, morality**.

irrugate (ir'roo"gayt) vt. to wrinkle. [< participial stem of L *irrugare* to wrinkle < *ir*- = *in*- pref., q.v., before *r* + < L *ruga* wrinkle < *rugare* to become wrinkled]. See **skin**. See **physique, appearance**.

isolophobia (īs"sō-lō-fōb'bi-ə) n. morbid fear of being alone, of loneliness. Recently, a sense of loneliness in the elderly has been linked to, and found predictive of, dimentia, often with onset within three years (Holwerda, T. J., et al, J. of Neurology, Neurosurgery, and Psychiatry, Dec. 10, 2012.) [It *isolare*; Medieval L *insulo*, pp. *-atus* to insulate < *insula* island + < G *phobos* fear]. adj. **isolophobic**. n. **isolophobe**. syns. **autophobia**, **eremophobia**, **monophobia**, **solophobia**, q.v. See **phobias**. See **loneliness, solitude, silence**.

isonogamia (īs"sō-nō-gam'mi-ə) n. marriage between persons of the same or nearly the same age. [< G *isonomos* equality of laws, or of people before the law < iso-, pref., equal, uniform < G *isos* equal + *nomos* law + *gamos* marriage]. ant. **anisonogamia**, **dysonogamia**, q.v. See **marriage**.

itinerant (ī-tin'nər-ənt) adj. traveling from place to place, e.g., one homeless, or a worker seeking work. [< late L *itinerant*-, pres.p. of *itinerari* journey < *itiner*-, pref., way]. n. **itinerancy**. n. **itinerant**. adv. **itinerantly**. vi. **itinerate** = to move from place to place; to make a circuit (L: *Solvitari ambulando*. = It is solved by wandering—said of itinerant scholars of medieval Europe). See **role**. See **work, activity**.

J

Jucundi acti labores.
(The recollection of past labors is pleasant.)
—Cicero. [L].

jabberwocky (jab'bur-wok-ee) n. meaningless speech or writing. [< "Jabberwocky", a nonsense poem by Lewis Carroll that was part of his novel, "Through the Looking Glass" (1871)]. Cf. **glossolalia**, etc. See **talk**.

jacent (jay'sent) adj. recumbent. [< L *jacere* to lie, lie down, lie flat, rest]. See **sleep, wakefulness**. See **tiredness, weakness**.

jactancy (jak'ten-see) n. boasting, bragging. [< L *jactatio* boast < *jactus* throw]. syns. **braggadocio, fanfaronade, gasconade, & rhodomontade**, q.v. See **talk**.

jactitation (jak-ti-tay'shun) n. 1. excessive twitching & restlessness. 2. loud or public bragging. (3. a false claim {law}.) [< L *jactitare* bring forward in public, boast < *jacere* throw]. See **nerve, muscle, motion, touch**. See **talk**.

jargoggle (jaar'gōg-gel) vi. to confuse, mix up. [?]. adj. **jargogogled**. Cf. **fuddle**. See **mentality, mentation, behavior**.

jeremiad (jer-ee-mī'ed) n. a woeful tirade; lament: often used sarcastically. [< "Lamentations of Jeremiah", a book in the Old Testament]. n. **Jeremiah** = a frequent or constant complainer. See **talk**. See **role**.

jobation (jō-bay'shen) n. tedious criticism; a rebuke, reproof, especially one of long and tedious character; a "talking to", a "lecture". [< the Bible: Job—an Old-Testament Wisdom book. (Dialectically rendered as *jawbation*, as if derived from *jaw*, *jawing*)]. vi. &vt. **jobe** = to rebuke, reprove, or reprimand, in a long and tedious harangue; to lecture. [< the ancient Hebrew patriarch, Job, in allusion to the lengthy reproofs addressed to Job by his friends. A **Job's comforter** is one with good intentions to comfort another in distress, but who succeeds only in exacerbating the situation]. See **talk**.

<u>joint, extremities, back</u>: acronyx, ankylosed, ankylosis, arthralgia, arthritis, arthrocele, arthrodynia, arthroendoscopy, arthrogryposis, arthroneuralgia, arthropathy, arthroplasty, arthrosclerosis, arthroscopy, arthroxerosis, callosity, callositas, charlie (charley) horse, chiropodist, chiropody, clavus, discalceate, Dupuytren's contracture, exostosis, exungulate, Heberden's nodes, heloma, heloma durum, heloma molle, keratoma, kyphosis, lassipedes, lordosis, Morton's neuroma, onychauxis, onychogryphosis/onychogryposis, osteoarthritis, osteoarthropathy, osteoarthrosis, osteochondropathy, osteopenia, osteoporosis, PLMD, podagra, podalgia, podarthritis, podiatrist, podiatry, pododynia, poroma, rheumatic, rheumatism, sacroiliitis, sciatica, spinal stenosis, spondyloarthropathy, spondylosis, steatopygous, sura, suralgia, surbate, surbater, tophaceous, tophus, tyloma, uratic arthritis.

<u>joint, extremities, back</u>: Subcategories

I. <u>Back</u>:
   1. Increased dorsal convexity of the thoracic spine: **kyphosis**
   2. Pain in lowermost back: **sacroiliitis**
   3. Ventral, anterior spinal curvature: **lordosis**
II. <u>Bone</u>:
   1. Reduced bone formation or increased reabsorption: **osteopenia**
   2. Reduced bone mass: **osteoporosis**
III. <u>Corn</u>: **callosity, callositas, clavus, heloma, heloma durum** (soft corn), **heloma molle** (hard corn), **keratoma, poroma, tyloma**
IV. <u>Foot & Leg</u>:
   1. A cause of sciatica: **spinal stenosis**
   2. Barefoot, barefooted; **discalceate**
   3. Calf of the leg: **sura**
   a. calf pain: **suralgia**
   4. Fat buttocks: **steatopygous**
   5. Foot doctor: **chiropodist, podiatrist**
   6. Foot doctoring: **chiropody, podiatry**
   7. Foot pain: **podalgia, pododynia, Morton's neuroma**
   8. Gouty pain in the great toe: **podagra**
   9. Inflammation of any of the tarsal or metatarsal joints of the foot: **podarthritis**

10. Muscle pain and spasm in the calf or anterior thigh: **charlie (charley) horse**
11. One who causes footsoreness: **surbater**
12. Periodic nocturnal leg movement: **PLMD**
12. Thigh, buttock, lateral leg pain: **sciatica**
13. Tired feet: **lassipedes**
14. To make or become footsore: **surbate**

V. Nails:
1. Ingrown fingernail or toenail: **acronyx**
2. Overgrowth and distortion of nails: **onychogryphosis/onychogryposis**.
3. Overgrowth of nails: **onychauxis**
4. To cut, trim the nails: **exungulate**

VI. Hand:
1. Contraction of palmar fascia causing finger flexion: **Dupuytren's contracture**
2. Nodules on the terminal finger joints in osteoarthritis: **Heberden's nodes**
3. Overgrowth and distortion of nails: **onychogryphosis/onychogryposis**
4. Overgrowth of nails: **onychauxis**

VII. Joints:
1. Affected with rheumatism: **rheumatic**
2. Any joint disease: **osteoarthropathy**
3. Chronic joint arthritis: **arthroxerosis**
4. Degenerative joint disease of bone and cartilage, and/or bone formation in cartilage: **osteochondropathy**
5. Degenerative joint disease of the spine: **spondylosis**
6. Disease of connective tissue, especially of joints and related structures: **rheumatism**
7. Disease of old age: **osteoarthritis, osteoarthrosis**
8. Medical examination of a joint's interior: **arthroendoscopy, arthroscopy**
9. Fused joint: **ankylosed**
10. Gout:
   a. arthritis: **uratic arthritis**
   b. gouty deposit: **tophus** (pl. = **tophi**)
   c. hard or gritty like tophi: **tophaceous**
11. inflammation of any of the tarsal or metatarsal joints of the foot: **podarthritis**

12. inflammatory disease of the joints of the spine: **spondyloarthropathy**
13. Joint disease: **arthropathy**
14. Joint inflammation: **arthritis**
15. Joint flexion or contracture: **arthrogryposis**
16. Joint pain: **arthralgia, arthrodynia, arthroneuralgia**
17. Joint stiffness or immobility or hardening: **ankylosis, arthrosclerosis**
18. Joint swelling: **arthrocele**
19. Plastic surgery of a joint: **arthroplasty**
20. Protruding bony growth: **exostosis**

jollop/jellop/jowlop (jol'ləp) n. an animal's (e.g., a fowl's, lizard's) dewlap or wattle (Wattle, properly, is restricted to animals.). Jollop is used comparatively and fig. in relation to persons. [apparently from jowl < ME *cholle* neck + lap, a hanging part, flap < OE *lappa*]. pp. **jolloped** = equipped with a jollop. Cf. **buccula, dewlap, wattle**, q.v. See **physique, appearance**.

juvenescent (joo-ven-es'sənt) adj. becoming youthful. • After a cosmetician's long labors the **grimalkin**, q.v., seemed to be *juvenescent*. [< L *juvenescere* to grow up; to get young again]. See **youth, younger generation**. See **physique, appearance**.

K

"I'm old enough to tell the truth. It's one
of the privileges of age."
—Georges Clemenceau.

kaino(to)phobia/caino(to)phobia (kayn"nō-fōb'bi-ə/kay-nōt"tō-) n. fear of novelty or of something new. [< G *kainos* new + -phobia, suff., fearing < G *phobos* fear]. adj. **kainophobic/cainophobic**. n. **kainophobe/cainophobe**. syns. **neophobia, centophobia**, q.v. Cf. **tropophobia** q.v. See **phobias**. See **mentality, mentation, behavior**.

Kaposi's sarcoma (kaa-pōs'sheez saar-kōm'mə) n.phr. a multicentric malignant vascular neoplasm affecting the skin and subcutaneous tissues and sometimes affecting other organs. Typically Kaposi's sarcoma occurs as an indolent tumor in elderly patients of Central European descent, especially men of Jewish or It ancestry. It is endemic in certain parts of equatorial Africa. It also occurs in immunosuppressed organ-transplant recipients, and in AIDS (acquired immune deficiency syndrome) patients. Herpes virus appears to have an etiologic role, particularly among immunosuppressed patients. It presents as one or more purple or dark blue macules (spots) that enlarge to become nodules or ulcers. (Merck Manual of Geriatrics). [< Moritz Kaposi Kohn, Austrian dermatologist, 1837-1902, and < G *karkinoma* < *karkinos* crab]. See **skin**.

Kegel's exercises (kayg'gəlss) n.phr. pelvic-muscle (mainly pubococcygeal) exercises for urinary incontinence from outlet incompetence, e.g., after radical prostatectomy, pelvic support disorders, urinary sphincter incompetence. [< the originating physician, Dr. Arnold Kegel (1894-1981), who was a gynecologist]. See **genitourinary**.

keratoacanthomas (ker'rə-tō-ay'kan-thōm'mə) n.pl. rapidly enlarging skin nodules, sometimes umbilicated, and with a smooth outline; they have a central keratin plug. They are usually benign, but are difficult to differentiate from squamous cell carcinomas. Left alone, untreated, they usually resolve spontaneously, but can leave a scar. [kerat(o)-, pref., denoting horny tissue or cells < G *keras*, horn + acantho-, pref., denoting relationship to a spinous process, or meaning spiny or thorny < *akantha* thorn + -*oma*, suff., tumor]. See **skin**. See **cancer, neoplasm, tumor**.

keratoma (ker-ə-tōm'mə) n. See **callosity**.

keratosis (ker-aa-tō'sis, ker-ə-) n. any lesion on the skin (epidermis) marked by the presence of circumscribed overgrowths of the horny layer. Keratosis is common in the elderly: **senile keratosis**., q.v., or **keratosis senilis**, q.v. [kerat(o)-, pref., < G *keras* horn, + -*osis* condition]. syn. = **keratoma** [kerato-, pref., < G *keras* horn + -*oma* tumor] = a **callosity**, q.v. See **skin**.

keratosis senilis (ker-aa-tōs'siss se-nil'liss) n.phr. See **senile keratosis**.

kilobytophobia (kil"lə-bīt'tə-fōb'bi-ə) n. morbid fear of learning about computers. Current statistics—< Pew Research Center/WSJ, 5/9/11 article: "My Grandparents R My BFF {Best Facebook Friends}" by Molly Baker—somewhat exonerate the elderly from kilobytophobia.

Currently, of those Americans 65+, 90% send/read email, 58% go online, 59% buy a product online, 34% use a social network; 29% send instant messages, 8% work on their own blog—4.4% of Facebook users are 65+, and some of them Skype. [kilo-, pref., a thousand, < G *khilioi* thousand + byte 1. a group of eight bits of computer information representing a unit of data, e.g., a number or letter, or 2. a unit of computer memory equal to that needed to store a single character; mid-20th C. < alteration of bite, a morsel, or an onomatopoeic acronym of "binary digit eight" + < G *phobos* fear]. adj. **kilobytophobic**. n. **kilobytophobe** (-bīt'tō-fōb). Cf. **cyberphobia, compuphobia**. See **phobias**. See **innovation, misoneism**.

kleptophobia/cleptophobia (klep"tō-fōb'bi-ə) n. morbid fear of thieves (or of becoming a thief). [< G *klepto* to steal + *phobos* fear]. adj. **kleptophobic**. n. **kleptophobe**. syn. **harpaxophobia**, q.v. See **phobias**.

klotho (klō'thō) n.1. a human gene that has to do with longevity. (It was first discovered by Japanese scientists in mice. Absence of Klotho's protein caused the rodents to develop arteriosclerosis, osteoarthritis, and emphysema—diseases common in elderly humans—and to die earlier). Changes in the "spelling" of the gene are associated with longevity and common age-related diseases in humans including coronary arterial disease and stroke. A Klotho allele, KL_VS, has been linked with a lower risk of coronary disease, stroke, and longer life. One hopes for two {one from each parent} "good" Klotho genes. (2. the name of one of the mythological G Fates—G *Moirae*—three sisters. Lachesis and Atropos were purported to spin the thread of life, whereas Klotho cut life's thread. Klotho could also renew lost life, as she did with Pelops, whose father, Tantalus, killed, cooked and served him for dinner to Zeus. Klotho brought Pelops back to life except for one of his shoulders, which had been eaten absentmindedly by Demeter, who was worriedly distracted about her daughter, Persephone, being in Hades. Klotho replaced Pelop's shoulder with one of ivory.) [< G *Klotho*]. Cf. **macrobian**, q.v. See **health, illness**.

kompology (kom-pol'lə-jee) n. (rare) braggadocio, boasting or vaunting speech. [< G *kompologia* < *kompos* boast + *-logia* speaking]. See **talk**.

kopophobia (kōp"pō-fōb'bi-ə) n. a morbid fear of exhaustion, overwork. [< G *kopos* fatigue + *phobos* fear]. adj. **kopophobic**. n. **kopophobe** (kō'pō-). syn. **ponophobia**, q.v. See **phobias**. See **tiredness, weakness**.

kvetch (kə-vetch') vi. (informal) to grumble, complain habitually, to whine, gripe all the time about most everything. [mid-20th C. < Yid. n. *kvetsh*, v. *kvetshn* to squeeze, punch < Ger. *Quetsche* crusher < MHG *quetschen* to crush < G *quetschen*]. n. **kvetch** or **kvetcher** = 1. someone who incessantly complains. 2. a complaint about something. See **talk**. See **mentality, mentation, behavior**. See **role**.

kyphosis (kī-fō'siss) n. abnormally increased convexity backward, posteriorly, of the thoracic spine's curvature as viewed from the side: humpback, or hunchback. **Osteoporosis**, q.v., is a frequent cause of kyphosis in the elderly. Kyphosis with exaggerated lordosis (swayback) in an older woman is called "**dowager's hump**". [G, humpback]. adj. **kyphotic** (-fot'tik). n. **kyphos** (kī'foss) = the hump itself in kyphosis. Cf. **lordosis**, q.v., & **scoliosis**. See **physique, appearance**. See **joint, extremities, back**.

L

"I have liv'd long enough: my way of lif/ Is fall'n into *the sear, the yellow leaf,*/ And that which should accompany old age,/ As honor, love, obedience, troops of friends,/ I must not look to have; but in their stead,/ Curses, not loud but deep, mouth-honor, breath,/ Which the poor heart would fain deny, and dare not."
—Shakespeare. **Macbeth**, V, iii, 22.

labefaction (la-bee-fak'shən) n. 1. a weakening, undermining, overthrowing—especially in reference to moral principles or the downfall of an established order. 2. used physically: a shaking or weakening. • *Labefaction* frequently accompanies **senescence**, q.v. [< L *labare* to totter + *facere* to make]. vt. **labefy** = to cause to totter (obs.). See **religion, theology, morality**. See **tiredness, weakness**.

labent (lay'bənt) adj. (obs.) slipping or falling. [< L *labent*- pres.p. of *labi* to fall]. See **religion, theology, morality**. See **tiredness, weakness**.

laconic (lə-kon'nik), **laconical** (lə-kon'ni-kəl) adj. using very few words; terse; concise. • He became increasingly *laconic* with age. [< G *lakonikos* of Laconia, Spartan < the reputation of the Spartans, who lived in Laconia (Lacedaemonia) for terseness]. adv. **laconically**. n. **laconicism**. n. **laconism**. See <u>talk</u>.

lagnesis/lagnosis (lag-nees'siss)/(lag-nōs'siss) n. 1. nymphomania. 2. satyriasis—"dirty-old-man" syndrome. [< G *lagneia* lust; coition— *lagneia furor* = extreme sex urge]. syn. **neanilagnia**, q.v. Cf. **shunam(m)itism**, q.v. See <u>sex, love</u>.

lalochezia (la-lō-keez'zi-ə) n. talking dirty to relieve tension; cursing or using foul language for its anxiolytic effect. [G *lalo-*, pref., denoting relationship to speech < *lalein* to babble, speak (*lalia* speech) + *chezo* to relieve oneself]. syn. **catarolysis**, q.v. See <u>talk</u>. See <u>sex, love</u>.

lalorrhea (lal-ō-rhee'ə) n. excessive flow of words. [< G *lalia* speech + *rhoia* flow]. See <u>talk</u>.

lamprophony (lam-prof'fə-nee) n. sonorous, loudness, and clarity of voice. • Age has caused the preacher to lose the *lamprophony* for which he was renowned. [lampro-, pref., < G *lanpro* bright, shining, + phon(o)-, comb. form, sound, < G *phone* sound, voice]. adj. **lamprophonic** (lam"prō-fon'nik). adv. **lamprophonicly** (lam"prō-fon'nik-lee). See <u>talk</u>.

languescent (lang-gwes'sənt) adj. becoming faint or tired. [< L *languens* languid, drooping, listless < *languere* to be tired, weary; weak, feeble (from disease); to be dull, languid, listless, without energy (fig.) + suff., -escent, beginning or inclined to be, becoming, < L –escent- pres.p. of verbs in –escere, expressing the beginning of action]. See <u>sleep & wakefulness</u>. See <u>tiredness, weakness</u>.

languid (lang'gwid) adj. lacking vigor, energy, or vitality; sluggish or slow-moving; feeble, apathetic; listless, indifferent. [< L *languidus* < *languere* be weak or faint]. adv. **languidly**. n. **languidness**. See <u>sleep & wakefulness</u>. See <u>tiredness, weakness</u>.

languish (lang'gwish) vi. 1. to undergo hardship as a result of being deprived of something, e.g. independence, freedom, or attention. 2. to decline steadily, losing vitality, strength, success. 3. to long, pine for something being denied. • Since being crippled and immobilized by arthritis, she *languished* perceptibly. [< OF *languiss-*, stem of *languir* < L *languere* be weak or faint]. n. **languisher.** n., adj. **languishing.** adv. **languishingly.** n. **languishment.** See **tiredness, weakness.** See **emotion.** See **role.**

languorous (lang'gər-əs) adj. lazily or pleasantly lacking vigor or vitality; listless and indifferent; sluggish, slow-moving, sullen. [< L *languidus* < *languere* be weak or faint]. adv. **languorously.** n. **languorousness.** See **tiredness, weakness.**

lao (low) adj. a respectful term, honorific used for older people. The term can apply equally to one's great-grandfather or the senior member of an assembly line or management team. • *Lao* Grandfather John, what do you advise? [Chinese]. See **old**

laolaiqiao/laolaiqiao Gaga (?/? gaa'gaa) n./n.phr. the terms refer to a new genre on Chinese video sites. In Mandarin, the reference is to old people doing young things that even young people might not do. Classic Gaga refers to meat garments, or otherwise odd costumes, and has the connotation of the English phrase "mutton dressed up as lamb", i.e., elders, e.g., wearing clothes more suited to youth. Gaga refers to an icon of modernity and youth. The idea behind the terms is that the young can better relate to the elderly, and can thereby relieve their loneliness. Gaga in the Huanese dialect means grandma. ("Week In Words": Erin McKean, Wall street Journal, 1/12-13/13.)

lapactic (la-pak'tik) n. a laxative, purgative. [< G *lapaktikos* < *lapasso* to empty]. syn. = **aperient**, q.v. See **gastrointestinal.**

laparoscopy (lap"pə-ros'kŏ-pee) n. examination of the interior of the abdomen by means of a laparoscope, an instrument comparable to an endoscope (or peritoneoscope) which, when inserted via a very small incision into the peritoneal cavity, permits it to be inspected, and instruments to be inserted. Many operative procedures on abdominal organs are currently performed laparoscopically in lieu of a laparotomy, i.e., sectioning of the abdominal wall (or flank). Laparoscopy can be "robotic assisted". [lapar(o)-, pref., denoting relationship to the loin or flank, or loosely in reference to the abdomen, < G *lapara* flank, + *skopein* to examine]. adj. **laparoscopic** (-kop'-pik). adv. **laparoscopically** (-kop'-pik-kəl-lee). See **gastrointestinal.** See **genitourinary.** See **therapy.**

lapsus calami (lap'sus kal'laa-mee) n.phr. slip of the pen; a mistake or inadvertence in writing. [L, *lapsus* blunder, error, fault + *calamus, -i* pen]. See **memory**. See **mentality, mentation, behavior**.

lapsus linguae (lap'soŏs lin'gwī) n.phr. slip of the tongue. [L, *lapsus* blunder, error, fault + *lingua, -ae* tongue]. syn. ***lubricum linguae***, q.v. See **memory**. See **mentality, mentation, behavior**. See **talk**.

lardy (laar'dee) adj. (obs.) fat. [< L *lar(i)dum, -i* lard, bacon fat]. syns. **adipose, pinguid**, q.v. Cf. **fubsy**; **abdominous, ventricous**; **pursy**, q.v. See **physique, appearance**.

larmoyant (laar-moy'yənt) adj. 1. tearful. 2. melancholic. [F, *larmoyant*, pres. p. of *larmoyer* to be tearful < *larme* tear]. syn. **lachrymose**. See **emotion**.

lassipedes (las-sip'pid-eez) n.pl. tired feet. [< L *lassus* tired, weary, fatigued, exhausted < *lassare* to fatigue, exhaust + *pes* foot]. See **tiredness, weakness**. See **jont, extremities, back**.

latibulize (la-tib'yoo-līz) vi. to hibernate. [< L *latibulum* hiding place, hide-out, lair, den; refuge]. Cf. **aestivate/estivate**; **torpor**, q.v. See **end-of-life, death**. See **sleep, wakefulness**. See **work, activity**.

latrinalia (la"tri-nayl'li-ə) n. talking dirty; using foul language, swearing, cursing. [< L *latrina*—derivation of the word latrine, a place for evacuation of bowels and bladder—contraction of *lavatrina* < *lavare* to wash + < G *lalia* a form of speech]. adj. **latrinalic**. Cf. **catarolysis**, **lalochezia**, q.v. See **talk**.

lécheur (leʃœr), f. ***lécheuse*** (leʃøz), n. 1. a gourmand, gourmandizer. 2. a devotee of oral intercourse. 3. a licker. [< F *lécher* to lick]. See **drink, food**. See **sex, love**. See **role**.

lector (lek'tor) n. 1. one who reads aloud to a religious congregation from the Bible. 2. a university lecturer. [L, reader < *lect-* pp. of *legere* to read]. See **role**. See **religion, theology, morality**. See **talk**.

lectual (lek'choo-əl) adj. bedridden. [< L *lectus* bed, couch; bier]. See **health, illness**.

legerity (lə-jer'ri-tee) n. nimbleness; agility. ● A loss of legerity (alegerity?) is a major complication of **agerasia**, q.v. [< F *legerèté* < *léger* light < L *leviarius* < *levis* light]. See **nerve, muscle, movement, touch**.

lenocinant (len-os'sin-ənt) adj. lewd. ● *Lenocinant* is an apt word to apply to a dirty old man. [< L *lenocinium* pandering, pimping; allurement, attraction; bawdy or gaudy clothes; flattery < *lenocinare* to be a pimp]. See **sex, love**.

lentigo maligna (len-teeg'gō maa-lig'nə) pigmented macules, often > 1 cm. in diameter, with an irregular border; they occur mainly on sun-exposed areas, particularly on the cheeks and forehead, and can have brown, black, red, and white areas; they expand radially. Development of nodules, and/or bleeding, is indicative of malignant (cancerous) conversion to **lentigo maligna melanoma** (mel-an-nō'mə). [L, freckle. + *maligna* spiteful, malicious, jealous, mean. + melan(o)-, pref., meaning black < G *melas*, gen., *melanos* black + -*oma* tumor]. See **skin**.

lentor (len'tawr) n. sluggishness (or tenacity). [< L *lentus* slow, sluggish, lingering]. See **tiredness, weakness**. See **health, illness**. See **work, activity**.

lepidic (le-pid'dik) adj. pertaining to scales. ● *Lepidic* skin on her hands and arms, particularly, was the price of many years playing golf in the sun. (2. pertaining to embryonic layers.) [< G *lepis*, gen. *lepidos* flake or scale]. aff. **lepid(o)-**, a combining form meaning scale or scaly. See **skin**.

lepidote (lep'pi-dōte) adj. covered with flaky scales, desquamating. ● Elders with **actinic keratosis**, q.v., are characteristically *lepidote*. [< G *lepis*, gen. *lepidos* flake or scale]. aff. **lepid(o)-**, a combining form meaning scale or scaly. See **skin**.

leptorrhine (lept'-tōr-rīn) adj. pertaining to a long, narrow nose. (The nose's shape, due mainly to gravitational effects, changes with age: The tip drops and the nose elongates and narrows in the elderly. [< lepto-, pref., slender, thin, or delicate, < G *leptos* slender, + rhin(o)-, comb., denotes relationship to the nose, < G *rhis* gen., *rhinos* nose]. See **nose, smell**. See **physique, appearance**.

leptosomatic (lep" tō-sō-mat'tik) adj. having a slender, light, or thin body. n. **leptosome** = a leptosomatic person. [< G *leptos*, thin, delicate, weak + *somatikos* bodily < *soma* body + -ic]. syn. **leptosomic**. See **physique, appearance**. See **role**.

lethe (lee'thee) n. oblivion, forgetfulness of the past. • ". . . a slow and silent stream,/ Lethe the river of oblivion . . ."—John Milton (1608-1674), "Paradise Lost". [G < classical mythology, a river in *Hades*, the underworld; all souls of the dead were required to drink from the river *Lethe* in order that they should completely forget the past: a draught (draft) of lethe]. See **memory**. See **end-of-life, death**.

lethiferous (lee-thif'ər-əss) adj. deadly, resulting in death, deadly; destructive. [< G *lethe*, q.v. supra, forgetfulness + < L *ferre* carry]. n. **lethiferousness**. See **end-of-life, death**.

lethologica (lee"thō-lōj'-ji-kə) n. inability to recall the precise word, *le mot juste,* for something; inability to recall words. • *Lethologica* is a characteristic of old age. [< G *lethe* forgetfulness + *logike* art of reason < *logos* word, reckoning]. n. **lethologiac**. Cf. **lethonomia**, q.v. See **memory**. See **role**.

lethonomia (lee"thō-nōm'mi-ə, leth"ō-) n. a tendency to forget, or inability to recall, names. [< G *lethe* forgetfulness + *nomos* name]. syn. **anomia**, q.v. Cf. **lethologica**, q.v. See **memory**.

levisomnous (le-vi-som'nəs) (obs., rare) adj. watchful, soon waked. [< L *levitas* lightness + *somnus* sleep]. n. **levisomnous** = light sleep. See **sleep, wakefulness**.

levophobia (leev"vō-fōb'bi-ə) n. morbid fear of the left, or of things to the left. [levo-, pref., denoting left, toward or on the left side < L *laevis* left + < G *phobos* fear]. adj. **levophobic**. • The old **cogger's**, q.v., politics were *levophobic*. n. **levophobe**. syn. **sinistrophobia**, q.v. ant. **dextrophobia**, q.v. See **phobias**.

lewdster (lood'stur) n. a lewd, i.e., offensively sexual, person. [< OE *lew(e)de* lay, i.e., not in holy orders]. adv. **lewdly**. n. **lewdness**. See **sex, love**. See **role**.

lexaphasia (leks-ə-fay'zhə, -zee-ə) n. word forgetfulness or misunderstanding. [< G *lexikon* of words < *lexis* word < *legein* speak

+ *aphatos* speechless (*a-*, priv. + *phatos*) < *phanai* speak]. adj. **lexaphasic**. See **memory**. See **talk**.

libido (li-bee'dō, li-bī'dō) n. 1. sexual drive. 2. in some theories, the psychic and emotional energy in people's psychological makeup that is related to basic human instincts, especially the sex drive. [early 20ᵗʰ C. < L, desire, lust]. adj. **libidinal** (lǝ-bid'i-nǝl). adv. **libidinally** (lǝ-bid'i-). See **sex, love**.

libidopause (lǝ-bid'dǝ-paws, -dō-paws) n. the time of life when the libido wanes and interest in sex declines, i.e., either in advanced age, or shortly after marriage; the word is used usually, if not exclusively, in connection with men. (Late in life, Sophocles, the Greek poet, declared his relief at being freed of sex, that "frenzied and savage master".) [< L *libido* desire, lust + *pausa* pause, stopping, cessation < G *pausein* to stop, cease]. Cf. **andropause, viripause**, q.v. See **sex, love**.

lichen simplex chronicus (lī'ken sim'pleks-chron'ni-kǝss) n.phr. an eczematous (characterized by papules {small circumscribed, superficial, solid elevations of the skin} and vesicles {small sacs containing liquid}) dermatitis due to repeated rubbing or scratching of the skin, and characterized by sharply demarcated, circumscribed, hyperpigmented, scaling, lichenified (thickened with accentuated markings) plaques of furrowed skin located most commonly on the face, neck, extremities, scrotum, vulva, and perianal region. It is common in the elderly. [< G *leichen* a tree-moss. + L, simple. + L, chronic]. syn. **neurodermatitis**. See **skin**.

limen (līm'men), pl. **limena** (lim'men-aa), n. a response threshold at which point a stimulus is sufficiently intense to effect a response. ● The old gentleman's hearing *limen* was not reached until someone yelled. (The "Limen of twoness" = the necessary distance between two points of contact on the skin for their recognition as two separate stimuli.) [L, threshold]. See **nerve, muscle, movement, touch.**

linguacious (lin-gway'shǝs) adj. (obs.) loquacious, talking a great deal. [< L *lingua* tongue]. See **talk**.

linsey-woolsey (lin'zee-wôol'zee) n. 1. (fig.) some strange medley; something disordered or nonsensical in speech or action. (2. dress material of coarse inferior wool woven on cotton warp {originally of wool & flax}). [15th C. < linsey, poss. < line, fine long flax separated from the tow, < OE *lin* < L *linum* + (obs.) *say* silk. + wool < OE *wull* < Gmc. *wullo* + a jingling termination]. See **talk**. See **mentality, mentation, behavior**.

lippitude (lip'pi-tood) n. (arch.) blepharitis ciliaris, i.e., a chronic inflammation of the hair follicles and sebaceous-gland openings of the margins of the eyelids; also called **bleareye**, **blearedness**, soreness or the eyes. • *Lippitude* is a problem associated with old age. [< L *lippitudo* running eyes, inflammation of the eyes < *lippus* blear-eyed, sore-eyed; blearedness]. n. **lippitudo** = inflammation of the sebaceous glands on the margin of the eyelids. See **eye**.

lipsanographer (hip"san-og'grə-fər) n. one who writes about relics, fig., about the elderly. • Her literary colleagues referred to her as "the *lipsanographer*" because of her writing so extensively about the elderly. [< G *lipsanon* a relic, remnant, < *leipein* to leave + -graph, suff., thing written in such a way, < G *graphos* written, writing + -er, suff., one versed in *graphos*]. n. **lypsanography**. adj. **lipsanographic** (-graf'fik). See **role**. See **old age**.

lipsanotheca (lip-san"nō-theek'kə) n. a shrine for holding relics. [<G *leipsanon* a relic, remnant < *leipein* to leave + *theke* a chest, shrine].

lirk/lerk/lurk (lirk) n. a fold in the skin; a wrinkle. [Sc & northern dial.]. v. **lirk** = to wrinkle. Cf. **rhagades**, **rugae**, **rugulosity**, q.v. See **skin**.

locust years (lōk'kəst years) n.phr. a period of economic hardship. • Meager retirement funds and increasing inflation often result in *locust years* for *les vieillards*, q.v. [collocation coined by Winston Churchill in reference to the financial recession of the mid-1930s in Britain < "the years that the locust hath eaten" < the Bible, Joel 2:25]. See **finance**.

log(o)-, pref., relating to speech or words. [< G *logos* word, discourse].

logagnosia (log"ag-nōs'see-ə) n. **aphasia**, q.v., **alogia**, q.v., or other central-nervous- system word defect; inability to speak, articulate. [log-, pref., q.v., + G *a-*, priv. + *gnosis* knowledge]. syns. **alogia**, **aphasia**. See **talk**. See **nerve, muscle, movement, touch**.

logagraphia (log"gaa-graf'fi-aa, log-gə-) n. inability to express ideas in writing. [log-, pref., q.v., + G *graphein* to write]. See nerve, muscle, movement, touch.

logamnesia (log"gam-neez'zhə, -neez'zee-ə) n. receptive aphasia, i. e., inability to understand written or spoken words, or tactile speech symbols, due to disease of the auditory and visual word centers in the temporal-parietal areas of the brain, as in word blindness; called also *impression aphasia, sensory aphasia, temporoparietal aphasia*, and *Wernicke's aphasia*. [log-, pref., q.v., + < G *amnesia* forgetfulness]. See memory. See talk. See nerve, muscle, movement, touch.

loganamnosis (log"gan-am-nōs'siss) n. an obsession with, mania for, trying to recall a forgotten word(s). [log-, pref., q.v., + < G *anamnesis* recollection + -osis, suff., a process, condition, or state, usually abnormal or diseased, < G suff., -*osis*]. See memory.

logaphasia (log"gaa-fay'zhə, -gə-fay'zee-ə)/**logophasia** (log'gō-fay') n. expressive aphasia, i.e. aphasia in which there is impairment of the ability to speak and write, due to a lesion of the cortical center of the brain. The patient understands written and spoken words, and knows what he wants to say, but cannot utter the words [log-, pref., q.v., + < G *phasis* speech]. syns. **ataxic aphasia, Broca's aphasia, motor aphasia, frontocortical aphasia**, and **verbal aphasia**. See talk. See nerve, muscle, movement, touch.

logasthenia (log"gas-thee'ni-ə) n. disturbance of that faculty of the mind that deals with the comprehension of speech. [log-, pref., q.v., + < G *asthenes* without strength + -ia, suff.]. See talk. See nerve, muscle, movement, touch.

logoclonia (log"gō-klōn'ni-ə)/**logoklony** (log'gō-klō"nee) n. spasmodic repetition of end-syllables of words. [logo-, pref., q.v., + < G *klonos* tumult + -ia, suff.]. See talk.

logodaedaly (log"gō-ded'də-lee)/**logodaeidale/logodaedalus** (-də-ləs), n. (obs.) verbal legerdemain, cunning. • The old **satyr**, q.v., employing with **dicacity**, q.v., an **equivoque**, q.v., said he would try *logodaedaly* to achieve his ends. [< logo-, pref., q.v., + *Daedalus* (G *daidalos* cunning). In G mythology, Daedalus was a craftsman and inventor who built a labyrinth on the island of Crete to house a half-bull, half-man monster: Minotaur. Daedalus made wings so that he could escape from Crete with his son, Icarus, but Icarus perished during the flight by flying, despite warning, too close to the sun, against his father's advice. The sun's heat melted his waxen wings.]. n. **logodaedalist**. Cf. **dicacity**, q.v. See **talk**. See **role**.

logokophosis (log"gō-kō-fōs'siss) n. (obs.) word deafness, auditory aphasia; inability to comprehend spoken language. [logo-, pref, q.v., + < G *kophosis* deafness]. Cf. **presbyacusis**. See **talk**. See **ear, hearing**.

logomania (log"gō-may'ni-ə) n. over talkativeness. [logo- pref., q.v., + < G *mania* madness]. adj. **logomanic** (-man'ik). adj. **logomaniacal** (-ma-nī'ə-kəl). n. **logomaniac**. Cf. **logomania**, **logorrhea**, **longiloquence**, **logomonomania**, **multiloquence**, **omniloquence**, **pleniloquence**, **polyloquence**, q.v. See **manias**. See **talk**.

logomonomania (log"gō-mon"nō-may'ni-ə) n. morbidly great loquacity. [logo-, pref., q.v., + < G *monos* one + -mania, suff, referring to an abnormal love for, or morbid impulse toward, some specific object, place, or action < *mania* madness]. adj. **logomonomanic** (-mən'ik). adj. **logomonomanical** (-mə-nī'ə-kal). n. **logomonomaniac**. syn. **logomania**, q.v. See **talk**. See **manias**.

logoneurosis (log"gō-noo-rōs'siss) n. any neurosis associated with a speech defect. [logo-, pref., q.v., + neuro-, comb., denoting nerve or relating to the nervous system < G *neuron* nerve + -osis, suff., condition]. adj. **logoneurotic** (-rot'tik). See **talk**. See **nerve, muscle, movement, touch**.

logopathy (log"gop'ə-thee) n. any disorder of speech arising from derangement of the central nervous system. [logo-, pref., q.v., + < G *pathos* illness]. See **talk**. See **nerve, muscle, movement, touch**.

logoplegia (log"gō-pleej'ji-ə) n. paralysis of the speech organs. [logo-, pref., q.v., + < G *plege* stroke]. See **talk**. See **nerve, muscle, movement, touch**.

logorati (log"gō-raat'tee) n.pl. people interested in or expert at words. ● The retired elderly, having more spare time, are more likely than the young to be *logorati*. [a neologism coined by William Safire < L *logos* word, after literati, directly or via It < L, *literati* lettered people, and digerati, people with expertise in computers, the Internet, and the

World Wide Web, < *digitalis* (any finger-like structure) < *digitus* finger, toe]. Cf. **wordsmith**. See <u>role</u>. See <u>talk</u>.

logorrhea (log"gə-ree'ə) n. excessive and incoherent talking, as seen in certain psychiatric disorders; "diarrhea" of the mouth. [logo-, pref., q.v., + < G *rhein* to flow]. adj. **logorrheic**. syns. & Cf. **longiloquence**, **logomania**, **logomonomania**, **logorrhea**, **multiloquence**, **omniloquence**, **pleniloquence**, **polyloquence**, q.v. See <u>talk</u>.

logospasm (log"gō-spaz'zəm) n. the spasmodic utterance of words. [logo-, pref., q.v., + < G *spasmos* spasm]. adj. **logospasmotic** (-mot'tik). adv. **logospasmotically**(-kəl-lee). See <u>talk</u>.

loneliness, solitude, silence: autophobia, burdalone, conticent, erem(i)ophobia, eremomania, isolophobia, monophobia, oikomania, silential, silentiary, solivagant, solophobia, taciturn, troglodyte, wallflower.

> **loneliness, solitude, silence**: Subcategories

    I.   <u>Fear</u>:
         1.   Fear of being alone, loneliness: **autophobia, erem(i) ophobia, Isolophobia, monophobia, solophobia**
         2.   Fear of oneself: **autophobia**
   II. <u>Silence</u>:
         1.   Abnormal interest in stillness: **eremomania**
         2.   Habitually saying little: **taciturn**
         3.   Keeper of silence: **silentiary**
         4.   Pertaining to or performed in silence: **silential**
         5.   Silent: **conticent**
  III. <u>Solitude</u>:
         1. Living in seclusion: **troglodyte**
         2.   One wandering alone: **solivagant**
         3.   Solitary person: **burdalone, wallflower**
         4.   Morbid desire to be at home: **oikomania**

longanimity (long"gan-im'mə-tee) n. (rare) 1. "Longanimity is an untired confidence of mind in expecting the good things of the life to come." (Blount, 1656). 2. suffering in silence over a period of time, while brooding on revenge. 3. patient bearing of injuries. • *Longanimity* is much more an elderly than a youthful trait. [< L *longus* long + *animus* soul, mind, spirit]. adj. **longanimous** (-gan'i-məs). See **mentality, mentation, behavior**.

longevity (lon-jev'i-tee) n. the condition or quality of being long lived. The oldest person alive today is said to be 116 years of age; the oldest person on record (Jeanne Calmet, who died in 1997) lived to be 122 years of age. Current life expectancy in the U.S. for Hispanics = 80 yrs., for blacks = 73 yrs., and for whites = 78 yrs. People aged 65 and over in the U.S., for the first time in history, will soon outnumber children less than five years of age, and elders' requiring pensions, health services, and long-term care will soon outnumber those adults still in the work force. A recent book, "The Longevity Project" by H. S. Friedman & L.R. Martin indicates the best childhood predictor of longevity is a personality considered conscientious and prudent, not one that is carefree. Parental divorce during childhood was found to be the single best predictor of early death—by five years on average—in adulthood. Having a high I.Q. or an advanced degree was unrelated to longevity. Adults who were physically active, gave to their community, had thriving, long-lasting careers, and a healthy marriage and family life were more likely to be long lived. A gene influencing longevity is **klotho**, q.v., and a chromosome end's length, its **telomere**, q.v., has important influence, also. [< L *longus* long + *aevum* age]. Cf. **biometry**, q.v. See **health, illness**. See **old age**.

longevous (lon-geev'vus) adj. (rare) living a long time, of great age; having lived to a great age. By disabling a single gene in worms, researchers have extended their lifespan by 6 to 10 times. Longevity of monkeys has been increased by caloric restriction. [L *longaevus*, of great age < *longus* long + *aevum* age]. syn. **macrobian**, q.v. See **old**. See **health, illness**.

longiloquence (lon-jil'lō-kwənz) n. long-windedness (in speaking). [< L *longe* at great length + *loqui* to say, speak, speak about, talk of, tell, declare]. adj. **longiloquent**. adv. **longiloquently** (-jil'lō-kwent"lee). Cf. **logomania**. See **talk**.

long in the tooth adj. phr. old, aged. [< the tendency of gums to recede with age thus giving the appearance of longer teeth]. See **old**.

lordosis (lor-dōs'siss) n. hollow back, saddle back, anteroposterior curvature of the spine, generally lumbar, with the convexity looking anteriorly. [G, *lordosis* a bending backward]. See **kyphosis**: **dowager's hump**. See **joint, extremities, back**.

lovertine (luv'ver-teen) adj. addicted to love-making. ● The **roué**, q.v., was noticeably *lovertine* although quite **long in the tooth**, q.v. [< OE *lufian* < *lufu* love < IE to love]. See **sex, love**.

lowering (lōr' or lowr'ing)/**louring** (lowr'ing) adj. 1. sullen, frowning, gloomy; angry. (2. being overcast and threatening storms, heavy rain.) [< ME *louring* < *louren* to frown; lurk]. adv. **loweringly**. vi. & n. **lower**. See **emotion**.

lubricum linguae (lub'ri-cum lin'guī) n.phr. slip of the tongue. [L, < *lubricare* to oil, grease, make smooth + *lingua* tongue; speech, language, dialect]. syn. *lapsus linguae*, q.v. See **memory**. See **mentality, mentation, behavior**. See **talk**.

luctiferous (luk-tif'fer-es) adj. sad and sorry. [< L *luctificus* causing sorrow, doleful, woeful < *luctus* sorrow, mourning, grief, distress; signs of sorrow]. Cf. **lypemanic, lypomanic, lypothymic**. See **emotion**.

lucubration (look"kyoo-bray'shen, -kye-bray-) n. 1. nocturnal study or meditation; literary work, especially of pedantic or elaborate character and requiring a great deal of study, work. 2. laborious work. ● Her neurologic deficit caused her considerable *lucubration* just in signing her name. 3. long hard study. vi. **lucubrate** (look'kyoo-brayt, -ke-brayt). [L, < *lucubrare* work by lamplight < *lux* light + -ation, suff.].

Luddite (lud'dīt) n. someone fanatically opposed to technological innovation, e.g., machines, computers that displace laborers. [< Ned Ludd, a **misoneist**, q.v., of 18ᵗʰ C. England. Luddites was the name taken by textile workers in England during 1811-1816. They destroyed machinery that was displacing them. Ned Ludd's identity is not clear, but he is said to have destroyed, in a fit of insanity, a knitting frame in 1779. In response to the Luddites, the British parliament passed the Frame Breaking Act which made the destruction of knitting frames punishable by death]. See **innovation, misoneism**. See **role**.

lugubrious (loo-goo'bri-es) adj. dismal, mournful, gloomy, especially in an exaggerated manner. ● The old **biddy's**, q.v., reaction was *lugubrious* to the point of embarrassment. [< L *lugubris* < *lugere* mourn]. adv. **lugubriously**. n. **lugubriousness**. n. **lugubriosity** (-os'si-tee). See **emotion**.

lupanarian (loo-pə-ner'ri-ən) adj. lascivious, lewd, and lubricious. [< L *lupanar*, n. a brothel + -ian, suff., belonging to, coming from, being involved in, etc., via F -*ian* < L -*ianus*]. See **sex, love**.

luscition (loos-si'shən) n. poor eyesight. [< L *luscitiosus* purblind, partly blind]. syn. **purblind**, q.v., See **eye**.

lutein/luteine (loot'tee-in/loo'teen") n. a carotenoid found in green, leafy vegetables such as spinach, kale, in egg yolk, animal fats, in the human corpus luteum (area of the brain), and in the macula (central vision area) of the eye. It's an antioxidant said to protect against high energy (blue and near-ultraviolet) light, oxidative stress, and macular degeneration in the aged. Six mgs./day is adequate in the diet. Some carotenoids have vitamin A activity and can be converted to retinal, an anti-oxidant. Excess lutein can cause bronzing of the skin, i.e., **carotenoderma**. [< L *luteus* yellow]. See **eye**.

luteolus (loo-tee'ō-ləs) adj. yellowish. • The *luteolus* cast to the **nonagenarian's**, q.v., skin certainly suggested jaundice. [L, yellowish < *luteus* yellow]. Cf. **icterical, flavescent, feuillemorte**, q.v. See: **color**. See: **skin**.

lypemania (lī-pee-may'ni-ə) n. melancholia. [< G *lype* pain, grief + -*mania*, suff., < G frenzy]. adj. **lypemanic** (-man'ik). syn. **lypomania, lypothymia**, q.v. Cf. **lypophrenia**. See **manias**. See **emotion**.

lypophrenia (lī-pō-freen'ni-ə) n. a vague feeling of sadness, seemingly without cause. [< G *lype* pain, grief + -phrenia, suff., denoting the mind (or the diaphragm) < G *phren* the diaphragm, heart, seat of emotions, mind]. adj. **lypophrenic** (-fren'ik). Cf. **lypemania, lypothymia**, q.v. See **emotion**.

lypothymia (lī-pō-thī'mee-ə) n. melancholia. [< G *lype* pain, grief + -thymi, suff., denoting mind, soul, or emotions < *thymos* the mind]. adj. **lypothymic**. Cf. **lypemania**, q.v. See **emotion**.

M

"I don't feel old. I don't feel anything until noon.
Then it's time for my nap."
—Bob Hope.

macilent (mas'sil-ənt) adj. lean, thin. • A *macilent* appearance; weight loss; sadness; eating, grocery-shopping, and food-preparation problems; along with abnormally low cholesterol and serum albumin levels all suggest malnutrition in the elderly. [< L *macer* lean & *macilentus* lean]. See **physique, appearance**.

mackabroin (mak'kə-broyn) n. (obs.) an old hag; a hideous old woman. [obscure]. See **old woman**.

macrobian (ma-krōb'bi-ən) adj. long-lived. [macro- pref., large, long, < G *macros* large + *bios* life]. n. **macrobiosis** (mak"krō-bī-ōs'siss) = **longevity**, q.v. n. **macrobiote** = an organism—e.g., a person—that or who is long-lived. Cf. **klotho**, q.v. syn. **longevous**, q.v. See **health, illness**. See **role**. See: **old**. See **old man**. See **old woman**. See **old person(s)**.

macrorhinia (mak"rō-rīn'nee-ə) n. excessive size of the nose. (The nose enlarges with age, as do the ears, **macrotia**, q.v., but the size of the eyes remains the same throughout life.) (Perhaps the best known literary example of *macrorhinia* is that of Cyrano, in the 1897 play, *Cyrano de Bergerac*, by Edmond Rostand.) [macr(o)-, pref., large, or of abnormal size or length < G *makros* large, long + *rhis* nose + -ia, suff.]. syn. **nasute**, q.v. Cf. **leptorrhine**, **rhinophyma**, q.v. See **nose, smell**.

macrotous (mak-rōt'tess) adj. having large ears, i. e., large pinnae or auriculae (external ears). • Ears are apt to be *macrotous* in the elderly since they do slowly enlarge with age, as does the nose (**macrorhinia**, **nasute**, q.v.), but the eyes remain the same size throughout life. [macro- pref., large, long < G *macros* large + ot-, pref., relating to the ear < *ous* ear]. n. **macrotia** (ma-krō'shə). See **ear, hearing**. See **physique, appearance**.

macular degeneration (mak'kyoŏ-laar, -kyə-lər) n.phr. deteriorative changes resulting in a decrease and loss of function of tissue in the *macula retinae* or *macula lutea* (yellow), an irregular yellowish depression of the retina, about 3 degrees wide, lateral to and slightly inferior to the optic disk, the origin of the optic nerve. [L *macula* spot, stain, blemish & *degereratio* degeneration]. The macula is the site of absorption of short wavelengths of light and of the most acute vision and color perception. Degeneration results in loss of visual acuity, blindness. Macular degeneration is associated with aging, **AMD** (**a**ge-related **m**acular **d**egeneration), and is of two types: wet and dry. High blood pressure and smoking are risk factors for AMG. (David Levine {1920-2010}, the noted artist and caricaturist, was a victim of macular degeneration and said, "I always knew I was a degenerate, but didn't know it was macular." See **eye**.

maculopathy (mak"kyoo-lop'pə-thee) n. a series of old-age-related pathologic changes in the macula accompanied by decreased visual acuity; **macular degeneration**, q.v. (There are "wet" and "dry" types.) [< L *macula* spot + -pathy, suff., meaning disease, < G *pathos* disease, suffering]. See **eye**.

madarosis (mad"də-rōs'siss) n. loss of hair, especially of the eyebrows or eyelashes. [G, *madarosis*, *madaros*, bald, *madaein* to fall off (of hair)]. See **eye**. See **hair**.

maffle (maf'əl) (obs., except dial.) vi. to speak indistinctly, mumble, or stutter; to blunder, bungle; to waste time. [Origin is uncertain. Cf. Du *maffelen*, to move the jaws]. vt. **maffle** = to confuse. ppl. adj. **maffled** = confused. See **talk**.

maggot (mag'gət) n. 1. (archaic) a whimsical, nonsensical, or perverse fancy, odd fad, crotchet. • There may be bats in our belfry, and we may be bugs about peace and quiet, but not all seniors have such *maggots*. (2. a larva, legless grub, of certain insects of the order Diptera, e.g., houseflies, mosquitoes, gnats.) [1. OE *maggot*, a variant of *maddock*? < the ancient folklore attributing odd or whimsical behavior to having maggots (the grub type) in the brain: "Are you not mad, my friend!? What time o' th'moon is 't? Have you not maggots in your brain?"—*Women Pleased*, John Fletcher (1584-1616) < N.W. Schur, q.v. Cf. "bats in the belfry"]. See **mentality, mentation, behavior**.

magniloquent (mag-nil'lə-kwənt) adj. boastful, pompous, full of hot air; employing impressive words and an exaggeratedly solemn and dignified style. [< L *magniloquos* < *magnus* great + -*loquus* speaking]. See **talk**.

magpie (mag'pī) n. 1. (fig., informal) an incurable chatterer. 2. (fig., informal) an enthusiastic or compulsive collector, especially of small objects. 3. a chattering bird of the crow family—by inference, an idle chatterer. (4. an Australian song bird.) [late 16ᵗʰ C. < *Mag*, shortening of the name *Margaret* + *pie* < 14ᵗʰ C.?]. See **talk**. See: **mentality, mentation, behavior**.

mah-jongg (maa-zhong', -jong') n. a game of Chinese origin played with 144 small decorated—featuring birds, flowers, Chinese characters—tiles of bone or ivory, and more recently of plastic. Usually there are four players, who, in the U.S., are typically elderly women. They sit around a square table; betting may or may not be involved. In very recent years the game has attracted young women, also. American mah-jongg is somewhat different from its Chinese progenitor. [Early 20ᵗʰ C. < Chinese dialect *ma jiang* sparrows]. See **work, activity**.

malacodermous (mal"lə-kō-dur'məs) adj. 1. soft-skinned. 2. (fig.) quick to take umbrage. [malaco-, pref., soft or softening < G *malakos* soft; *malakia* a softness, + derm-, a combining form signifying skin < *derma* skin]. See **skin**. See **mentality, mentation, behavior**.

malactic (mə-lak'tik/ maa') n. an **emollient**, q.v., medication. adj. softening, emollient. [malac(o)-, pref., < G *malakos* soft]. See **skin**. See **therapy**.

malapert (mal'ə-purt) adj. boldly disrespectful to a person of higher standing, e.g., to an elder; impudent in speech or behavior. • The *malapert* teenager's behavior toward her dowager grandmother was despicable. [< OF not experienced < L *malus* bad + *expertus* pp. of *experiri* try out, alt. < ME *apert*, arch., insolent]. n. **malapert**. n. **malapertness** (mal"ə-purt'ness). adv. **malapertly**. See **mentality, mentation, behavior**.

malnoia (mal-noy'yə) n. a vague feeling of mental discomfort. • *Malnoia* was also to feature in her closing years. [mal-, pref., ill or bad < L *malus* evil + < G *nous* mind—as in the G *paranoia* out of one's mind]. See **mentality, mentation, behavior**.

mammothrept (mam'mō-thrept) n. 1. a child brought up by its grandmother. 2. a spoiled child. [G, raised by one's grandmother]. See **youth, younger generation**. See **role**.

manducable (man-dyook'kə-bəl) adj. chewable or edible. [< L *manducare* to chew]. See **mouth, gums, teeth**. See **drink, food**. **-mania** (mayn'ni-ə) suff. excessive enthusiasm for or attachment to. [G *mania* loss of reason, frenzy, madness < *mainesthai* to rage].

manias (may'ni-əs) pl.n. emotional disorders characterized by great psychomotor activity, excitement, a rapid passing of ideas, exaltation, and unstable attention. [< G *mania*, frenzy, madness]: **aidoimania, alcoholomania, clinomania, coimetromania, cretomania, dipsomania, dromomania, ecdemomania, ecomania, edeomania, enosimania, entheomania, eremiomania, ergasiomania, ergomania, erotomania, gynecomania, hamartomania, hieromania, logomania, logomonomania, lypemania, methomania, misomania, monomania, necromania, nosomania, nostomania, oenomania, oikomania, onomatomania, opsomania, phaneromania, pharmacomania, philopatrodomania, poriomania, posiomania, satyromania, sideromonomania, thanatomania**.

manias: Subcategories

I.   Abnormal Interest in, or a craving for:
1. Cemeteries, graves: **coimetromania**
2. Certain words: **onomatomania**
3. Alcohol: **alcoholomania, dipsomania, methomania, posiomania**
4. Sin: **hamartomania**
5. Stillness: **eremiomania**
6. Wine: **oenomania**
7. Traveling by railroad: **sideromonomania**

II. Belief:
1. Abnormal belief that one is inspired: **entheomania**
2. Belief one has sinned unpardonably: **enosimania**
3. Incorrect belief one has a certain disease: **nosomania**

III. Compulsion, obsession, preoccupation:
1. Compulsive wandering: **ecdemomania, poriomania**
2. Longing for or compulsive traveling: **dromomania**

3. Obsessive over talkativeness: **logomania, logomonomania**
4. Obsessive picking at scabs or growths on the skin: **phaneromania**
5. Religious insanity: **hieromania**
6. Preoccupation with death: **thanatomania**
7. Preoccupation with dead bodies: **necromania**
8. Preoccupation with one subject, idea: **monomania**
9. Preoccupation with visiting cemeteries, graves: **coimetromania**
10. Trying frantically to recall a certain word: **onomatomania**

IV. Desire, craving:
1. Abnormal desire to be at home: **ecomania, oikomania**
1. Craving for a certain food or seasoned food: **opsomania**
3. Craving for alcohol: **alcoholomania, dipsomania, methomania, posiomania**
4. Excessive desire to stay in bed: **clinomania**
5. Overeagerness to be at work: **ergasiomania, ergomania**
6. Strong or abnormal sexual desire:
   a. in man or woman: **aidoimania, edeomania, erotomania**
   b. in a man: **cretomania, gynecomania, satyromania**
7. Uncontrolled desire to take or administer drugs: **pharmacomania**
8. Wanderlust: **poriomania**

IV. Extreme:
1. Extreme homesickness: **nostomania, philopatrodomania**
2. Over talkativeness: **logomania, logomonomania**

V. Hatred:
1. Hatred of everything: **misomania**

VI. Melancholia: **lypemania**

VII. Neurosis:

1. neurosis dependent on home environment: **ecomania**, **oikomania**

manqué, -e (f.) (măкe, -ə) adj. unfulfilled, might-have-been, missed, unsuccessful, abortive, frustrated in fulfillment of one's ambitions. • She was an operatic diva *manquée*. [F pp. of *manquer* fail, lack < L *mancus* maimed]. See **mentality, mentation, behavior**.

mansuetude (man'swee-tood) n. tameness, gentleness, mildness, meekness. [< L *mansuetudo* mildness, gentleness]. See **mentality, mentation, behavior**.

marasmus (mə-ras'məss) n. a wasting away of the body. [< G *marasmos, marainein* to decay]. adj. **marasmic**. See **health, illness**. See **physique, appearance**.

marcescent (maar ses'sənt) adj. withering, but not falling off (said of parts of plants)—can apply fig. to the aged. • Although increasingly *marcescent* in his old age, he's happy to maintain the status quo. [< L *marcere* to wither + -escent, suff., beginning or inclined to be, becoming < –escent- pres. p. of verbs in –escere, expressing the beginning of action]. n. **marcescence** (-ses'enz). adj. **marcescible**, q.v. See **physique, appearance**. See **skin**. See **health, illness**.

marcescible (maar-ses'si-bəl) adj. tending to wither or fade. [< L *marcescere* to fade]. See **physique, appearance**. See **skin**. See **health, illness**.

marplot (mawr'plot) n. an offensive meddler whose interference compromises the success of an undertaking. • The **elder-care hostel**, q.v., recognized her as a *marplot* in their attempted projects. [< Marplot, a character in the "Busy Body", a play by Susannah Cantivre (1669-1723), < American Heritage Dictionary, ed. 4]. See **mentality, mentation, behavior**.

marriage: alphamegamia, anilojuvenogamia, anisonogamia, deuterogamist, digamous, disespoused, dysonogamia, endogamy, isonogamia, nomogamosis, opsigamy, opsimatria, opsipatria, opsiproligery, seneucia, sororate, *veuf*, *veuvage*, *veuve*, *vidua*, viduage, viduation, *viduité*, viduity, *viduus*

marriage: Subcategories

I. Childbearing:
    1. Ability to have children late in life: **opsiproligery**
    2. Bearing a child late in a woman's life: **opsimatria**.
II. Fatherhood: Becoming a father late in life: **opsipatria**
III. Marriage:
    1. A second marriage for a widow, widower, or someone who marries a second time or remarries: **deuterogamist**.
    2. Married a second time: **digamous**
    3. Divorced: **disespoused**
    4. Marriage between:
        a. those highly suitable for each other: **nomogamosis**
        b. those of equal or nearly equal age: **isonogamia**
        c. those late in life: **opsigamy**
        d. those unequal in age: **anisonogamia**, **dysonogamia**
        e. an older woman and a young man: **anilojuvenogamy**
        f. an old man and a young or adolescent woman: **alphamegamia**
    5. Marriage within a specific social group: **endogamy**
    6. Marrying a wife's sister after a wife dies: **sororate**
IV. Unmarried: **viduus**
    1. Spinster: *vidua*
V. Widowhood:
    1. Widow: *veuve, vidua*
    2. Widower: *veuf, viduus*
    3. Widowerhood: *veuvage*
    4. Widowhood: **seneucia**, *veuvage*, viduage, viduation, *viduité*, viduity

mataeology/mateology (may"tee-ol'lə-jee/-lō-jee) n. vain, in the sense of unsuccessful or unprofitable, discourse. [< G *mataios* vain + *logos* discourse]. n **mataeologian** (-ō-lōj'jee-ən). n. **mataeologue** (may'ti-ō-logj, -ə-log). adj. **mataeological** (-ō-loj'ji-kəl). See **talk**. See **role**.

matriarch (may'tree-aark) n.1. a woman who is recognized as being the head of a family, community, or people. 2. a woman, usually a grandmother, who is highly respected by her family and to whom the family turn for advice and help. 3. a woman who holds a position of dominance, authority, or respect. [< L *matr-* mother, after patriarch]. adj. **matriarchal** (may"tree-aar'kal). adj. **matriarchic** (may"tree-aar'kik). n. **matriarchalism** (may"tree-aar'kal-ism). See **old woman**. See **role**.

matronolagnia (may"trən-ō-lag'ni-ə) n. attraction to older women, especially mature women (i.e., matrons) who are married or widowed and who have borne children. [< L *matrona* < *matr-* mother + < G *lagneia* lust; coition]. adj. **matronolagnic**. See **sex, love**.

maunderer (mawn'dur-ər) n. 1. someone who wanders aimlessly, moving, acting in a vague, rambling, meandering, or incoherent way. 2. a grumbler, mutterer; an incoherent, confused, rambling speaker. vi. & vt. **maunder**. [via L *maenander* < G *maiandros* a winding < *Maiandros*, the G name for the Menderes River—in what is now north-western Turkey—noted for its tortuous course, and, notably, as the model on which the ubiquitous Greek-key design is based]. See **mentality, mentation, behavior**. See **talk**. See **role**. See **standing, walking, wandering**.

mawkish (maw'kish) adj. overly and offputtingly sentimental or maudlin. • She's the *mawkish* great aunt who's always crying and talking about who's in her will. [< Old Norse *maðkr*]. adv. **mawkishly**. n. **mawkishness**. See **emotion**.

Medea's cauldron/caldron (me-dee'əss kawl'drən) n.phr. in Greek mythology, the large metal pot used by Medea, a sorceress and princess of Colchis (modern Georgia), at the eastern end of the Black Sea, to brew a magic potion, which, when applied in prescribed fashion to an old man, could restore, rejuvenate him by many years. She did this to Aeson, the father of her lover, Jason, whom she helped obtain the golden fleece. (After slitting Aeson's throat, Medea then put his corpse in a pot and Aeson came to life as a young man. She promised the daughters of King Pelias of Colchis that she would do the same for their father. They slit his throat, but Medea refused then to perform her magic, so Pelias remained dead.) [G, *medea* genitals or cunning]. See **therapy**.

medomalacophobia (meed"dō-mal"lə-kə-fōb'bi-ə) n. morbid fear of losing an erection during sexual intercourse. [< G *medea*, (pl.), the genitals {or cunning}, (*medos* {sing.}, the bladder) + *makakia* a softness + -phobia, suff., fearing < G -*phobia* < *phobos* fear]. adj. **medomalacophobic**. n. **medomalacophobe**. See: **genitourinary**. See **phobias**. See **sex, love**.

megillah (mə-gil'ləh) n. any long-winded account, especially one concerning a minor matter benefiting from much greater condensation. [H, scroll, particularly the Book of Esther, Ecclesiastes, the Song of Solomon, the Book of Ruth, or the Book of Lamentations. In Yid., *megillah* is usually preceded by *ganz* (gaants) = whole or complete, thus *ganz megillah* = an exhaustive account]. See **talk**.

megrims (mee'grimss) n.pl. a spell of depression, melancholy, or low spirits. (**megrim** n.s. 1. a migraine headache. 2. {archaic} a sudden change of mind, or something about which someone is enthusiastic {often used in the plural}). [variant of **migraine**, via F < G *hemikrania* < *hemi-* half + *kranion* skull]. adj. = **migranous**. See **emotion**. See **health, illness**. See **mentality, mentation, behavior**.

meibomian cyst (mī-bōm'mee-ən) n.phr. a sty or **chalazion**, q.v., or **hordeolum**. [< L *hordeolus* sty]. Inflammation of a meibomian gland. (A meibomian sty, a more common type, drains through the conjunctival surface of the lid, while a **zeisian** sty, one involving a zeisian gland, drains onto the surface of the skin at the edge of the lid.) • *Meibomian cysts* are more common in the elderly. [< Heinrich Meibom, German anatomist]. syns. **chalazion**, **hordeolum**, q.v. See **eye**.

melanocyte (mel'lə-nō-sīt, me-lən'ō-sīt) n. cells of the epidermis that synthesize the pigment **melanin**. Melanin determines skin and hair color. It's the decrease in melanin with age that results in graying of the hair (British English = grey, greying), in some degree, in about 50% of people by 50 years of age. [< G *melas* black + -cyte-, suff., denoting a cell < G *kytos* hollow vessel]. adj. **melanocytic** (mel"lə-nō-sit'tik). See **color**. See **hair**.

melanoma (mel-ə-nōm'mə) n. a highly malignant skin tumor that readily metastasizes (spreads to other organs). There are four types: 1. superficial spreading melanoma is the most frequent type, and the most common type in the elderly; it's a pigmented plaque, with an irregular border, variable pigmentation, often with areas of red, white, black, and brown, and usually asymptomatic. 2. Nodular melanoma presents as a darkly pigmented papule that is apt to enlarge rapidly. 3. Lentigo (freckle) melanoma is nodular, changes color or ulcerates after long standing. 4. Acral (tip)-lentiginous (freckle) melanoma presents as a pigmented, usually macular (macula = spot, stain) lesion on the nail bed, palm, sole, or finger. Melanomas are especially frequent in the elderly. [melan(o)-, pref, meaning black, or denoting relationship to melanin < G *melas*, gen. *melanos*, black +-*oma*, suff., tumor]. See **skin**.

memory: **AAADD**, *aide-mémoire*, **amnesia**, **anamnesis**, **anamnestic**, **anomia**, *apomnemoneumata*, **cache**, **cache memory**, **CRAFT**, **CRAT**, **CRS**, **CRTLA**, **cryptomnesia**, **dysmnesia**, **dysnomia**, **ecmnesia**, **eidetic**, **eidetic image**, **enchiridion**, *ex capite*, **hippocampus**, **hypermnesia**, *lapsus calami*, *lapsus linguae*, **lethe**, **lethologica**, **lethonomia**, **lexaphasia**, **loganamnosis**, *lubricum linguae*, **metaforgotten**, **mneme**, **mnemonic**, **mnemonist**, **Mnemosyne**, **mnemotechnist**, **neomnesia**, **nepenthe**, **nepimnemic**, **neoroplasticity**, **nominal aphasia**, **onomatomania**, **OSIF**, **paleomnesia**, **panmnesia**, **paramnesia**, **parapraxis**, **Pelmanism**, **philalethe**, **prefrontal cortex**, **prosopagnosis**, **prosopolethy**, **Proustian experience**, **pseudomnesia**, **rememble**, **revenant** (adj.), **senior moment**, **SM**, **telamnesia**, **zeigarnik**.

memory: Sub-categories

I. Memory:
    1. Definition: **mneme**
    2. Goddess of memory: **Mnemosyne**
    3. Memoirs: *apomnemoneumata*
    4. Memory aid: *aide-mémoire*, **anamnestic**, **mnemonic**, **mnemotechnist**, **Pelmonism**
    5. Memory renewal or preservation by brain exercise: **neuroplasticity**
    6. Store of computer memory: **cache**, **cache memory**
    7. A forgotten, outmoded word, sometimes resurrected: **metaforgotten**
    8. Immediate things (working memory): **prefrontal cortex** (brain site of working memory)

II. Bad, impaired memory:
    1. General:
        a. confused memory: **paramnesia**
        b. impaired memory: **dysmnesia**
        c. no memory: **amnesia, lethe, lexaphasia**
        d. temporary memory lapse: **senior moment, SM**
    2. Inability to remember:
        a. a f---ing thing: **CRAFT**
        b. anything: **CRAT**
        c. drug used to forget: **nepenthe**
        d. names: **anomia, dysnomia, lethonomia, nominal aphasia**
        e. words: **lethologica, onomatomania**
        f. facts: **prosopagnosis**
        g. faces: **prosopolethy**
        h. hidden, subconscious memories: **cryptomnesia, nepimnemic**
        i. s--t: **CRS**
        j. the three-letter acronym: **CRTLA**
        k. things happening long ago: **telamnesia**
        l. immediate things (working memory): **prefrontal cortex** (brain site)
        l. things in succession (interrupted memory): **AAADD**

III. Good, excellent:
    1. For long-past events: **paleomnesia**
    2. For recent events: **neomnesia, ecmnesia, hippocampus** (brain site of recent memory)
    3. From memory: *ex capite*
    2. Total memory: **panmnesia, mnemonist**
    3. Vivid memory: **eidetic, eidetic image, hypermnesia**

IV. Obsessive memory:
    1. Obsession recalling a word: **loganamnosis, onomatomania**

V. Slip:
    1. Of the tongue: **lapsus linguae, lubricum linguae, parapraxis**
    2. Of the pen, writing, typing, texting: *lapsus calami*
    3. Oh s--t I forgot: **OSIF**

VI. Remembering: **rememble**
1. An uncompleted task: **zeigarnik**
2. Handbook: **enchiridion**
3. Medical past history: **anamnesis**
4. Something long forgotten: **revenant**, **Proustian experience**
5. Things that never happened, false memory: **pseudomnesia**

VII. Role:
1. One who loves to forget: **philalethe**
2. One skilled in remembering: **mnemonist**, **mnemotechnist**

mensch (mensh), pl. = **menschen** (var. = **mensches**); ({inf.}**mensh**, {inf.} pl. vars. = **menshen, menshes**). n. (inf.) someone good, kind, decent, solid, honorable, generously human, and compassionate. [mid 20th C. < Yid. < OHG *mennisco* manly, human]. See **role**.

mentality, mentation, behavior (See **intelligence**, also): **a dog in the manger, abderite, abulia, acedia, adamantine, afforient, ageism, agelast, agonist,** *agonistes*, **alogism, amadelphous, anaclitic, anagapesis, anhedonia, anosodiaphoria, anosognosia, antinomian, apanthropia/apanthropy, aphilophrenia, apodictic/ apodeictic, apolaustic, aponoia, aprosexia,** *apud se*, **arrectness, astucious, ataraxia, athetise, atrabilarian, atrabilious, attercop, autognosis, autophobia, autoptic, azygophrenia, benignant, blinkered, bluenose, braggadocio, brass-collar, Briareus,** *cacoethes carpendi*, **cantankerous, captious, carphology, cathect, cathexis, churlish, coagitabund, cognition, cognitive dysfunction, comity,** *compos mentis*, **conation, congruence, conservative, conspue, contumacious, contumelius, cosset, crabbed, crocidismus, curmudgeon,** *distrait*, **douceur, drimble/drumble, dudgeon, dysbulia, dyspepsia, dysphoria, dysphoriant, dysteleology, dystropia/dystropy, ebriection, egotheism, eleemosynary,** *empressement*, **encephalophonic, encraty, ensynopticity, epicaricacy, erethism, errabund, esclandre, euthymia, evagation, evancalous, faff, fart around/ about, feckless, feisty, fey, filiopietistic, finifugal, flatulopetic, floccilegium, floccillation, flounder, footle, fractious, frampold, franion, froward, fuddle, fumacious, fusty, grinch,** *habitué* **(-e), halcyon, hamartithia, hesternopathic/–pothic, heteroclitic, heteroclite, horbgorgling, huggermugger/hugger-mugger,**

hyperprosexia, hypobulia, *idée fixe*, immorigerous, *impotentia*, indocible, indocile, inductile, intractable, intransigent, iracund, irascible, jargoggle, kaino(to)phobia, kvetch, linsey-woolsey, *lapsus calami*, *lapsus linguae*, longanimity, *lubricum linguae*, maggot, magpie, malacodermous, malapert, malnoia, *manqué*, mansuetude, marplot, maunderer, megrims, miccrolipet, misocainea, misologist, misology, misomania, mixty-maxty, mizmaze, Morton's fork, mulligrubs, mumpsimus, Munchausenism, muzzy, nasute, nebulochaotic, neurobics, neuroplasticity, nocebo, nolition/nolleity, nononeiric, nonplus/ non-plus, nosocomephrenia, obdurate, obnubilation, obstruent, obtrude, officious, oligophrenia, oneiric, oppugnant, oscitancy, *outré*, overslaugh, paedomorphism/pedomorphism, palinoia, pallid, parapraxia, paraprosexia, parsimony, patharmosis, pathocryptia, Pecksniffian, pertinacious, pervicacious, pettifoggery, pharisaical, phlegmatic, picaresque, pickmote, Pickwickian, piffle, pococurante, porlockian, prepresbyophrenia, protervity, Prufrockian, pump head, purblind, querulous, quiescence, quixotic, recalcitrant, recrudescence, recusant, refractory, renitent, repine, rhytiscopia, rudesby, ruminate, Schadenfreude, senior moment, serotine, *shpilkes*, skeuomorph, smellfungus, splenetic, spoffish, spry, staunch, sthenobulia, stomachous, sundowning, swivet, synoikismos, tardigrade, tenebrous, tetchy, tilmus, *Torschlusspanik*, tracasserie, *traditionaliste*, traduce, truculent, umbrageous, unwitting, vade mecum, vagarious, vagary, vecordious, velitation, verjuice, versute, waspish, wastrel, whiffle, widdendream, wowser, zoilism.

mentality, mentation, behavior: Subcategories

I. Behavior:
  1. Normal:
    a. generous, kind, benevolent; nor literal: **Pickwickian**
    b. in a state of rest, inactivity: **quiescence**
    c. mutual consideration, civility: **comity**
    d. pertaining to one engaged in a struggle: *agonistes*
    e pleasant to embrace: **evancalous**
    f. selecting one over another: **overslaugh**
    g. one who frequents a particular place: *habitué*, -e

2. Abnormal:
   a. abnormal or eccentric behavior: **dystropia/ dystrophy, fey**
   b. act sluggishly: **drimble/drumble**
   c. aimless plucking motion at bedding, etc.: **carphology,   c r o c i d i s m u s , floccilegium, floccillation, tilmus**
   d. bossy: **officious**
   e. breaking out, becoming active again of hostile feelings: **recrudescence**
   f. crafty, wily, cunning: **versute**
   g. description of adult behavior in terms of child behavior: **paedomorphism/pedomorphism**
   h. erratic: **errabund**
   i. erroneous, faulty, blundering action: **parapraxia**
   j. exacerbation of confusion, disruptive behavior at sundown: **sundowning**
   k. excessive bragging: **braggadocio**
   l. excessive sexuality: **hyperprosexia, paraprosexia**
   m. extreme politeness: *empressement*
   n. faltering of will: **dysbulia**
   o. fault finding, complaining: **kvetch, querulous**
   p. hedonist: **franion**
   q. hypocritically & unctuously benevolent: **Pecksniffian**
   r. ill-bred: **churlish**
   s. ill-tempered, peevish, irascible, spiteful: **splenetic**
   t. impotence, weakness: *impotentia*
   u. impudent: **malapert**
   v. impulsive, idealistic, romantic, impractical: **quixotic**
   w. inability to sit still, fidgets: *shpilkes*
   x. inattentive: **aprosexia**
   y. insolent: **contumelius**
   z. insubordinate: **contumacious**
   aa. intrusive, interrupting: **porlockian**
   bb. loss of will, volition, ability to decide: **abulia**

cc. meddler whose interference compromises an undertaking's success: **marplot**
dd. meekness: **mansuetude**
ee. obstinate, obstructing, hindering, opposing, stubbornly resistant, inflexible: **obstruent**, **oppugnant**, **recalcitrant**, **refractory**, **renitent**, **stomachous**, **truculent**
ff. over dependent on another: **anaclitic**
gg. perplexed, bewildered: **nonplus/non-plus**
hh. persistently resolute: **pertinacious**
ii. perverse behavior: **froward**, **maggot**
jj. perversity, petulance, impudence, peevishness: **protervity**
kk. pompous, inflated: **flatulopetic**
ll. producing a feeling of discomfort: **dysphoriant**
mm. prone to make mistakes: **hamartithia**
nn. puttering around aimlessly: **horbgorgling**
oo. quarrelsome: **cantankerous**, **fractious**, **frampold**
pp. quibbling, nit picking: **pettifoggery**
qq. quick to take offence (soft-skinned): **malacodermous**
rr. reject, spurn: **athetise**, **conspue**
ss. resentment: **dudgeon**
tt. said or done unintentionally: **unwitting**
uu. secret, clandestine: **huggermugger/hugger-mugger**
vv. self-righteously hypocritical: **pharisaical**
ww. sense of annoyance: **tracasserie**
xx. slow-moving, sluggish: **tardigrade**
yy. timid, cautious, indecisive, *manqué*: **Prufrockian**
zz. to act foolishly, trifle: **footle**; **piffle**
ab. to confuse, perplex, mix up: **fuddle**, **jargoggle**
bc. to disparagingly abuse someone: **traduce**
cd. to dither, fumble: **faff**
de. to drink too much: **fuddle**
ef. to impose oneself or one's opinions: **obtrude**

fg. to make mistakes: **flounder**

gh. to vacillate like the wind: **whiffle**

hi. tries to prevent others from having or doing something that he or

ij. she can't have or do: **a dog in the manger**

jk. typical of rogues or scoundrels: **picaresque**

kl. undecipherable handwriting: **crabbed**

lm. unpredictable, erratic in behavior; unpredictable or eccentric change, action, or idea: **vagarious**; **vagary**

mn. unacceptable behavior performance: *outré*

no. unswervingly loyal politically: **brass-collar**

op. unpleasant scene, cause a disturbance: **esclandre**

pq. upset at trifles; bustling; fussy: **spoffish**

qr. useless, ineffective: **feckless**

rs. wandering: **errabund**

st. waste time by behaving foolishly: **fart around/about**

tu. wastes money, is profligate: **wastrel**

uv whimsical behavior: **maggot**

vw. whine: **kvetch**

3. Undefined, uncertain:

a. behave secretly: **huggermugger/huggermugger**

b. coming together as one: **synoikismos**

c. eccentric: **heteroclitic**

d. handbook or other thing carried constantly about the person: **vade mecum**

e. minor conflict, slight skirmish, controversy: **velitation**

f. old fashioned, conservative in style, etc.: **fusty**

g. personality late in occurring, developing, flowering: **serotine**

h. refusing to submit to authority, dissenting: **recusant**

i shunning the end (of anything, but especially life itself): **finifugal**

j. spoil, pamper: **cosset**

k. stinginess, frugality, careful use of money: **parsimony**

I.   woolgathering, yawning, inattentiveness: **oscitancy**

II. Emotion:
1. Angry: **stomachous**
2. Breaking out, becoming active again of hostile feelings, discontent: **recrudescence**
3. Easily angered: **iracund, splenetic**
4. Easily irritated, annoyed; sharp in retort: **waspish**
5. Fear of oneself, of being alone, loneliness: **autophobia**
6. Fear of something new: **kaino(to)phobia**
7. Feeling of being unloved: **aphilophrenia**
8. Feeling of discomfort: **dysphoria**
9. Fond of smoking: **fumacious**
10. Inability to be happy: **anhedonia**
11. Joyfulness: **euthymia**
12. Lacking in color, intensity, spirit: **pallid**
13. Self awareness: **autognosis**
14. Sense of life passing one by: *Torschlusspanik*
15. Soft-skinned: **malacodermous**
16. State of discomposure, anxiety, agitation: **swivet**
17. Take offence easily: **umbrageous**
18. Taking pleasure in others' suffering, misfortune: **Schadenfreude, epicaricacy**
19. Unusual emotional activity, investment in a person or thing: **cathect, cathexis**
20. Upset or annoyed easily, oversensitive: **tetchy**

III. Mental state, ability:
1. Normal or increased:
   a. able to take a general view of something: **ensynopticity**
   b. before the onset of senility: **prepresbyophrenia**
   c. harmony felt when various aspects of one's life are in agreement: **congruence**
   d. having a bad temper, gloomy, irritable: **dyspepsia**
   e. in one's senses: *apud se, compos mentis*
   f. renew or retain memory by mental activity: **neuroplasticity**
   g. self awareness: **autognosis**
   h. sharp, acute (of mind): **nasute**

        i. Unusual concentration of mental activity on a particular thing. person, or idea: **cathect, cathexis**

2. Decreased:

    a. absence of mental ability, mentation: **aponoia**

    b. absence of willing: unwilling: **nolition/ nolleity**

    c. clouded or confused mental state: **obnubilation, cognitive dysfunction**

    d. discordant, nonsensical: **linsey-woolsey**

    e. feeblemindedness: **oligophrenia**

    f. foolish, senseless, as in one's dotage: **vecordious**

    g. hazy, confused: **nebulochaotic**

    h. in a state of confusion: **widdendream** (in a widdendream)

    i. inattentive, absentminded: *distrait*

    j. lack of purposefulness: **dysteleology**

    k. breakdown: **ebriection**

    l. maze, confusion, bewilderment: **mizmaze**

    m. mental wandering, digression: **evagation**

    n. mixed up, confused; a mishmash: **mixty-maxty**

    o. moment of absent mindedness, befuddlement: **senior moment**

    p. resisting discipline or instruction: **indocile**

    q. short-term cognitive loss after cardiac surgery: **pump head, cognitive dysfunction**

    r. slip of the pen, writing, typing, etc.: *lapsus calami*

    s. slip of the tongue: *lapsus linguae, lubricum linguae*

    t. state of confusion, wandering: **afforient, muzzy**

    u. unaware of what is happening: **unwitting**

    v. unteachable: **inductile, indocible**

IV. <u>Mood</u>:

1. Apathetic, of a sluggish temperament; nonchalant: **phlegmatic; pococurante**

2. Apathy, boredom, sloth, indifference: **acedia**

3. Brisk and active: **spry**

4. Dark, gloomy mood (adj.): **tenebrous**

5. Depression: **megrims, mulligrubs**
   a. depressed from a long hospital stay: **nosocomephrenia**
6. Disease disbelief; unwilling to believe in (or talk about) one's illness: **anosognosia, pathocryptia**
7. Disease indifference: **anosodiaphoria**
8. Easily irritated, annoyed; sharp in retort: **waspish**
9. Excessive irritability, excitability, or sensitivity: **erethism**
10. Fractious: **crabbed**
11. Gloomy, dismal: **atrabilious**
12. Gloomy hypochondriac: **atrabilarian**
13. Imperturbable calmness: **ataraxia**
14. Intense alertness: **arrectness**
15. Kind & gracious: **benignant**
16. Loss of will, volition, ability to decide: **abulia**
17. Mental adjustment to one's disease: **patharmosis**
18. Messy disorder: **huggermugger/hugger-mugger**
19. Mutual consideration, civility: **comity**
20. Not yielding to treatment: **refractory**
21. Of an irritable temperament: **irascible**
22. Pensive: **coagitabund**
23. Sense of annoyance: **tracasserie**
24. Someone yearning for the good old days; clinging to the past: **hesternopathic/–pothic, fusty/fustiness**
25. Sourness of temperament: **verjuice**
26. Spirited: **feisty**
27. Stubbornly unyielding, not persuadable: **obdurate**
28. Sweetness: **douceur**
29. Tranquil, golden, joyful, peaceful: **halcyon**
30. Yearning for the good old days: **hesternopathic/-pothic**

V. Role:
   1. A bad-tempered, venomous person: **attercop**
   2. A conservative: *traditionaliste*
   3. A malcontent, fault-finder, grumbler: **smellfungus**
   4. A simpleton, dimwit: **abderite**
   5. An eccentric: **heteroclite**
   6. Enthusiastic or compulsive collector (fig., inf.): **magpie**
   7. Fault finder: **pickmote**
   8. Ill-mannered, loud-mouthed bore: **rudesby**

9. Irritable person: **curmudgeon**
10. Might have been: *manqué*
11. One engaged in a struggle: **agonist**
12. One unresponsive to other or new ideas, opinions, approaches: **blinkered**
13. One upset by small things: **miccrolipet**
14. One who doesn't laugh: **agelast**
15. One who hates logical argument: **misologist**
16. One who refuses to obey authority: **recusant**
17. Person refusing to correct a known error: **mumpsimus**
18. Puritanical spoilsport: **wowser**
19. Someone ruining others' enjoyment: **grinch**
20. Wanderer: **maunderer**

VI. Talent:
  1. Someone totally *au fait*: **Briareus**
  2. Strong will power: **sthenobulia**

VII. Thought patterns, attitude:
  1. Desirable:
    a. charitable: **eleemosynary**
    b. coming together as one: **synoikismos**
    c. engaging different parts of the brain to do familiar tasks: **neurobics**
    d. firm in attitude, loyalty: **staunch**
    e. perspicacious: **astucious**
    f. prolonged expectation of the good or bearing of injuries: **longanimity**
    g. reverence for ancestors, tradition: **filiopietistic**
    h. self-restraint: **encraty**
    i. to chew over, meditate, ponder: **ruminate**
  2. Neutral:
    a. based on one's own perception: **autoptic**
    b. compulsion to repeat until perfect: **palinoia**
    c. dedicated to pleasure: **apolaustic**
    d. faith & divine grace alone will see one through: **antinomian**
    e. mental effort having to do with striving: **conation**
    f. not relating to dream(s): **nononeiric**
    g. relating to dream(s): **oneiric**
    h. someone excessively moral: **bluenose**

i. supporter of traditional ideas and values: **conservative**, *traditionaliste*
j. talkative: **amadelphous**
k. thought: **cognition**
l. unyielding, firm, inflexible, obstinate, not easily led: **adamantine**, **immorigerous**, **intractable**, **intransigent**, **pervicacious**

3. Undesirable:
a. age prejudice: **ageism**
b. aversion to society, people: **apanthropia/ apanthropy**
c. calculated to entrap, caviling: **captious**
d. compulsion to find fault: : *cacoethes carpendi*
e. destructive, nagging criticism: **zoilism**
f. difficulty in making decisions: **hypobulia**.
g. disease disbelief; unwilling to believe in (or talk about) one's illness: **anosognosia**, **pathocryptia**
h. disease indifference: **anosodiaphoria**
i. fixed idea, monomania: *idée fixe*
j. hatred of everything: **misomania**
k. hatred of logical argument: **misology**
l. hatred of the new: **misocainea**
m. having fixed ideas, attitudes, etc.: **blinkered**
n. illness caused by sugestion, e.g., of drug side affects: **nocebo**
o. indisputably true: **apodictic, apodeictic**
p. lack of interest in former loved ones: **anagapesis**
q. mixed up, confused; a mishmash: **mixty-maxty, cognitive dysfunction**
r. neurosis due to being single: **azygophrenia**
s. neurotic preoccupation with facial wrinkles: **rhytiscopia**
t. refers to hearing, noises, talk, voices in one's head: **encephalophonic**
u. secret, clandestine: **huggermugger/hug- ger-mugger**
v. self-deification: **egotheism**
w. telling fabulous, but false (**commentitious**, q.v.), stories: **Munchausenism**

x. to complain, grumble, lament: **kvetch,
    repine**
y. totally unable to see: **purblind**
z. two lines of reasoning leading to the same
    unpleasant conclusion: **Morton's fork**
aa. typical of rogues or scoundrels: **picaresque**
bb. unreasonable, illogical statement, thought:
    alogism
cc. unresponsive to stimulus: **refractory**
dd. vague mental discomfort: **malnoia**
ee. woolgathering, yawning, inattentiveness,
    being unfocused: **oscitancy**
ff. yesterday's design, idea copied today
    without regard to function: **skeuomorph**

mephitic (me-fit'tik, mə-) adj. of gases, etc., smelling unpleasant, foul, or poisonous; noxious emanation, noisome stench. • He identified a certain *mephitic* odor in that badly maintained nursing home. [L, *mephitis*, *-is* malaria]. adj. **mephitical** (-əl). adv. **mephitically**. n. **mephitis** (-fī'-). See **nose, smell**. See **gastrointestinal**.

mesothelioma (mees"sō-theel"lee-ōm'mə) n. a malignant tumor derived from mesothelial tissue, i.e., peritoneum, pleura, or pericardium, and appearing as large sheets of cells having sarcoma-like or adenoma (gland)-like patterns. Pleural (lung lining) mesotheliomas have been linked to asbestos exposure. [mes(o)-, pref., in the mid, mediate, or moderate < G *mesos* middle + epithelium < ep(i)-, pref., upon, above, or beside < *epi* on + < G *thele* nipple + -oma, suff., meaning tumor or neoplasm or the part indicated by the stem to which it is attached < G *-oma*, noun-forming suff.]. See **neoplasm, cancer, tumor**.

metaforgotten (met"tə-for-got"tən) n. a neologism indicating an outmoded word that has "faded into the mists of antiquity", as defined by William Safire, who gives as examples *washboard*, and *dial phone*—"On Language" column, New York Times, 5/24/2009. Some metaforgotten words are resurrected, e. g., *washboard*, n., which can be used attributively, to indicate prominent, sculptured-like trans-abdominal muscles—currently clipped to *abs*—that result from strenuous abdominal-muscle exercise and dieting. Another is *Cellphone*—increasingly shortened to *cell*—is a retronym of *phone*, an abbreviation of *telephone*. • *Metaforgottens* not infrequently occurred in conversation as the elders reminisced. [met(a)- (meth-, before an aspirate), pref., later; beyond, transcending; change < G *meta* with, after, (with the sense of) change + forgotten]. See **memory**.

metanoia (met-ə-noy'ə) n. a profound change, usually spiritual, a transformation; a conversion. [< G, change of mind; repentance]. See **religion, theology, morality**.

methomania (meth"ō-may'ni-ə) n. morbid desire for alcoholic beverages. [< G *methe* strong drink + *mania* frenzy]. adj. **methomaniacal** (-mə-nī'ə-kəl). n. **methomaniac**. syns. **alcoholomania**, **dipsomania**, **posiomania**, q.v. Cf. **oenomania**, q.v. See **manias**. See **drink, food**. See **role**.

Methuselah (mə-thoŏ'zə-lə, me-) p.n. 1. a very **old man**, q.v.; old and long lived. (2. alt. **methuselah**, a wine bottle that holds the equivalent of eight normal bottles, about 208 fluid oz. or 6 liters.) [< Bible (Gen. 5: 21-27): Methuselah supposedly lived for 969 years and was an ancestor of Noah]. syns. **patriarch**, **whitebeard**, **progenitor**, q.v. See **old man**.

metrona (me-trōn'nə) n. a young grandmother. [? < L *metr-*, pref., mother.? < L *metro-*, pref., uterus < G *metra* womb]. See **old woman**.

microbiophobia (mīk"krō-bī"ō-fōb'bi-ə) n. morbid fear of germs. [< G *micros* small + *bios* life + *phobia* fear]. adj. **microbiophobic**. n. **microbiophobe**. syns. **bacteriophobia**, **bacillophobia**, q.v. Cf. **my**(or i)**sophobia**, q.v. See **phobias**.

micrographia (mī-krō-graf'fi-ə) n. writing with very small letters, sometimes getting smaller and smaller, as occurs in **Pakinson's disease**, q.v. [< G *mikros* small + *grapho* to write]. n. **micrographer** (-krog'grə-fər) = one who writes small or increasingly smaller. See **nerve, muscle, movement, touch**. See **role**.

microlipet (mīk"krō-lip'pit) n. someone who gets all worked up about trivial things. [micro-, pref, denoting smallness < G *mikros* small, +?]. See **mentality, mentation, behavior**. See **role**.

micturition (mik-tur-i'shən) n. 1. urination, the passage of urine. 2. the desire to urinate or frequency of urination. • His *micturition*, characteristic of so many elderly men with prostate hypertrophy, was frequent, urgent, interrupted, small-streamed, and prolonged. [< L *micturio* the desire to make water < *micturire* to urinate]. n.phr. **frequency of micturition** or **micturition frequency** = micturition at short intervals due to decreased bladder capacity resulting from increased urine residual, rather than to increased daily volume of urinary output. [< L *frequens* repeated, often, constant]. vi. **micturate** = to urinate, pass urine. syns. **miction, voiding, urinating,** (slang, offensive) **pissing, peeing, taking a leak.** See **genitourinary**.

miosis (mī-ōs'siss) n. 1. the period of decline of a disease in which the intensity of the symptoms begins to diminish. 2. contraction of the pupil. (The elderly have smaller pupils, and therefore have less effective dark adaptation: Their pupils don't dilate as much in darkness so they can see less.) (3. sometimes incorrectly used as an alternative spelling of "meiosis", which relates to cellular division.) [G, *meiosis* a lessening]. adj. **miotic.** n. **miotic** = an agent causing the pupil to contract. See **eye**. See **health, illness**.

misocainea (mī-sō-kīn'nee-ə, -kayn'nee-) n. hatred of new things, e.g., new ideas. [G < *miseo* to hate + *kainos* new]. syn. **misoneism,** q.v. See **innovation, misoneism**. See **mentality, mentation, behavior**.

misologist (mī-sol'lə-jist) n. one who hates reason, logical argument, discussion, or enlightenment. n. **misology.** adj. **misological** (mī''sō-log'i-kəl). [< G *misologia* < *misein* to hate + *logos* word, reason, reckoning]. See **mentality, mentation, behavior**. See **role**.

misomania (mī-sō-may'ni-ə) n. hatred of everything. [G < *miseo* to hate + *-mania*, suff., < G frenzy]. adj. **misomaniacal** (-mə-nī'ə-kəl). n. **misomaniac.** See **manias**. See **mentality, mentation, behavior**.

misoneism (mī''sō-nee'iz-əm) n. hatred of new things. [G < *miseo* to hate + *neos* new]. n. **misoneist.** adj. = **misoneistic** (-nee-iz'tik). syn. **misocainea,** q.v. Cf. **Luddite,** q.v. See **innovation, misoneism**. Se **role**.

mixty-maxty (miks'tee-maks'tee) adj. mixed up; confused. [< L *mixtus*, pp. of *miscere* to mix + max (shortening of maximum) < *maximus* greatest < *magnus* great]. n. **mixty-maxty** = a mishmash. See **mentality, mentation, behavior**.

mizmaze (miz'mayz) n. a maze; confusion, bewilderment. [< miz? + maze, shortening (aphesis) of amaze < OE *amasian* stupefy, stun]. See **mentality, mentation, behavior**.

mneme (nee'mee) n., pl. = **mnemes** (nee'meess) 1. the continuing effect of an individual's past experience in explanation of his present conduct, feelings. 2. the effect of race in explanation of a current population's characteristics. [< G *mneme* memory]. See **memory**.

mnemonic (nee-mon'nik) n. &. adj. a device—a word, name, poem, etc.—intended to remind one of something else, e.g., a string tied around a finger to remind one to keep an appointment. • The need for *mnemonics* increases with ole age. [< G *mnemon* mindful]. See **memory**.

mnemonist (nee-mon'nist) n. someone skilled in memorizing, and adept at not forgetting. [< G *mneme* memory + -ist, suff., practicing a specific skill or profession (or a specific belief or school of thought) < -*istes* < -*izo*/-ize + -*tes*, suff., agent). adj. **mnemonistic**. syn. **mnemotechnist**, q.v. See **memory**. See **role**.

Mnemosyne (nee-mos'nee) n. the ancient Greek goddess of memory. Zeus and Mnemosyne were the parents of the muses, who were initially three, then extended to nine by the poet Hesiod ("Theogony"), and later each muse was given a specific art by bureaucratic Romans: Calliope (epic poetry), Clio (history), Euterpe (lyric poetry, song), Erato (erotic poetry, song), Melpomene (tragedy), Polymnia (sacred poetry, song), Terpsichore (choral dance), Thalia (comedy), and Urania (astronomy). [< G *Mnemosune*]. See **memory**.

mnemotechnist (nee-mō-tek'nist) n. someone skilled in the art and techniques of memorization and memory retention. [< G *mneme* memory + *tekhne* art, craft + -ist, suff.]. adj. **mnemotechnik** = skillful in the art and techniques of memorization and memory retention. syn. **mnemonist**, q.v. See **memory**. See **role**.

moider (moy'dər)/**moyder, (moidher, moyther, moidur, moidar, mither, myther, meyther, meither**) vt. 1. to worry, confuse, distract. 2. to smother, to crowd. 3. to work (used with "away"). vi. 1. to talk incoherently or foolishly. (2.{dialect} to work). [obscure,? related to muddle]. See **talk**.

moirologist (moy-rol'lə-jist) n. a hired mourner. [< G *moira* fate, death + *logos* word]. See **role**. See **end-of-life, death**.

molys(o)mophobia (mo-liz"mō-fōb'bi-ə) n. a morbid fear of infection. [< G *molysma* filth, infection + *phobos* fear]. adj. **molys(o)mophobic**. n. **molysmophobe**. syn. **mysophobia**. Cf. **bacteriophobia, bacillophobia, microbiophobia**, q.v. See **phobia**. See **health, illness**.

monadnock (mə-nad'nok) n. (1. an isolated hill or mountain that, having resisted erosion, rises above a plain.) 2. (fig.) things or persons standing out in spite of difficulties or in contrast to their surroundings. • The wellderly, q.v., are *monadnocks* among their generation. [< Mount Monadnock, a peak in New Hampshire, the name of which, in Algonquian, means isolated mountain]. See **role**.

monepic (mon-ep'pik) adj. consisting of one word or one-word sentences. [mon(o)-, pref., one, single, alone < G *monos* one + *epicos* < *epos* word, song]. See **talk**.

monomania (mon"nə-mayn'nee-ə) n. a form of mental disorder characterized by preoccupation with one subject or idea. • *Monomania* is more likely in the elderly. [mon(o)-, pref., one or single < G *monos* single + *mania* madness]. n. **monomaniac**. adj. **monomaniacal** (-mə-nî'ə-kəl). See **manias**.

monophobia (mōn"nō-fō'bi-ə) n. morbid fear of being alone, of loneliness. [mon(o)-, pref., one or single < G *monos* single + *phobos* fear]. adj. **monophobic**. n. **monophobe**. syns. **autophobia, eremophobia, isolophobia, solophobia**, q.v. See **phobias**. See **loneliness, solitude, silence**.

moribund (mawr'ri-bund) adj. 1. in a dying state, nearly dead. 2. having lost all purpose or vitality; no longer effective. 3. becoming obsolete. [< L *moribundus* < *mori* to die]. n. **moribundity** (-bund'di-tee). adv. **moribundly**. See **end-of-life, death**. See **tiredness, weakness**.

morose (mə-rōss', maw-) adj. gloomy, sullen, withdrawn. [< L *morosus* peevish < *mos* will, disposition, manner, inclination + *-osus, -ose*, suff.]. adv. **morosely**. n. **morosity** (-ros'si-tee). n. **moroseness**. See **emotion**.

Morton's fork (mawr'tonss fawk) n.phr. a situation involving a choice between two equally undesirable outcomes, or a choice between two equally unpleasant alternatives—a dilemma—or two lines of reasoning leading to the same unpleasant conclusion. ● The hazard of the surgical operation vs. that of the experimental drug's side effects presented yet another *Morton's-fork* situation for the **octogenarian**, q.v. (In Greek mythology, Orestes faced such a situation when, having interpreted Apollo's oracle telling him to slay his mother, Clytemnestra, who murdered his father, he was committing a mortal sin by killing her.) [< John Morton (c. 1420-1500), initially Archbishop of Canterbury, was then (1487) Lord Chancellor, thus English King Henry VII's tax collector, and ultimately was a Cardinal. His policy was to collect Henry's tax from both rich and poor by arguing that those living luxuriously obviously had money to spare, and those living frugally must have accumulated savings, and thus were also able to pay. More currently, similar situations are called: "between the devil and the deep blue sea", "between a rock and a hard place", and "catch 22"]. See **finance**. See **mentality, mentation, behavior.**

Morton's neuroma (mawr'tonss noo-rō'mə) n.phr. a new growth of nerve cells and fibers occurring in the nerves between the toes, usually 3rd & 4th, and causing prominent foot pain. It is more common in the elderly, especially in women who have chronically worn high heels, or in athletes who have worn tight shoes or whose feet were subjected to chronic trauma, such as occurs in basketball players, runners. Age-related atrophy of the metatarsal foot pad may increase risk of the condition. See **cancer, neoplasm, tumor**. See **joint, extremities, back**. See **nerve, muscle, movement, touch**.

mossback (moss'bak) n., n.pl. **–backs** or **–back**, 1. an offensive term (insult) for a person, male or female, regarded as old fashioned, conservative, or reactionary. (2. an old turtle, shellfish, or fish with algae growing on its back.) [< OE *mos* bog < Gmc. *mos-*, pref.; previously the term was applied to a rustic or backwoods type person]. syns. **duffer**, **gaffer**, q.v. See **old man**. See **old person(s), people**. See **old woman**.

moss-grown (moss'gron") adj. 1. old-fashioned, out of date, *démodé*. (2. covered with moss). [< OE *mos* bog < Gmc. *mos-*, pref.]. See **innovation, misoneism**. See **past, time**.

motatorios (mō-tə-tawr'ri-əss) adj. constantly active. [< L *motio* motion < *motare* to keep moving, shifting]. See **work, activity**.

mouth, gums, teeth: agomphious, amasesis, bruxism, crassilingual, dedentition, dentigerous, dentophobia, dentulous, edentate, edentulous/edentulate expuition, gerodontics, gerodontology, manducable, odontophobia, prosthodontics/ prosthodontia, rheum, sialoquent, slaver, slubber-degullion, thegosis, xanthodontic/xanthodontous, xerostomia.

mouth, gums, teeth: Subcategories

I. Dentistry:
    1. Dentistry using false teeth: **prosthodontics/ prosthodontia**
    2. Morbid fear of dentists: **dentophobia, odontophobia**
    3. Senior-citizen dentistry: **gerodontics, gerodontology**
II. Saliva:
    1. A spitting: **expuition**
    2. Dryness of the mouth: **xerostomia**
    3. One who slobbers his clothing: **slubber-degullion**
    4. Spraying saliva when speaking: **sialoquent**
    5. To drool, dribble saliva: **slaver**
    6. Watery discharge from the mouth: **rheum**
III. Teeth:
    1. Chewable, edible: **manducable**
    2. Having teeth: **dentigerous, dentulous**
    3. Inability to chew: **amasesis**
    4. Loss of teeth: **dedentition**
    5. Sharpening teeth by grinding them: **thegosis**
    6. Teeth grinding: **bruxism**
    7. Toothless: **agomphious, edentate, edentulous/ edentulate**
    8. Yellow-toothed: **xanthodontic/xanthodontous**
IV. Tongue:
    1. Thick tongued, distorted pronunciation due to a thick tongue: **crassilingual**

mulligrubs (mul'-li-grubz) n.pl. 1. grumpiness; colic, stomach-ache; low spirits, depression. 2. an ill-tempered person. n.s. 1. applied to a person: a **mulligrubs**. 2. a fit of **mulligrubs**. [< *mulliegrums*, "a grotesque arbitrary formation"—Oxford English Dictionary—apparently

< *megrims*, variant of migraine, low spirits < F *migraine* headache].
See **mentality, mentation**. See **gastrointestinal**. See **role**.

multiloquent (mul-til'lō-kwənt) adj. loquacious, gabby, talkative. [<
multi-, pref., many, multiple, more than one or two < L *multus* much,
many + *loqui* speak, talk, say, speak about, tell]. adv. **multiloquently**.
n. **multiloquence**. syn. **longiloquent**, **pleniloquet**, q.v. Cf.
logomania. See **talk**.

mumpsimus (mump'si-məs) n. 1. a person who refuses to correct
an error, habit, or practice even though knowing it has been shown to
be wrong. 2. an unswerving bigot. [< a pigheaded 16th C. priest who
always said *mumpsimus* when reciting the Mass even though he had
been shown many times that *sumpsimus*—now indicative of a correct
expression that takes the place of a popular but incorrect expression—
was correct. The L *sumpsimus* means "we have received", i.e., the
host, bread consecrated in the Eucharist]. See **mentality, mentation,
behavior**. See **role**.

Münchausenism (mun'chow"zən-iz-əm) n. telling **commentitious**,
q.v., fabulous, or fantastic adventure stories. [< the tall tales told by
Baron Karl Hieronymus von Münchausen, 1720-1791]. **Münchausen
syndrome** (a clinical-medicine term) is the fabrication by a malingerer
of a clinically convincing, but false, story and simulation of disease.
Münchausen-by-proxy refers to a malingerer doing the same, but
via someone else, e.g., a child, or a demented elder in whom illness
or disease is seriously claimed and simulated.) Cf. **pathomimesis**,
pathomimicry, q.v. See **talk**. See **mentality, mentation, behavior**.

musard (moo'zərd) (F = myzar) n. an absent-minded dreamer or fool.
[< F *musarder* to dawdle, idle]. See **role**. See **intelligence**.

mussitation (mus"si-tay'shən) n. 1. muttering, murmuring,
grumbling to oneself, or in a very low voice. 2. silently imitating the
lip movements of people who are speaking; moving the lips as if
speaking, but without making a sound. The elderly are more prone to
fulfill both definitions. [< L *mussitare* freq. of *mussare* to mutter]. See
talk.

muzzy (muz'zee) (-**zi-er** & -**zi-est**) adj. 1. thinking in a confused,
muddled way, especially as a result of illness or drinking. 2. vague,

blurred, and confused. [Early 18th C. <?]. n. **muzziness**. adv. **muzzily**. See **mentality, mentation, behavior**.

mydriatic (mid-ri-at'tik) adj. 1. causing mydriasis, i.e., dilation of the pupil. 2. an agent, e.g., mydriatic drops, that dilate the pupil. [G, *mydriasis* dilation of the pupil(s)]. n. **mydriasis**. See **eye**.

myopia (mī-ō'pee-ə) n. 1. shortsighted, lacking foresight, narrow-minded. 2. short sightedness, near sightedness, a condition in which, in consequence of an error in refraction or of elongation of the globe of the eye, parallel light rays are focused in front of the retina rather than on it. [myo-, pref., relating to muscle < G *mys* muscle + *ops* eye]. adj. **myopic** (-op'ik). n. **myope** = one who is shortsighted. Cf. **gerontopia**, **senopia**, q.v. See **eye**. See **role**.

my(or **i**)**sophobia** (mīs"sō-fōb'bi-ə) n. morbid fear of contamination. (In re: spelling, **my-** rather than **mi-** is preferred: G *mysos* = defilement, while G *miseo* = hatred.) [< G *mysos* defilement + *phobos* fear]. adj. **mysophobic**. n. **mysophobe** (mī'sō-). syn. **molys(o) mophobia**, q.v. Cf. **bacteriophobia**, **bacillophobia**, **microbiophobia**. See **phobias**.

mythopoeic (mith-ō-pee'ik) adj. anything related to myth making, or giving rise to a myth. [< G *mythopoios* making stories < *mytho-* the combining form of *mythos* + *-poios*, suff., making < *poiein* to make]. (n. **mythomania** = a psychiatric term for excessive exaggeration or lying to an abnormal degree; it's not just a craze for reading or hearing myths, stories.) Cf. **confabulation**, **commentitious**, q.v. See **talk**.

myxedema (miks-e-deem'mə) n. hypothyroidism (Gull's disease) that is characterized by a relatively hard edema (swelling) of subcutaneous tissue, skin dryness, loss of hair, subnormal temperature, hoarseness, muscle weakness, and, after a tendon jerk, slow return of a muscle to its neutral position; it is caused by removal or loss of functioning thyroid tissue. ● In the elderly, *myxedema* is not as common as in the young, but non-*myxedematous* hypothyroidism is increasingly frequent in the elderly. [myx(o)-, pref., relating to mucus < G *myxa* mucus + *oidema* swelling—the G hero, Oedipus, (G. *oidema* swelling + *pous* foot), who, as a neonate, had his feet pierced by his father and as a consequence had swollen feet.)]. adj. **myxedematous** (-dem'mə-təs). See **blood, circulation, glands**. See **physique, appearance**.

N

"Growing old is no more than a bad habit, which a busy
man has no time to form"—André Maurois.

narcolepsy (naar'kō-lep-see) n. paroxysmal sleep; sleep epilepsy; hypnolepsy; a sudden uncontrollable disposition to sleep occurring at irregular intervals, with or without obvious predisposing cause, usually involving an abnormality in sleep-stage sequencing. [narco-, pref., relating to stupor or narcosis < G *narkoun* to benumb, deaden + *lepsis* seizure]. adj. **narcoleptic**. syns. **hypnolepsy**, **hypnopathy**, q.v. See **sleep, wakefulness**.

nashgab (nash'gab)/**gabnash** (gab'nash) n. prattle; chatter. [Sc.]. n. **nashgab** = a pert chatterer. See **talk**. See **role**.

nasute (nay'syoot) adj. 1. having a large nose. 2. having a keen sense of smell. 3. sharp, astute. [< L *nasutus* big-nosed; satirical, sarcastic & *nasute* sarcastically < *nasus* nose; sense of smell; sagacity; anger; scorn; nozzle, spout]. syn. **macrorhinia**, q.v. See **nose, smell**. See **mentality, mentation, behavior**.

natter (nat'tər) vi. 1. (informal) chatter idly, rapidly. 2. (informal) grumble irritatingly. • When the elderly matron was accused by her husband of *nattering*, she recalled Vice-President Spiro Agnew's labeling his political opponents "nattering nabobs of negativism", a phrase created by his speech writer, William Safire. [early 19th C. <?]. n. **natter** = rapid idle chatter, grumbling, gossiping, irritating chatter. ppl. adj. **nattering** = idly chattering; grumbling irritatingly. See **talk**.

nazzard (naz'zərd) n. (obs., except as dial.) an insignificant or feeble person. [of obscure origin]. adj. **nazzardly** = poor, ill-thriven. See **tiredness, weakness**. See **role**.

neanilagnia (nee-an"i-lag'ni-ə) n. a yen, desire for nymphets—a "trophy wife" may possibly satisfy this yen. • The **pornogenarian's**, q.v., neanilagnia was risible. [< G *neos* new + *lagneia* lust; coition— *lagneia furor* = extreme sex urge]. syn. **lagnesis**, q.v. Cf. **shunam(m) itism**, q.v. See **sex, love**.

neanimorphism (nee-an"i-mawr'fiz"əm) n. looking younger than one's years. [< G *neos* new + *morphe* form]. adj. **neanimorphic**. syn.

agerasia, q.v. ant. **geromorphism**, q.v. Cf. **paedomorphism**, q.v. See youth, younger generation. See physique, appearance.

nebulochaotic (neb"yoo-lō-kay-ot'tik) adj. hazy, chaotic, confused. [< L *nebula* mist, fog, vapor; cloud; smoke; darkness, obscurity + < G *khaos* void, abyss]. See mentality, mentation, behavior.

necrologist (nek-rol'ə-jist) n. an obituary writer. [necro-, pref., death, the dead, dead body < G *nekros* corpse + -logy, suff., science, study < *logos* word, reason]. n. **necrology** = a list of persons recently dead; an obituary. adj. **necrologic** (–loj'jik). adj. **necrological** (-loj'ik-). adv. **necrologically** (-loj'jik-). See role. See end-of-life, death.

necromania (nek"rō-may'nee-ə) n. morbid preoccupation with dead bodies. [necr(o)-, pref., denoting relationship to death or to a dead body, cells, tissue < G *necros* dead + *mania* madness]. See end-of-life, death. See manias.

necromimesis (nek"rō-mi-mees'siss) n. feigning death; the delusion of being dead. [necro-, pref., death, the dead, dead body < G *nekros* corpse + *mimetikos* < *mimesis* < *mimeisthai* imitate < *mimos* mime]. adj. **necromimetic** (-mi-met'tik). syn. **necromorphous**, q.v. See end-of-life, death.

necromorphous (nek"rō-mawr'fəss) adj. feigning death to deter someone, e.g., an aggressor. [necro-, pref., death, the dead, dead body < G *nekros* corpse + *morphe* form]. n. **necromorph** (nek'-rō-mawrf) = one who feigns death. Cf. **necromimetic**, q.v. See end-of-life, death. See role.

neomnesia (nee-om-nee'zee-ə, -nee'zha) n. good memory for recent events. [< G *neos* new + *mneme* memory]. See memory.

neopharmaphobia (nee"ō-farm"mə-fōb'bi-ə) n. morbid fear of new medicines or drugs. [neo-, pref., meaning new or recent, < G *neos* new, + *pharma*, a contraction of *pharmacon* medicine + *phobos* fear]. adj. **neopharmaphobic**. n. **neopharmaphobe** (-farm'mə-). Cf. **pharmacophobia** (-kō-fōb'bi-ə), q.v. See phobias. See therapy.

neophobia (nee"ō-fōb'bi-ə) fear of anything new. [neo-, pref., denoting new, modern, later, recast, lately found, or invented < G *neos* new + -phobia, suff., fearing < G *-phobia* < phobos fear]. adj. **neophobic**.

syn. = **kaino(to)phobia** or **caino(to)phobia**, **centophobia**; **tropophobia**, q.v. See **phobias**. See **innovation, misoneism**.

nepenthe (nə-pen'thee) n. the name of an ancient Egyptian drug taken to drown cares and sorrows and to forget woes. The word nepenthe now is used in a generalized sense indicative of any drug having that effect; a tranquilizer. • With so many aches and pains at her advanced age, she relied on a tranquilizer, her *nepenthe*. [< G *nepenthes* soothing herb < *ne-* not + *penthos* grief. (Nepenthe is mentioned in the Odyssey as given by Polydamna, wife of Egypt's King Thonis, to Helen, daughter of Zeus and Leda, and wife of Menelaus, king of Sparta. Helen and Paris, son of King Priam of Troy, fled to Egypt. Their elopement resulted in the 10-year Trojan War and the destruction of Troy by the Greeks.) ("Quaff, oh, quaff this kind nepenthe,/ and forget this lost Lenore!—Edgar Allen Poe, "The Raven")]. See **therapy**. See **memory**.

nephalism (nef'fal-iz-əm) n. total abstinence from alcoholic drinks. The aged, more easily affected unfavorably by alcohol, are more apt to be teetotalers. [G *nephein* to drink no wine]. n. **nephalist**, a teetotaler. See **drink, food**. See **role**.

nepimnemic (nep"pim-neem'mik) adj. childhood memory retained in the subconscious. [< G *nepios* (adj.) infant + *mneme* memory]. See **memory**. See **youth, younger generation**.

nerve, muscle, movement, touch: **akathisia**, **anisosthenic**, **apraxia**, **ataxia**, **calando**, **charlie horse**, **CIMT**, delirium, **dysaphia**, **dyscheiria**, **dysdiadochokinesia**, **dyserethism**, **dysergia**, **dysesthesia**, **dysgeusia**, **dysgraphia**, **dyskinesia/dyscinesia**, **dysmetria**, **dysmimia**, **dysmyotonia**, **dysphasia/dysphrasia**, **dyssynergia**, **dystonia**, **ebriection**, **effleurage**, **gelotripsy**, **herpes zoster**, **hobble**, **hypaesthesia/hypesthesia**, **hyperthermalgesia**, **hypothermalgesia**, **impotentia**, **jactitation**, **limen**, **logagnosia**, **logagraphia**, **logamnesia**, **logaphasia/logophasia**, **logasthenia**, **logoneurosis**, **logopathy**, **logoplegia**, **micrographia**, **Morton's neuroma**, **neurobics**, **palikinesia/palicinesia**, **palsy**, **pandiculation**, **paralysis agitans**, **paresis**, **paresthesia**, **parkinsonism**, **Parkinson's/Parkinson's disease**, **sarcopenia**, **senile delirium**, *shpilkes*, **stereotypy**, **torpid**, **tremor**, **vertiginous**, **zoster**.

nerve, muscle, movement, touch: Subcategories

I. Sensation:
   1. Any sense:
      a. diminished sensation: **hypaesthesia/ hypesthesia**
      b. impairment of *any* sense, but especially of touch: **dysesthesia**
      c. impaired sensibility to stimuli: **dyserethism**
      d. of a body part's numbness: **torpid**
   2. Heat:
      a. decreased sensitivity to heat: **hypothermalgesia**
      b. increased sensitivity to heat: **hyperthermalgesia**
   3. Pain:
      a. from neuralgia: **Morton's neuroma**
      b. from shingles: **herpes zoster**
   4. Peculiar:
      a. morbid or perverted sensation: **paresthesia**
   5. Taste:
      a. impaired sense of taste: **dysgeusia**
   6. Threshold:
      a. threshold of response: **limen**
   7. Touch:
      a. impaired sense of touch: **dysaphia**, **dysesthesia**
      b. impaired sense of on which side the body is touched: **dyscheiria**

II. Muscle movement & tone:
   1. Movement:
      a. excessive twitching, restlessness, inability to sit still: **jactitation**, *shpilkes*
      b. gradual slowing of movement: **calando** (used fig.)
      c. impaired ability to express thought by gesture: **dysmimia**
      d. impaired sense of limb movement, direction: **dysdiadochokinesia**
      e. motor-restlessness neurosis: **akathisia**
      f. slight or incomplete paralysis: **paresis**
      g. to limit movement: **hobble**

2. Involuntary movement:
   a. fixed, patterned, meaningless repeated speech or movements with mental impairment: **stereotypy**
   b. inability to stop a muscle movement at a desired point: **dysmetria** (a form of **dysergia**, q.v. below)
   c. inharmonious muscle action in voluntary movement: **dysergia**
   d. loss of muscle coordination: **ataxia, dyssynergia**
   e. repetition of movements: **palikinesia/ palicinesia**
   f. involuntary trembling, shaking: **tremor**
3. Speech:
   a. lack of coordination in speech & failure to arrange words understandably: **dysphasia / dysphrasia**
   b. speech paralysis: **logoplegia**
4. Tone, force:
   a. abnormal muscle tonicity, either hyper- or hypo-: **dysmyotonia, dystonia**
   b. of unequal force: **anisosthenic**
5. Voluntary, purposeful movement:
   a. incapacity to execute voluntary purposeful movements: **apraxia** (despite good musculature), **dyskinesia/dyscinesia**
   b. inharmonious voluntary-muscle action: **dysergia**
   c. stretching and yawning: **pandiculation**
   d. voluntary muscular inability to move part or all of the body: **palsy**

III. Writing:
   1. Impaired writing ability: **dysgraphia**
   2. Writing with very small letters, sometimes getting smaller and smaller (Parkinson's disease): **micrographia**

IV. Central nervous system incapacity:
   1. Dizziness: dizzy, revolving; vacillating: **vertiginous**
   3. Mental deficiency:
      a. delirium: an acute old-age syndrome characterized by disorientation, restlessness,

insomnia, hallucinations, aimless wandering, etc.: **senile delirium**
  b. mental breakdown due to too much boozing: **ebriection**
  c. mental disorder with confusion, loss of attentiveness, inattention, incoherent speech, reduced consciousness, sensory misperception, hyperactivity: **delirium**
4. Mental exercise:
  a. engaging different parts of the brain to do familiar tasks: **neurobics**
5. Parkinson's: **Parkinson's/Parkinson's disease, paralysis agitans, parkinsonism**
6. Speech:
  a. any speech disorder due to a central nervous system derangement: **logopathy**
  b. any neurosis associated with a speech defect: **logoneurosis**
  c. fixed, patterned, meaningless repeated speech or movements with mental impairment: **stereotypy**
  d. impairment of the ability to speak or write: **logaphasia/logophasia**
  e. inability to speak, articulate; aphasia; agnosia: **logagnosia**
  f. inability to understand spoken or written words, speech, or tactile speech symbols: **logamnesia**
  g. lack of coordination in speech and failure to arrange words understandably: **dysphasia/dysphrasia**
  h. mental disorder with confusion, loss of attentiveness, inattention, incoherent speech, reduced consciousness, sensory misperception, hyperactivity: **delirium**
  i. speech incomprehension: **logasthenia**
7. Writing:
  a. impairment of the ability to speak or write: **logaphasia/logophasia**
  b. inability to express ideas in writing: **logagraphia**

9. Other:
   a. impotence: **impotentia**
   b. localized muscular cramp: **charlie horse**
   c. loss of muscle: **sarcopenia**
   d. massage via gentle rubbing with the palm: **effleurage**
   e. nerve-point massage: **gelotripsy**
   f. painful vesicular rash, usually along one side of the chest: **zoster**
   g. stroke prediction: **CIMT**

nestor (ness'tawr) n. an old man, a patriarch, worthy to be revered for his wisdom. In Homer's Iliad, Nestor, having outlived two generations, is represented as an elder statesman who often gave advice, sometimes ineffectually. [G < *Nestor,* such a man in the Iliad, who was king of Elian Pylos]. See **old**. See **old man**.

neuraminidase inhibitors (noor"-ram-in'ni-dayz) n.phr. drugs (trade names = Tamiflu and Relenza) used, usually effectively, in early treatment of influenza so as to shorten its course and avert its complications. ● Influenza particularly affects the elderly; immunization is less effective in this age group, but *neuraminidase-inhibitor* treatment is advised in both older adults and children. [neur(o)-, pref., denoting relationship to a nerve or nerves, or to the nervous system, < G *neuron* nerve, + amine, an organic compound containing nitrogen + -ase, suff., denoting an enzyme; it is suffixed to the name of the substance upon which the enzyme acts—neuraminidase is a major enzyme of influenza virus]. syn. **sialidase**. See **therapy**.

neurobics (noo-rōb'bikss) n.pl. (used as a singular) engaging different parts of the brain to do familiar tasks, e.g., brushing one's teeth or dialing the phone with one's non-dominant hand, or exercising on an elliptical trainer with one's eyes closed—a danger in the elderly! Such mentally-stimulating endeavors are said to strengthen the pathways on the opposite side of one's brain and to stave off Alzheimer's disease. [a term coined by Lawrence Katz < neuro-, pref., denoting nerve, neural < G *neuron* nerve + *bios* life]. See **nerve, muscle, movement, touch**. See **mentality, mentation, behavior**.

neurodermatitis (noor"rō-derm-mə-tît'tiss) n. See **lichen simplex chronicus**.

neuroplasticity (noor"rō-plas-tis'si-tee) n. the brain's ability to rewire itself throughout life by creating neural connections in response to mental activity. On this premise, cognitive training and brain exercises (brain or cerebral gym or gymnastics) have been developed, particularly via Internet software, in order to improve memory, attention skills, and cognitive reserve. E.g., there is a software program, DriverSharp (from Posit Science) which trains elderly drivers to regain age-degraded capability to rapidly grasp and act on what their eyes see, so they become better drivers. Neuroplasticity is based on relatively new scientific discovery. [neuro-, pref., denoting nerve, neural < G *neuron* nerve + *plastikos* moldable < *plastos* pp. of *plassein* to form, mold + -ity, suff., expressing state or condition < L –*itatem*]. Cf. **neurobics**. See **memory**. See **mentality, mentation, behavior**.

neurotrophins (noo-rō-trō'fən prō'teen) pl.n. two proteins in the cochlea of the inner ear that tend to degenerate with age, and are important in relaying sound messages from the inner ear to the brain. It may be possible to replace them therapeutically. [< neuro-, pref., denoting nerve or relating to the nervous system < G *neuron* nerve + -trophin (trofin), suff., denoting an affinity for the structure or thing indicated by the stem to which it is affixed < *trophe* nourishment]. See **ear, hearing**.

nid-nod (nid-nod) vi.&vt. to nod when sleepy [obscure]. See **sleep, wakefulness**.

nihilarian (nī"hi-lair'ree-ən) n. a person who deals with, concentrates on, things of no importance. [< L *nihil* nothing]. See **role**.

Noachian (nō-aak'ki-ən) adj. pertaining to the Biblical Noah; extremely old. See **old**.

nocebo (nō-seeb'bō) n. illness caused by suggestion—placebo's "evil twin". The **nocebo effect** refers to experiencing the side effects of a drug, medical procedure, or treatment just from being aware of, or being informed of, its existence. E.g., knowing that heart attack can be a drug's side effect and thinking one might be having such an attack. Rarely the nocebo effect can even result in fatality. Thus, it's possible that forewarning patients of possible side effects can result in their causation. Nocebos work by way of a neuropeptide (cholecystokinin) that heightens pain sensation. A blocking drug will cause the pain of a nocebo to diminish. It's appropriate to treat a manifest nocebo with a placebo—< Health Journal by Melinda Beck, Wall Street Journal, 11/18/08. [< a neologism based on the antithesis of a placebo < L, I shall please < *placere* to please. (*Placebo* is the first word in the Vulgate, i.e., for the public, text of Psalm 114:9, used in the Roman Catholic service for the dead)]. See **mentality, mentation, behavior**. See **health, illness**.

noctivagant (nok-tiv'və-gənt) adj. wandering by night. [< L *noctivagus* night-wandering]. n. **noctivagant** = one who wanders by night. syn. **noctivagator**, q.v. See **standing, walking, wandering**. See **role**.

noctivagation (nok-tiv"ə-gay'shən) n. wandering around at night. [< L *noctivagus* (adj.) night-wandering < *nox* night + *vagari* to wander]. n. **noctivagator**. syn. **noctivagant**, q.v. See **standing, walking, wandering**. See **role**.

nocturia (nok-tyoo'ri-ə) n. urinating at night, often because of increased nocturnal secretion of urine, or the increased urinary frequency associated with decreased residual urinary-bladder capacity, due, in turn, in men, to obstructive prostatic enlargement, hypertrophy, which is frequent in older men, or to constipation resulting in a dilated rectum that presses on the prostate and urinary bladder. [< noct(o)-, pref., meaning night, nocturnal < L *nox* night + < G *ouron* urine]. See **prostatism**. See **genitourinary**.

noetic (nō-et'-tik) adj. of or pertaining to the mind or intellect; typical of, coming from, or understood by, the human mind. • Unfortunately, she's *noetically* impaired. [< G *noetikos* < *noetos* < *noeo* apprehend, or < *noetikos* < *noein* to think < *nous* mind]. adv. **noetically**. n. **noesis** (nō-ee'sis), a G n.pl. used as a sing.= intellectual activity, the exercise of reason. n. **noetics** = the science of the intellect. See **intelligence**.

nolition (nō-li'shən)/(rare) **nolleity** (nol-lee'i-tee) n. (obsolete) unwillingness, i.e., the antonym of volition, the absence of willingness. [< L *nolo* to be unwilling to, as in *nolo contendere* = I will not contest it, i.e., the law, thus, guilty]. See **mentality, mentation, behavior**.

nominal aphasia (nom'mi-nəl aa-fay'zhə, -fay'zi-ə) n.phr. **aphasia**, q.v., marked by the defective use of names of objects. Cf. **anomia**, **dysnomia**, **lethonomia**, q.v. See **talk**.

nomogamosis (nōm"mō-gə-mōs'siss) n. marriage between persons highly suitable for each other. [< G *nomos* law + *gamos* marriage]. See **marriage**.

nonagenarian (nōn"nə-jen-ayr'ri-ən) n. someone in his/her ninth decade, i.e., nineties. [< L *nonagenarius* nonagenarian, someone in his/her nineties]. See old man. See **old person(s)**. **See old woman.**

nononeiric (non"ō-nī'rik) adj. not relating to, experienced in, or similar to a dream or dreams. [< non-, pref., not, without, the opposite of < L *non* + G *oneiros* dream]. See **mentality, mentation, behavior**.

nonplus/non-plus (non-pluʂ'/non'plus) vt. (-plussing or –plusing; -plusses or -pluses; -plussed or -plused) to reduce to hopeless perplexity, bewilderment, what to do. [L, *non plus* no more]. adj. **nonplussed**. n. **nonplus** = (dated) a state of confusion, perplexity, standstill, and nervousness. See **mentality, mentation, behavior**.

noodge/nudzh/nudge (nooj) vt.&vi.: vt. to pester or nag. & vi. to whine. [< Yid. *nudyen* to pester, bore < Polish *nudzie*. The word's variant spelling, "nudge", was influenced by the E word "nudge". A related word, **nudnik** = a boring pest. First recorded use was 1960 (Anu Garg)]. n. **noodge** = one who pesters, annoys with unremitting complaining. See **talk**. See **role**.

nose, smell: anosmia, anticholinergic, antihistamines, caprylic, dysosmia, emunctory, epistaxis, feculent, frowsty, frowzy, fusty, hyposmia, leptorrhine, macrorhinia, mephitic, nasute, olfaction, osmesis, osmesthesia, otorhinolaryngologist, ozostomia, pseudosmia, rheum, rhinopathy, rhinophyma, rhinorrhea, rhonchisonant, rosacea, vibrissa.

nose, smell: Subcategories

I. Nose:
    1. Content:
        a. a bristle, long hair growing in the anterior nares: **vibrissa**
        b. excretory, cleansing: **emunctory**
        c. watery discharge from the nose: **rheum**
    2. Disease: **rhinopathy**
        a. nosebleed: **epistaxis**

      b. vascular dilation and hypertrophy of the nose: **rosacea**

      c. runny nose: **rhinorrhea**

  3. Doctor: an ear, nose, and throat doctor: **otorhinolaryngologist**

  4. Size, enlarged:

      a. normal: having a large nose: **nasute, macrorhinia**

      b. abnormal: enlargement of the nose due to connective tissue and sebaceous gland hypertrophy: **rhinophyma**

      c. lengthened and narrow: **leptorrhine**

  5. Snoring: **rhonchisonant**

  6. Treatment of runny nose:

      a. antagonistic to parasympathetic action: **anticholinergic**

      b. histamine-antagonist drugs: **antihistamines**

II. Smell:

  1. Ability to perceive and distinguish odors: **osmesthesia**

  2. Absent or impaired sense of smell: **anosmia**

  3. Diminished sense of smell: **hyposmia**

  4. False smell-perception: **pseudosmia**

  5. Foul breath: **ozostomia**

  6. Foul smelling: **mephitic, feculent**

  7. Having a keen sense of smell: **nasute**

  8. Having a rancid animal odor: **caprylic**

  9. Impaired sense of smell: **dysosmia**

  10. Musty, having a stale smell, ill smelling, **fusty**, q.v.: **frowsty, frowzy**

  11. Smelling of damp dust, mildew, or age: **fusty**

  12. The act of smelling: **olfaction, osmesis**

nosocomephobia (nōs"sō-kōm"mǝ-fōb'bi-ǝ) n. morbid fear of hospitals. [noso-, pref., relating to disease < G *nosos* disease + < L *comes* a companion; concomitant, consequence < *com-* together & *eo*, pp. of *itus* to go + < G *phobos* fear]. adj. **nosocomephobic**. n. **nosocomephobe**. See <u>phobias</u>.

nosocomephrenia (nōs"sō-kōm"mǝ-free'ni-ǝ) n. depression from a prolonged hospital stay. [noso- pref., relating to disease < G *nosos* disease + < L *comes* a consequence; a companion; concomitant

< *com-* together & *eo*, pp. of *itus* to go + -phrenia, suff., denoting the mind (or the diaphragm) < *phren* seat of emotions, mind, the diaphragm, heart]. adj. **nosocomephrenic**. See **mentality, mentation, behavior**. See **health, illness**.

nosomania (nōs"sō-may'ni-ə) n. The incorrect belief of a patient that he has some special disease. [noso- pref., relating to disease < G *nosos* disease + *mania* frenzy, madness]. adj. **nosomaniacal** (-mə-nī'ə-kəl). n. **nosomaniac**. See **manias**. See **health, illness**.

nosophobia (nōs"sō-fōb'bi-ə) n. morbid fear of disease or of becoming ill. [noso-, pref., relating to disease < G *nosos* disease + -phobia, suff., fearing < G *-phobia* < *phobos* fear]. adj. **nosophobic**. n. **nosophobe**. syn. **pathophobia**, q.v. See **phobias**. See **health, illness**.

nosothymia (nos"sō-thīm'mi-ə) n. depression due to serious illness.
• *Nosothymia* is a not infrequent finding in the elderly; it should be treated as in other age groups. [noso-, pref., relating to disease < G *nosos* disease + -*thymia*, suff., denoting a condition of mind < G *thymos* 1. mind, spirit, or 2. thymus gland.] See **emotion**.

nostalgic (nōs-tal'jik) n. one who recollects sentimentally with mixed feelings of happiness, sadness, and longing about a person, place, or event; one who is homesick. [< G *nostos* home-coming + *algos* pain]. n. **nostalgia** (-jə). adj. **nostalgic**. adv. **nostalgically**. See **old man**. See **old person(s)**. See **old woman**. See **role**.

nostology (nos-tol'lə-jee) n. 1. the scientific study of old age, aging and its effects; study of senility. 2. the science of caring for the elderly. [< G *nostos* return home: from the former idea that later life is like a return to early years + *logos* word, study, discourse]. adj. **nostologic** (-tō-loj'jik). adv. **nostologically** (-tō-loj'ji-). n. **nostologist** = one who cares for the elderly or scientifically studies them. syn. **gerontology**, q.v. See **old age**. See **role**. See **therapy**.

nostomaniac (nos-tō-may'ni-ak) n. one exhibiting aggravated nostalgia, an obsessive or abnormal interest in nostalgia especially as an extreme manifestation of homesickness, mania to return home. [< G *nostos* return, homecoming + *mania* frenzy]. n. **nostomania**.

adj. **nostomaniacal** (-mə-nī'ə-kəl). Cf. **hesternopathic**, *laudator temporis acti*, **preterist**, q.v. See **manias**. See **role**.

nous (nows, nows—properly noos according to Alexander Pope: "Thine is the genuine head of many a house,/ And much divinity without a noos.") n. mind, intellect, intelligence; colloquially, common sense, horse sense; as slang: savvy, gumption. [via G philosophy, G, intelligence]. See **intelligence**.

nunc dimittis (noŏnk dee-mit'tis) n.phr. 1. willingness, readiness to die. 2. the canticle, Nunc Dimittis: Lord, now lettest thou sing *nunc dimittis*, i.e., Be willing to depart from life. Therefore, to receive one's *nunc dimittis* is to receive permission to die.) [L, now lettest thou {thy servant}go, i.e., depart this life < Luke 2, 29-32, starting in L with *"Nunc dimities servum tuum, Domine."*]. See **end-of-life, death**.

nuncupate (nun'kyoo-payt) vt. 1. to declare orally. 2. to make, declare an oral (non- written) will, last testament. 3. to dedicate, inscribe. [< L *nuncupatio* name, appellation; public pronouncing (of vows) < *nuncupare* to name, call; to take or make (a vow) publicly; to proclaim publicly—probably based on the phrase *nomen capere*, lit., to take a name, fig., to utter a name publicly]. adj. **nuncupative**, appearing almost always as "nuncupative will": a last will & testament spoken aloud to a witness(es), rather than written. See **talk**. See **finance**. **end-of-life, death**.

nutation (nyou-tay'shən) n. involuntary nodding of the head; specifically, habitual or constant nodding of the head. adj. **nutant**. [< L *nutare* to keep nodding; to sway to and fro, totter; to hesitate, waver]. See **sleep, wakefulness**.

nyctalopia (nik"təl-ōp'pi-ə) n. night blindness. [nyct(o)-, pref., night, nocturnal < G *nyx* night + *alaos* obscure + *ops* eye]. ant. = **hemeralopia**. Cf. **amaurosis**, **cecity**, **cecutiency**, **idiopia**, **luscition**, **occecation**, **purblind**, q.v. See **eye**.

O

"Old age is not for sissies."
—attributed to the actress, Betty Davis.

Seniores priores, i.e., Elders first!—which is used in reminding the young of the precedence due seniority. [L].

OBA a chat and text-message initialism = o̲ld b̲attle a̲xe—an offensive term for an unpleasant, querulous, demanding, criticizing, shrewish old woman. [Netlingo.com]. See **old woman**.

obambulate (ob-amb'byoo-layt) vt. (rare) to walk about, wander in an aimless fashion. [< L *obambulare* to prowl all over, prowl about; walk about, wander < *ob* in the way, against, toward; for the sake of, in the interest of, etc. + *ambulare* to traverse, travel; walk, take a walk]. syn. **oberration**, q.v. See **standing, walking, wandering**.

obdurate (ob'door-ət) adj. stubbornly unyielding to persuasion or influence; disinclined to be persuaded by emotion or sympathy, or to feel pity. [< L *obduratus*, pp. of obdurare to be hard < *durus* hard]. n. **obduracy** (ob'door-). n. **obdurateness** (ob'door-ət"ness). adv. **obdurately**. See **mentality, mentation, behavior**.

oberrate (ob'ber-ate) vt. (obs., rare) to wander, roam, lose one's way; to err, make a mistake. n. **oberration**. [< L. *oberrare* to ramble about, wander around < *ob* in the way, against, toward; for the sake of, in the interest of, etc., + *errare* to wander, lose one's way, stray, roam; waver, err, make a mistake]. syn. **obambulate**, q.v. See **standing, walking, wandering**.

obganiate (ob-gan'-ni-ayt) vi. (obs., rare) to irritate or trouble one with reiteration. [< L *obgannire* to yelp or growl]. n. **obganiator**. n. **obganiation**. syn. **verbigerate**, q.v. See **talk**. See **role**.

obituary (ō-bi'choo-air"ree) pl. **–ies** n. 1. a notice of a death or deaths, esp. in a newspaper. 2. an account of the life of a deceased person. 3. (attributive) of or serving as an obituary. [< L *obituaries* < *obitus* death < *obire obit-* to die < *ob-* + *ire* to go]. adj. **obituarial** (-bi"choo-air'i-əl). n. **obituarist** = a death-notice writer. See **end-of-life, death**. See **role**.

objurgate (ob'jər-gayt") vt. (literary) to chide or scold somebody angrily. [< L *objurgate-*, pp. of *objurgare* to quarrel against < *jurgium* quarrel]. n. **objurgation** (ob"jər-gay'shən). n. **objurgator** (ob'jər-gay"tər). adj. **objurgative** (ob-jur'gə-tiv). adj. **objurgatory** (ob-jur'gə-tawr"ee). adv. **objurgatively** (ob-jur'gə-tiv"lee). adv. **objurgatorily** (o b-jur'gə-tawr"ri-lee). See **talk**. See **role**.

obloquy (ob'lə-kwee) n. 1. (formal or literary) statements that severely criticize or defame somebody. 2. a state of disgrace brought about by being defamed. [< L *obloquium* talking against < *ob* in the way, against, toward; for the sake of, in the interest of, etc., + *loqui* to talk]. See **talk**.

obmutescence (ob-myoo-tes'ənz) n. obstinate silence; taciturn; the act of becoming unable to speak or of keeping silent. [< L *obmutescere* to become silent; hush up; cease < *mutus* dumb]. adj. **obmutescent**. ant. **logomania**, q.v. See **talk**.

obnubilate (ob-n{y}oob'bil-layt) vt. 1. to obstruct vision as if by clouds. 2. to befog or confuse. [< L *obnubilo*, pp. –*atus* overcloud, befog < *nubes* a cloud]. n. **obnubilation** (-ay'shən) = a clouded or confused mental state. See **eye**. See **talk**. See **mentality, mentation, behavior**.

obsequies (ob'sə-kweez) n.pl. (n.s. **obsequy**) rites or ceremonies carried out at a funeral. [< L *obsequiae*, an alteration (influenced by *obsequiun* compliance) of *exequiae* those following out (to the grave) < *exsequi* follow out < *sequi* follow]. See **end-of-life, death**.

obsolagnium (ob-sō-lag'ni-əm) n. waning sexual desire due to age. [< L *obsolescere* to wear out, become obsolete, lose value + < G *lagneia* lust]. See **sex, love**.

obsolescent (ob-sō-les'sənt) adj. becoming obsolete or disappearing from use or existence by being replaced by something new. [< L *obsolescere* wear out < *solere* be accustomed]. n. **obsolescence**. vi. **obsolesce**. See **Innovation, misoneist**.

obstipation (ob-sti-pay'shən) n. 1. extreme constipation; intestinal obstruction. (2. the act of stopping up.) [< L *ob* against + *stipoare* to crowd, cram, pack]. syn. **coprostasia**, q.v. See **gastrointestinal**.

obstruent (ob-stroo'ənt) adj. (lit. & fig.) producing an obstruction, hindering. [< L *obstruere* to pile up, block up, stop up; (with dative) to block or close against]. See **mentality, mentation, behavior**. See **health, illness**.

obtrude (ob-trood') vi.&vt. to impose oneself or one's opinions on other people. vt. to push something out or forward. vi. to appear or be present in a way that is unwelcome but can not be ignored.

[< L *obtrudere* thrust against < *trudere* to thrust]. n. **obtruder**. n. **obtrusion**. adj. **obtrusive**. adv. **obtrusively**. See **talk**. See **mentality, mentation, behavior**. See **role**.

occecation (ok-see-kay'shən) n. becoming blind; blindness. [< L *occaecare* to blind, make blind; to darken, obscure; to hide; to numb < *caecare* to blind]. See **eye**.

octogenarian n. someone in his/her eighth decade, eighties. [< L *octogenarius* octogenarian]. See **old person(s)**. See **role**.

odontophobia (ō-dont"tō-fōb'bi-ə) n. a morbid fear of dentists. [< G *odous* (*odont-*) tooth + -phobia, suff., fearing < G -*phobia* < *phobos* fear]. adj. **odontophobic**. n. **odontophobe**. See **phobias**. See **mouth, gums, teeth**.

odynophobia (ō-din"ō-fō'bi-ə) n. fear of pain. [odyn(o)-, pref., pain < G *odyne* pain + *phobos* fear]. adj. **odynophobic**. n. **odynophobe** (-din'ō-). syn. **algophobia**, q.v. See **phobias**. See **pain**.

oenomania (ee"nō-may'ni-ə)/**enomania**/**oinomania** n. abnormal interest in, desire for wine. • He justified his *oenomania* for red wine by belief in the benefits of **resveratrol**, q.v. [< G *oinos* wine + *mania* frenzy]. adj. **oenomaniacal** (-mə-nī'ə-kəl). n. **oenomaniac**. See **manias**. See **drink, food**. See **role**.

officious (ə-fish'həs) adj. 1. characteristic of somebody who is eager to give unwanted help or advice; aggressively asserting one's authority; bossy. (2. unofficial or informal, especially in political or diplomatic dealing.) [< L *officiosus* < *officium* doing work < *opus* work + *facere* to do]. adv. **officiously**. n. **officiousness**. See **mentality, mentation, behavior**.

Ogygian/ogygian (ō-jij'jee-ən) adj. (1. pertaining to King Ogyges (ō-jī'jees), or to a terrible flood during his reign.) 2. very old: **superseptuagenarian**, q.v.; incomparably ancient; antediluvian; primeval. [< G *Ogygos*, a mythological king of Attica or Boeotia, the most ancient king of Greece, during whose reign a great flood or deluge occurred. Comparable floods are associated with Noah, Deucalion (the Greek Noah), and Dardanus]. n. **Ogygian** (literary) = someone over seventy. See **old person(s), people**.

oikofugic (oy-kō-fyooj'jik) adj. obsessive wandering. [< G *oikos* household + L *fuga* flight, disappearance < *fugere* to escape, run away from flee; disappear + -ic, suff., of or relating to < L *-icus*, suff. < G *-ikos*, suff.]. n. **oikofuge** = one who wanders (away from home). See **standing, walking, wandering**. See **role**.

oikomania (oyk"kō-mayn'ni-ə) n. 1. abnormal desire to be at home, to stay at home. 2. any neurotic disorder supposed to result from something unpleasant or dreadful in one's home environment. [< G *oikos* house, household, habitation + *mania* frenzy]. adj. **oikomaniacal** (oyk"kō-ma-nī'ə-kəl). n. **oikomaniac**. syn. **ecomania**, q.v. See **manias**. See **loneliness, solitude, silence**.

old: This category is comprised of adj(s)., adj.phr(s)., & vi(s). Headwords are in **bold**; foreign words are in *italic*; foreign headwords are in ***bold and italic***; words in standard type are exdictionary. Only words in **bold** or ***bold & italic*** are included in the dictionary.

adamic, advanced in years (or age), ***aetate provectus***, age-old, **age**, **aged**, aging, ancestral, ancient, antebellum, **antediluvian**, **antiquarian**, **antiquated**, antique, **archaic**, ***arriere garde***, as old as Adam, as old as Methuselah, as old as the hills, as old as time, **ayne**, been around, blue-rinse, bygone, cast-aside, cast-off, **centenary**, **centennial**, classic, classical, **coetaneous**, **coeval**, creaky, crumbling, dated, decayed, **decrepit**, dilapidated, disintegrated, disused, doddering, ***démodé***, ***d'un certain age***, Edwardian, **eigne**, elder, elderly, **emeritus -a**, enduring, experienced, **fogram/fogrum**, fossil, fossilized, full-of-years, **fusty**, **gerocomical**, **gerontal/gerontic**, getting on or along (in years), gone, Gothic, gray/grey (British), gray-haired, grizzled, hairy, Helladic, Hellenic, **hoary**, immemorial, inveterate, Jacobean, lasting, *lao*, **longevous**, **long-in-the-tooth**, long-lived, long-standing, **macrobian**, mature, medieval, mellow, moldering, moss-grown, moth-eaten, musty, **Noachian**, not-getting-any-younger, obsolescent, obsolete, of advanced years, **Ogygian/ogygian**, **oldfangled**, old and gray, old-fashioned, old-hand, old-hat, oldie, old-time, old-world, one-time, out-dated, outmoded, out-of-date, out-of-the-arc, over-the-hill, *paleo-* (G pref. = ancient), **paleoanthropic**, **paleography**, ***passé***, past-it, past-one's-prime, patriarchal, practiced, prehistoric, **prelapsarian**, primal, primeval, primitive, primordial, **raddled**, ramshackle, **relict**, retired, ripe, rooted, rusty, **sear**, **senescent**, senile, **senior**, shot, **Silurian**, **spavined**, stale, superannuated, superseded, time-honored, time-worn, traditional, unused, **venerable**, veteran, **vetust**, Victorian, vintage, well-established, well-versed, white-haired, worn back number, *vieil-lle*, *vieillot* -otte, vieux. [old is < OE *eald*]. See **physique, appearance**.

old: Subcategories

I. <u>Advanced in age</u>:
   1. Having lived long, old: **aged, senior**
   2. Of advanced age: *aetate provectus*
II. <u>Extremely old (over seventy {!?})</u>:
   1. Incomparably ancient; antediluvian; primeval: **adamic**; **antediluvian**; **Ogygian/ogygian** (pertaining to King Ogyges, or to a terrible flood during his reign); **paleoanthropic**; **prelapsarian**
   2. Fig., extremely, terribly old; pertaining to the Biblical Noah: **archaic, Silurian; Noachian**
   3. Of a century: **centenary, centennial**
   4. Pertaining to a relic or survivor of a vanished species, race, etc., (can be used fig.): **relict**
III. <u>Getting old</u>:
   1. Approaching an advanced age: **senescent**
   2. Oldish, quaint; old (F): *vieillot* -otte
   3. To age: **age**
IV. <u>Impaired function due to age</u>:
   1. In poor condition, especially old, overused, or not working efficiently: **decrepit**
   2. Old and silly; aged and worsened by debauchery: **raddled**
   3. Old; decrepit; broken-down (fig.): **spavined**
V. <u>Long-lived: of great age; having lived to a great age</u>: **longevous, macrobian**
VI. <u>Of the same age</u> (not necessarily old): **coetaneous, coeval**
VII. <u>Old, elderly</u>:
   1. An extremely polite (**empressement**, q.v.) way of saying someone, especially a woman, is elderly: *d'un certain age* (lit. of a certain age)
   2. Eldest: **ayne, eigne**
   3. Old, aged: **long-in the-tooth, senior, vieux**
   4. Old, ancient, antique: **vetust**
   5. Senile, or old, or relating to an old man: **gerontal/ gerontic**

      6. Smelling of damp dust, mildew, or age: **fusty**

VIII. Old in appearance, color:
1. Gray, white, with age; having hair of such color: **hoary**
2. Withered, dried up (lit., of flowers, leaves, etc.; fig., of the aged): **sear**

IX. Outdated, old fashioned:
1. Aged; out of date, antiquated (F): *vieil -lle*
2. Ancient, outmoded, out of date: **archaic, oldfangled** (informal)
3. Extremely out of date or badly in need of updating or replacing. **antiquated**
4. Old-fashioned and conservative in style, etc.: **fusty**
5. Old fashioned, old hat, *passé*: **arriere garde**, *démodé*, **fogram/fogrum**
6. Past, gone; outdated, outmoded; faded; vanished: *passé*

X. Pertaining to a dealer in, collector, scholar of antiques: **antiquarian**

XI. Retired (usually of academicians) due to age: *emeritus -a*

XII. Study or writing about ancient things: **paleography**

XIII. Venerable, respected: hoary:
1. A respectful term, honorific used for older people: *lao* (low).
2. Respected in retirement: *emeritus -a*
3. Worthy of respect as a result of great age, wisdom, etc., extremely old: **venerable**

XIV. Treatment of the aged: **gerocomical**

old age: This category is comprised of nouns, n.phrs., & vis. Headwords are in **bold** type; foreign words are in italic; foreign headwords are in both **bold & italic**; words in standard type are exdictionary.

advancing or advanced years, *aetate provectus*, **age**, agedness, **ageism/agism**, **agerasia**, allotted span, ancientness, **anecdotage**, **anility** (women only), **antiquity**, **archaeolatry**, **archaism**, **archaist**, **archaizer**, **aureate years**, autumn of (one's) life, **babyboomer**, burden of years, **caducity**, **centennial**, debility, decline, declining years, decrepitude, **desuetude**, **dotage**, dust or cobwebs of antiquity, **elder-care hostel**, **elderliness**, **eugeria**, **evening of (one's) life**, feebleness, **fogydom**, (old) fogyism, FOX03A, frailty, geezerhood, geezersphere, gerascophobia, geriatric center, geriatrician, geriatrics, gerodontics, gerodontist, geromorphism, gerontocomium, gerontocracy, gerontology, gerontophilia, gerontophobia, geroscience, golden age, gold years, golden years, gray power, gray rights, grayness, harvest years, hibernacle, hoariness, hunkerousness, immune scenescence, infirmity, lipsanographer, lipsanography, longevity, maturity, mellowness, nostology, oldness, paracme, pensionable age, perennate, presbyatrician, presbyatrics/presbytiatrics, presenium, progerin, quinquennium, relic, relict, retirement age, ripe old age, second childhood, senectitude, senescence, senex -is, senilism, senility, senior, seniority, senium, September, shibui, silver alert, silver surge, sirtum 1/SirT1/SIRT1, superannuated, telomere, threescore years and ten, time immemorial, venerableness, vieilleries, vieillesse, vir magno jam natu, winter of (one's) life, years.

(For an AARP benefit at Radio City Music Hall, the actress, Julie Andrews, then celebrating her 69th birthday in 2009, sang a new version of the hit song,"These Are My Favorite Things" from the musical and movie, "The Sound of Music", which won the Academy of Motion Pictures' "Best Movie of 1965" award. The 2009 altered lyrics, typifying the problems of **old age**, follow:

> Maalox and nose drops and needles for knitting,/ Walkers and handrails and new dental fittings,/ Bundles of magazines tied up in string,/ These are a few of my favorite things. Cadillac's and cataracts and hearing aids and glasses,/ Polident and Fixodent and false teeth in glasses,/ Pacemakers, golf carts, and porches with swings,/ These are a few of my favorite things. When the pipes leak,/ When the bones creak,/ When the knees go bad,/ I simply remember my favorite things,/ And then I don't feel so bad. Hot tea and crumpets and corn pads for bunions,/ No spicy hot food or food cooked with onions,/ Bathrobes and heating pads and hot meals they bring,/ These are a few of my favorite things. Back pains, confused brains, and no need for sinnin',/ Thin bones and fractures and hair that is thinnin',/ And we won't mention our short, shrunken frames,/ When we remember our favorite things. When the joints ache,/ When the hips break,/ When the eyes grow

*dim,/ Then I remember the great life I've had,/ And then I
don't feel so bad.*

Ms. Andrews received a standing ovation that lasted over four minutes
from the crowd and had repeated encores.

In Shakespeare's Romeo and Juliet, Juliet, annoyed, impatient with
her doddering old nurse to tell her, Juliet, of Romeo's plan to marry
her says, "Old folks, many feign as they were dead. /Unwieldy, slow,
heavy, and pale as lead.")

old age: Subcategories

I.   An announcement of interest to elders: **silver alert**
II. Appearance in old age:
    1. Beauty revealed only by time: *shibui*
    2 Having white, gray hair &/or complexion: **hoariness**
    3. Someone surviving unchanged: **relict**
    4. The condition of appearing older than one's age,
       presenile: **geromorphism**
    5. Youthful appearance in an older person: **agerasia**
III. Extreme old age:
    1. The condition or quality of being long lived: **longevity**
    2. Survivor from the past: **relic**
    3. The state of being very old, ancient: **antiquity**
IV. Increasing proportion of elders to other age groups:
    babyboomer, silver surge
V.   Old-age dentist; old-age dentistry: **gerodontist;
    gerodontics**
VI. Old-age doctor; old age medical specialty; old age
    science, & study of old age: **geriatrician, presbyatrician;
    geriatrics, presbyatrics/presbytiatrics; gerontology,
    geroscience, nostology**
VII. Old-age entitlements: **gray rights**
VIII. Old-age failings:
    1. The state of failings, silliness associated with old age:
       dotage
    2. The weakness, feebleness of old age; decrepitude:
       caducity
IX   Old age itself: **elderliness**

X.   Old-age morbid fear: **gerascophobia, gerontophobia**
     Old-age genes:
     1. An old-age, longevity gene: **FOXO3A, Sirtum 1/ SirT1/SIRT1**.
XI. Old-age government, political influence: **gerontocracy**
     1. Political & consumer influence of the aged: **gray power**.
XII. Old-age happiness: **eugeria**
XIII. Old-age home, residence: **elder-care hostel, geriatric center, gerontocomium, hibernacle**
XIV. Old-age ideas, things: *vieilleries*.
     1. Something ancient, outmoded, no longer in use, e.g., a word or phrase: **archaism**
     2. State of disuse, neglect: being outmoded: **desuetude**
XV. Old-age love:
     1. Morbid love of old persons: **gerontophilia**
XVI. Old-age medical problems:
     1. Progressive immune-system dysfunction: **immune scenescence**
     2. Protein that accumulates with age: **progerin**
     3. The state of failings, silliness associated with old age: **dotage**
XVII. Old-age opposition to progress: **hunkerousness**
     1. The state of being old, old-fashioned: **fogydom**, (old) **fogyism, relict**
XVIII. Old-age persistence:
     1. To persist from season to season: **perennate**
     2. Increased-longevity genetic factor: **telomere**
XIX. Old-age prejudice: **ageism/agism**
XX. Old-age retirement:
     1. Made inactive, obsolete, retired, disqualified: **superannuated**
XXI. Old-age roles:
     1. One who is an elder: **senior**
     2. One who makes things to appear older than they are: **archaizer**
     3. One who uses archaic expressions: **archaist**
     4. One who writes about relics: **lipsanographer**
XXII. Old-age synonyms: *aetate provectus*, **aureate years, evening of (one's) life, golden years, September, senescence, geezerhood, geezersphere, golden years, harvest years, senectitude, senility, senium,** *vieillesse*

XXIII. <u>Old-age talkativeness, garrulousness</u>: **anecdotage**
XXIV. <u>Old-age veneration</u>:
    1. Worship of anything archaic: **archaeolatry, hoariness**
XXV. <u>Old-age writing</u>:
    1. Writing about relics (fig., old age): **lipsanography**
XXVI. <u>Old womanish</u>:
    1. Lacking in strength; faltering; imbecilic: **anility**
XXVII. <u>Period of 50 years</u>: **quinquennium**
XXVIII.<u>Premature ageing</u>: **senilism**
XXIX. <u>Pre-old age, period before old age</u>: **paracme, presenium, senescence**
XXX. <u>Something's one-hundredth anniversary</u>: **centennial**
XXXI. <u>To age</u>: **age**
XXXII. <u>Young-appearing elder, youthful appearance in old age</u>: **agerasia**

old as . . . / **as old as** . . . / **an old** . . . / **old** . . . adv(s)., n.phr(s), & sentences: old as the hills/ as old as Methuselah, as old as Panton Gates—a corruption of Pandon Gates at New-castle-on-Tyne/ An old man's eagle mind—Yeats, *Last Poems*; *An Acre of Grass*, st.4. An old parrot does not mind the stick—*Senex psittacus negligit ferulam* [L]/ Old men are garrulous by nature—Cicero, *De Senectute*, XVI. Old age: the crown of life, our play's last act—Cicero, *De Senectute*, XXIII. Old dogs will not learn new tricks. Old lady of Threadneedle Street—cognomen for the Bank of England: Gillray, 1797. Old Man Eloquent—refers to Isocrates, so called by Milton. Old persons do not readily fall into new ways. See **old**. See **old age**. See **old man**. See **old person(s)**. See **old woman**.

old birkie (birk'i) n. a Scottish term for an aggressive, crusty, self-assertive, independent old person. [? < ON *berkja* to bark, boast]. See **old person(s)**. See **role**.

old boy, old girl n.phr. British collocations for an alumnus/alumna of a secondary school; term of intimacy; can be used familiarly, generally. See **old man**. see **old woman**.

old buzzard (buz'zərd) n. 1. (slang & derogatory) an unprepossessing old man. (2. North American vulture, e.g. turkey vulture, or European buteo.) [< OF *busard*, alt. < *buson* < L *buteonem* falcon + -ard, suff., somebody characterize by a given quality < OF < Gmc.]. See **old man**.

old duffer (duf'fər) n.phr. (informal insult) an old man who is a slow-witted learner or incompetent at something. [mid-18th C. duffer = one who sells trash as valuable, pretending it to be smuggled, stolen, etc.; a peddler, hawker, faker of sham articles < duff vt., slang, to fake up goods, give a look of newness, etc., to—origin unknown]. See <u>old man</u>.

oldfangled (ōld-fang'gəld) adj. (informal) antiquated or out of date. [< newfangled < pp. of OE *fon* capture]. See <u>old</u>.

old fart n.phr. (offensive, indecent, taboo collocation) an old unpleasant person. (**fart** n. an expelling, accompanied by sound, of bowel gas from the anus; a **crepitus**, q.v.) [< OE *feorting*, a verbal noun, < Gmc.]. See <u>old person(s)</u>.

<u>old man (men)</u>: This category is comprised of both nouns and adjs. The latter are indicated by (adj.) after the word. Headwords are in **bold** type; foreign words are in italic; foreign headwords are in both ***bold*** & ***italic***; words in standard type are exdictionary; underlining indicates a term applicable to both genders. The bold-type word, **old**, before a word indicates its constant use with that word, while (old) indicates inconstant use. (All <u>old man</u> nouns would qualify in the <u>role</u> category, but are not listed there.) See <u>old person(s)</u>, also.

abuelo, *alter Kocker*, <u>aval</u> (adj.), **avuncular**, **bodach**, <u>(old) **buffer**</u>, **old buzzard**, <u>**centenarian**</u>, (old) **codger**, **cogger**, <u>**congener**</u>, <u>(old)</u> <u>**coot**</u>, (old) **coprolite**, **crambazzle**, <u>(old) **crony**</u>, <u>**curmudgeon**</u> (typically a man), <u>dinosaur</u>, dirty old man, <u>**dotard**</u>, <u>**dott(e)rel**</u>, **doyen**, **old duffer**, <u>**old fart**</u>, <u>**fogram/fogrum**</u>, **old fogy**, <u>(old) **fossil**</u>, <u>(old) **fuddy-duddy**</u>, **gaffer/gaffer-**, (old) **geezer**, **gerontal** (adj.), **gerontarchical** (adj.), *Gerousia*, <u>(old) **gnoff/gnof/gnoffe/gnooffe/**</u> <u>**gnuffe/knuffe**</u>, **gnome**, old goat, <u>**golden ager**</u>, **graybeard**, <u>**grisard/**</u> <u>**grizard**</u>, **grognard**, **hoarhead**, **hunker**, **hunks**, <u>**macrobiote**</u>, **Methuselah**, <u>**mossback**</u>, **nestor**, Noah, <u>**nonagenarian**</u>, <u>**nostalgic**</u> (n.), <u>**octogenarian**</u>, <u>**Ogygian**</u> (adj.), <u>**old** *birkie*</u>, <u>**old boy/old girl**</u>, **old buzzard**, old dog, **old duffer**, <u>**old fart**</u>, **old soak**, <u>**oldster**</u>, <u>**old timer**</u>, <u>**old thing**</u>, **OM**, <u>**padnag**</u>, **patriarch**, <u>**pensioner**</u>, **pornogenarian**, <u>**preterist**</u>, (old) **rake**, <u>**relic**</u>, <u>**relict**</u>, (old) **roué**, <u>(old)</u> <u>**rudesby**</u>, (old) **satyr**, <u>**sedens**</u>, <u>**sedentary**</u> (adj.), <u>**senescent**</u> (adj.), *senex*, senior, septuagenarian, sexagenarian, Silenus, Silurian (adj., n.), skinflint, snowbird, *Struldbrug*, supercentenarian, superseptuagenarian, Teiresias/ Tiresias, twichild, *veuf*, *veuvage*, *viduus*, *vieux*/*vieil*, *vir magno jam natu*, waffle, wellderly, whitebeard, WOG. N.B. some of the above terms are not limited to the elderly, e.g., grisard, avuncular, sedens; see definitions.

old man: Subcategories

I. Age of an old man by decade: 60's = sexagenarian, 70's = septuagenarian, > 70s = superseptuagenarian, 80's = octogenarian, 90's = nonagenarian, 100 = centenarian, > 100 = supercentenarian

II. Beard & hair:
   1. A gray-haired man: grisard/grizard, graybeard
   2. Gray- or white-haired old man: hoar head
   3. Small, shriveled, ugly old man with a beard: gnome
   4. White-bearded old man: whitebeard

III. Extremely old progenitor: Methuselah, nestor, patriarch

IV. Desirable, good, or neutral qualities in an old man:
   1. An alumnus, intimate or familiar, or general term: old boy
   2. Elderly rustic old man: gaffer/gaffer-
   3. Grandfather: *abuelo*
   4. Having gray hair: grisard/grizard
   5. Living where born: sedens
   6. Man who is long lived; long-lived men: macrobiote, Ogygian; wellderely; and see I. above: Age of an old man by decade.
   7. Most senior, respected, male member of a group: doyen, nestor
   8. Old-fashioned, passé, or conservative man resisting novelty: fogram/fogrum
   9. Old man: OM (old man)
   10. Old man who recollects sentimentally, with mixed feelings about the past, or is homesick: nostalgic (n.)
   11. Old, wise prophet: Teiresias/Tiresias
   12. One who sits a lot: sedentary
   13. Self-assertive, independent, crusty, aggressive old man: old *birkie*
   14. Uncle-like: avuncular

15. Wise old man: **WOG** (<u>w</u>ise <u>o</u>ld <u>g</u>uy)
V. <u>Government by old men</u>: **gerontarchical** (n. = **gerontarchy**), *Gerousia*
VI. <u>Oversexed</u>: (old) **rake**, (old) **roué**, (old) **satyr**, **pornogenarian**
VII. <u>Pensioned old man</u>: **pensioner**
VIII. <u>Pertaining to a grandfather</u>: <u>aval</u>
IX. <u>Physical deterioration</u>:
    1. Slow-witted, incompetent old man: **old duffer**
    2. Worn out, dissipated old man: **crambazzle**
    3. Worn out, slow, decrepit old man: <u>padnag</u>, <u>Struldbrug</u>
X. <u>Someone of the same (old) age; or of similar age</u>: <u>congener</u>; **old boy**
XI. <u>Synonyms for old man</u>: **centenarian**, **gerontal/gerontic** (adj.), <u>golden ager</u>, **graybeard**, <u>(old) buffer</u>, **old buzzard**, <u>(old) coot</u>, <u>(old) crony</u>, (old) **geezer**, <u>oldster</u>, <u>old-thing</u>, <u>old timer</u>, <u>relic</u>, <u>relict</u>, <u>senescent</u>, <u>senex</u>, <u>senior</u>, <u>Silurian</u>, <u>snowbird</u>, <u>twichild</u>, *vieillard*, *vieux/vieil*, *vir magno jam natu*
XII. <u>Undesirable, bad, disagreeable, or inappropriate qualities in an old man</u>:
    1. Canny, stubborn, unappealing old man (Yid.): *alter kocker*
    2. Drunken old man: **old soak**, **Silenus**
    3. Eccentric old man: (old) **codger**
    4. Goblin-, churl-, specter-like old man (Gaelic): **bodach**
    5. Heartedly disliked old man: <u>waffle</u>
    6. Loud-mouthed, ill-mannered, turbulent, boorish man: <u>rudesby</u>
    7. Man indulging unrestrainedly in pleasantries, vices: (old) **rake**, (old) **roué**
    8. Mean-spirited, churlish, cantankerous, crotchety, humorless, unpleasant old man: **coprolite**, <u>curmudgeon</u>, <u>old fart</u>, <u>(old) gnoff/gnof/gnoffe/ gnooffe/gnuffe/knuffe</u>, **hunks**
    9. Miser: <u>(old) skinflint</u>
    10. Old-fashioned, dull, elderly man: <u>(old) **fuddy-duddy**</u>
    11. Old-fashioned, progress-opposing, reactionary, dull, conservative man: (old) **fogy**, **hunker**, <u>mossback</u>, <u>preterist</u>
    12. Old feeble-minded man: <u>dotard</u>, <u>twichild</u>
    13. Phony male flatterer: (old) **cogger**

14. Senile, gullible man: **dott(e)rel**
15. Slow-witted or incompetent old man: **old duffer**
16. Small, shriveled, ugly old man with a beard: **gnome**
17. Very old man living in the past, unchangable: <u>(old)</u> **fossil**
18. Unprepossing old man: **old buzzard**

XIII. <u>Veteran (old) soldier</u>: **grognard**
XIV. Widower: **veuf, viduus**

<u>old person(s)</u>: This category is comprised of both nouns and adjs. The latter are indicated by (adj.) after the word. Headwords are in **bold** type; foreign words are in *italic*; foreign headwords are in both **bold** & ***italic***; words in standard type are exdictionary; underlining indicates a term applicable to both genders. The bold-type word, **old**, before a word indicates its constant use with that word, while (old) indicates inconstant use. (All **old man** nouns would qualify in the **role** category, but are not listed there.) ancestor(s), **<u>ancientry</u>**, **<u>aval</u>** (adj.), blue-rinse set or crowd (especially applicable to old women), <u>(old)</u> **<u>buffer</u>**, **<u>centenarian</u>**, **<u>congener</u>**, <u>(old)</u> **<u>coot</u>**, <u>(old)</u> **<u>crony</u>**, **<u>curmudgeon</u>** (typically a man), dinosaurs, **<u>dotard</u>**, **<u>dott(e)rel</u>**, elders, elders-and-betters, **<u>fogram/fogrum</u>**, forebears, <u>(old)</u> **<u>fossil</u>**, <u>(old)</u> **<u>fuddy-duddy</u>**, **<u>geezersphere</u>**, **<u>gerontic</u>** (adj.), <u>(old)</u> **<u>gnoff/gnof/ gnoffe/gnooffe/gnuffe/knuffe</u>**, **<u>golden ager</u>**, grandparent(s), **<u>grisard/ grizard</u>**, **<u>longevous</u>** (adj.), **<u>macrobiote</u>**, medievalists, **<u>mossback</u>**, **<u>nonagenarian</u>**, **<u>nostalgic</u>** (n.), **<u>octogenarian</u>**, **<u>Ogygian</u>**, **old *<u>birkie</u>***, **<u>old fart</u>**, **<u>oldster</u>**, **<u>old thing</u>**, **<u>old-timer</u>**, older generation, **<u>padnag</u>**, **<u>pensioner</u>**, **<u>preterist</u>**, **<u>relic</u>**, **<u>relict</u>**, <u>(old)</u> **<u>rudesby</u>**, **<u>sedens</u>**, **<u>sedentary</u>** (n.), **<u>senescent</u>**, **<u>senex</u>**, **<u>senior</u>**, senior citizens, **<u>septuagenarian</u>**, **<u>sexagenarian</u>**, **<u>Silurian</u>**, **<u>skinflint</u>**, **<u>snowbird</u>**, ***<u>Struldbrug</u>***, **<u>supercentenarian</u>**, **<u>superseptuagenarian</u>**, the elderly, **<u>twichild</u>**, ***<u>veuvage</u>***, ***<u>les vieillards</u>***, **<u>waffle</u>**, **<u>wellderly</u>**. N.B., some of the above terms are not limited to the elderly, e.g. **grisard, old thing, sedens, skinflint**; see their definitions.

<u>old person(s)</u>: Subcategories

I. Beard & hair:
    1. Gray-haired person: **<u>grisard/grizard</u>**
II. Extremely old:
    1. Incomparably ancient: **<u>Ogygian</u>** (adj.), **<u>Silurian</u>** (adj. & n.)
    2. Surviving trace of a person: **<u>relic</u>**

3. Collective: those very old: **ancientry**

III. Desirable, good, or neutral qualities:
1. Aggressive, independent old person: ***old birkie***
2. A person who is a friend of long standing: (old) **crony**, **old thing**
3. Grandparents: **aval** (adj.)
4. Living where born: **sedens**
5. Long-lived: long-lived person: **longevous** (adj.), **macrobiote**
6. Old person living in the past: **preterist**
7. Old person who recollects sentimentally, with mixed feelings about the past, or is homesick: **nostalgic** (n.)
8. One who sits a lot: **sedentary**
9. Person's age by decade, etc.:
   a. person in his/her sixth decade: **sexagenarian**
   b. person in his/her seventh decade: **septuagenarian**
   c. person older than seventy years of age: **superseptuagenarian**
   d. person in his/her eighth decade: **octogenarian**
   e. person in his/her ninth decade: **nonagenarian**
   f. person one-hundred-year of age: **centenarian**
   g. person greater than 110 years of age: **supercentenarian**

IV. Physical deterioration:
1. Old feeble-minded person: **dotard**, **dott(e)rel**, **twichild**
2. An old, decrepit shuffling person: ***Struldbrug***

V. Retired person:
1. Old person receiving a regular stipend: **pensioner**
2. Old retired northerner who moves south in winter to live: **snowbird**

VI. Role:
1. Miser: (old) **skinflint**
2. Old person who recollects sentimentally, with mixed feelings about the past, or is homesick: **nostalgic** (n.)
3. One who is widowed: ***veuvage***
3. Sits a lot: **sedentary**
4. Someone of the same (old) age: **congener**

5. Surviving person (especially a widow {archaic}: **relict**
VII. Synonyms for an old person or persons collectively: **ancientry**, **(old) buffer**, **geezersphere**, **gerontic** (adj.), **goldenager**, **oldster**, **old-timer**, **padnag**, **senescent** (n.), **senex**, **senior**, **Silurian**, **twichild**, *les vieillards*
VIII. Undesirable, bad, disagreeable, or inappropriate qualities:
    1. Eccentric or unreasonably stubborn old person: (old) **coot**
    2. Mean-spirited, churlish, cantankerous old person: **curmudgeon**, (old) **gnoff/gnof/gnoffe/gnooffe/gnuffe/knuffe**
    3. Miser: (old) **skinflint**
    4. Old-fashioned, progress-opposing, reactionary, dull, conservative person: (old) **fuddy-duddy**, **fogram/fogrum**, **mossback**
    5. Set completely in his/her ways: (old) **fossil**
    6. Uncivil, loud-mouthed, ill-mannered person: (old) **rudesby**
    7. Unpleasant old person: **old fart** (grossly offensive)
    8. Very disliked old person: **waffle**
IX. Well persons, > 100 years of age: **wellderly**

old soak n.phr. an old drunkard. [slang term < OE *socian* an earlier form of suck, OE < IE *sucan* to take liquid]. syn. **Silenus**, q.v. See **old man**.

oldster (old'ster) n. someone who has reached an advanced age. Older than 65 years of age is generally considered old, and is generally the U.S. retirement age, but this may change as longevity increases. The term is likely to be offensive. [early 19th C., and bottomed on "youngster". < OE *eald* old + -ster, suff.]. ant. youngster. See **old person(s)**.

old thing n.phr. a British vocative used familiarly. Perhaps it should be uemployed circumspectly in the case of those over 40 years of age, or perhaps when used strategically when confronted by "onomastic aphasia", i.e. meaning inability to remember a name—"Winged Words" by Philip Howard, q.v. The term is used more frequently in reference to men. syn. = *mon vieux*, q.v. See **old as . . .** /as old as . . . /an old . . . /old . . . See **old person(s)**.

old woman (women): This category is comprised of both nouns and adjs. The latter are indicated by (adj.) after the word. Headwords are in **bold** type; foreign words are in italic; foreign headwords are in both ***bold** & italic*; words in standard type are exdictionary; underlining indicates a term applicable to both genders. The bold-type word, **old**, before a word indicates its constant use with that word, while (old) indicates inconstant use. (All old woman nouns would qualify in the role category, but are not listed there.) See old person(s), also.

abuela, **anicular** (adj.), **anile** (adj.), ***Ardipithecus ramidus***, aval (adj.), **babushka**, **beldam**, blue-rinse (adj.—applying almost exclusively to women), (old) buffer, **catamaran**, centenarian, congener, **crone**, (old) crony, curmudgeon (typically a man), **dinosaur**, dotard, dott(e)rel, **dowager**, **doyenne**, (old) **dragon**, **Elli**, **fag-ma-fuff**, old fart, fogram/fogrum, (old) fossil, (old) fuddy-duddy, (old) **fustilugs**, **gammer**, (old) gnoff/gnof/gnoffe/ gnooffe/gnuffe/knuffe, golden ager, grandam(e), **grimalkin**, grisard/grizard, (old) hag, (old) **harpy**, **harridan**, **hellhag**, **mackabroin**, macrobiote, **matriarch**, **metrona**, mossback, nonagenarian, nostalgic, **OBA**, octogenarian, Ogygian (adj.), **old biddy**, old *birkie*, old boy/old girl, old coot, old fart, oldster,

old-thing, old-timer, padnag, pensioner, preterist, relic, relict, **rixatrix**, **rounceval**, **rudas**, (old) rudesby, sedens, sedentary (adj.), senescent, **seneucia**, senex, senior, septuagenarian, sexagenarian, (old) **shrew**, Silurian (adj., n.), (old)skinflint, snowbird, *Struldbrug*, supercentenarian, superseptuagenarian, **termagant**, twichild, *veuvage*, **veuve**, *vidua*, *vieille*, **virago**, (old) **vixen**, waffle, **wallydrag**, wellderly, **Xanthippe**, **zaftig** (adj.).

N.B., some of the above terms are not limited to the elderly, e.g. **grisard**, **metrona**, **Xanthippe**, **vixen**; see definitions.

old woman (women): Subcategories

I. Age of an old woman by decade: 60's = sexagenarian, 70's = septuagenarian, 80's = octogenarian, 90's = nonagenarian, 100 = centenarian, > 100 = supercentenarian
II. Appearance:
    1. Disreputable, unkempt old woman: (old) **wallydrag**
    2. Fat, unkempt, frowsy, old woman: (old) **fustilugs**
    3. Frumpy, spiteful old woman: **grimalkin**

4. Full-figured, pleasingly plump, buxom: **zaftig**
5. Having gray hair: **grisard/grizard**
6. Hideous old hag: **mackabroin**
7. Ugly old woman, hag: **beldam**, **rudas**

III. Desirable, good, or neutral qualities in an old woman:
1. An alumna, intimate, or familiar or general term: **old girl**
2. Garrulous old woman: **fag-ma-fuff**
3. Living where born: **sedens**
4. Most senior, respected, woman of a group: **doyenne**
5. Old-fashioned, passé, or conservative woman resisting novelty: **fogram/fogrum**
6. Old woman who recollects sentimentally, with mixed feelings about the past, or is homesick: **nostalgic** (n.)
7. Respected or rich old woman or old widow: **dowager**
8. Woman who is long lived; long-lived men: **macrobiote**, **nonagenarian**, **octogenarian**, **Ogygian**; **well-derely**

IV. Grandmother:
1. Pertaining to grandmother(s): **aval**
2. Russian grandmother: *babushka*
3. Spanish grandmother: *abuela*
4. Young grandmother: *metrona*

V. Hair:
1. A gray-haired woman: **grisard/grizard**,

VI. Old woman who is head of a family: **matriarch**

VII. Oldest woman (or man) hominid: *Ardipithecus ramidus*

VIII. Synonyms (old woman): **babushka**, **beldam**, **old biddy**, **crone**, **dowager**, **Elli**, **gammer** (comparable old man = **gaffer**, q.v.), **golden ager,** **grandam(e)**, (old) **buffer**, **old-thing**, *vieille*,
1. Old-womanish: **anicular** (adj.), **anile** (adj.)

IX. Undesirable, bad, disagreeable, or inappropriate qualities:
1. Bad-mouthed old woman: **rounceval**
2. Evil old woman: **hellhag**
3. Fierce, formidable old woman: (old) **dragon**
4. Frumpy, spiteful old woman: **grimalkin**
5. Heartedly disliked old woman: **waffle**
6. Loud-mouthed, ill-mannered, turbulent, boorish woman: (old) **rudesby**

7. Mean-spirited, churlish, bad-tempered, cantankerous, unpleasant old woman: **old fart**, (old) **gnoff/gnof/ gnoffe/gnooffe/gnuffe/knuffe**, **harpy**, **harridan**,
8. Miser: (old) **skinflint**
9. Nagging, quarrelsome old woman: (old) **catamaran**, **curmudgeon**, (old) **shrew**, **Xanthippe**
10. Old-fashioned, dull, elderly woman: (old) **fuddy-duddy**
11. Old-fashioned, progress-opposing, reactionary, dull, conservative woman: **mossback**, **preterist**
12. Old feeble-minded woman: **dotard**, **twichild**
13. Scolding, shrill, shrewish, brawling, nagging, nasty old woman: **rixatrix**, **termagant**
14. Senile, gullible woman: **dott(e)rel**
15. Turbulent, mannish woman: **virago**
16. Unpleasant, shrewish old woman: **OBA** (old battle axe)
17. Very old woman living in the past, unchangable: (old) **fossil**
18. Vindictive, bad-tempered old woman: (old) **vixen**

X. Widow & Widowhood: **seneucia**, *veuvage*, *veuve*, *vidua*

olfaction (ōl-fak'shən) n. 1. smell. 2. the act of smelling. The sense of smell wanes with old age. This may contribute to lack of interest in eating and maintaining a proper diet, using large amounts of salt or sugar, and inability to smell the ethyl mercaptain added to natural gas that makes gas leaks apparent. [< L *olfacio*, pp. *olfacere*, to smell]. adj. **olfactory** (ol-fak'tō-ree). syn. **osmesis**, q.v. See **hyposmia**, **anosmia**. See **nose, smell**.

oligophagous (ol-i-gof'ə-gəss) adj. eating only certain foods. [olig(o)-, pref., a few or a little < G *oligos* few + -phage, -phagia, -phagy, suffs., eating or devouring < *phagein* to eat]. See **drink, food**.

oligophrenia (ol'li-gō-freen'ni-ə) n. feeblemindedness. [olig-, oligo-, pref., a few or a little < G *oligos* few + -phreni, suff., denoting relationship to the 1. mind. (2. diaphragm) < G *phren* mind; seat of the emotions, heart; diaphragm]. syn. **dementia**, q.v. See **intelligence**.

oligoria (ol-i-gawr'ri-ə) n. disinterest in former friends or hobbies. [**?** < olig(o)-, pref., few, small < G *oligos* small, *oligoi* few + *agora* marketplace + –*ia*, a L & G suff. denoting a state or condition]. See **mentality, mentation, behavior**.

oligotrophia (ol"i-gŏ-trō'fi-ə)/**oligotrophy** (ol"i-gŏt'trō-fee) n. lack of nourishment, deficient nutrition. [olig(o)-, pref., a few or a little < G *oligos* few + *trophe* nourishment]. See **drink, food**. See **health, illness**.

OM a chat- and text-message initialism = old man. [< NetLingo, The Internet Dictionary: netlingo.com. (NetLingo does not list OW, which would, logically, = old woman.)]. See **old man**.

ombrosalgia (omb"brŏ-sal'ji-ə) n. aches and pains felt when it rains. [< G *ombros* rain + -*algia*, suff., denoting a painful condition < *algos* pain]. See **pain**.

omniana (om-ni-an'nə) pl.n. notes, jottings, or scraps of information about anything. • The elderly recluse's *omniana* relating to his hobby ultimately became unmanageable. [omni-, pref., all-, of all things, of all ways or places < L *omnis* all + -*ana*, suff., a collection of objects or information about a topic, person, or place < neuter pl. of L -*anus* relating to]. See **past, time**. See **work, activity**.

omniloquence (om-nil'lō-kwənz) n. talking about everything. [< L *omnis* all + *loqui* to talk]. See **talk**.

oneiric (ō-nī'rik) adj. relating to, experienced in, or similar to a dream or dreams. • It's said that the aged have enhanced, detailed *oneiric* recall compared to the young. [< G *oneiros* dream]. See **mentality, mentation, behavior**. See **sleep, wakefulness**.

onology (ō-nol'ō-jee, -ə-jee) n. foolish talk. [< G *onos* jackass + *logos* word, talk < *legein* to speak. (*onos* also means vessel)]. See **talk**.

onomatomania (on"nō-mat"tō-may'ni-ə) n. 1. An abnormal impulse to dwell upon certain words and their supposed special significance. 2. to try frantically to recall a particular word or name. [< G *onomo* name + *mania* frenzy]. adj. **onomatomaniacal** (-ma-nī'ə-kəl). n. **onomatomaniac**. syn. **loganamnosis**. Cf. **lethologica**, q.v. See **memory**. See **manias**.

ontogeny (on-toj'jə-nee) n. the life history of an individual organism—e.g., a person—from fertilization of an ovum to maturity as distinguished from phylogeny, the evolutionary development of a species. [< G *on* being + *genesis* origin]. adj. **ontogenic**. See <u>past, time</u>.

onychauxis (on"ni-kawks'siss) n. simple marked overgrowth of finger nails or toe nails without deformity. ● *Onychauxis* is frequently seen in the elderly who have difficulty trimming toenails, especially. [onych(o)-, pref., nail < G *onyx* nail + *auxe* increase < *auxein* to increase]. See <u>joint, extremities, back</u>. See <u>physique, appearance</u>.

onychogryphosis/onychogryposis (ōn"ni-kō-gri-fōs'siss/ -pō'siss) n. gross hypertrophy, thickening, and distortion of the nails producing a hooked or incurved clawlike (ram's horn) deformity. This occasionally happens in old age, along with much more common changes of dryness (**xerosis**, q.v.), brittleness, flattening, ridging, **onychauxis**, q.v., etc.—**Onycryptosis** (ōn"nee-krip-tōs'siss) = an ingrown nail. [onycho-, pref., denoting relationship to the nails < G *onyx*, gen. *onychos*, nail + *gryposis* a crooking, hooking]. See **joint, extremities, back**. See **physique, appearance**.

Opa Gefaengnis (ō-paag'e-fang'niss) n. a prison for old men, i.e., a "grandpa prison", or "granddad bandits", in Singen, a city in southern Germany near the Swiss border. It opened in 2007. All inmates were convicted of crimes committed after retirement. (20% of Germany's prison inmates are over 60 years of age, and Europe is said to be in the midst of a "gray crime wave" with the percentage of prisoners > 60 years of age increasing prominently. Often the crimes are minor, such as shoplifting; Britain has a number problem similar to that of Germany.) [Ger., *Opa* grandpa + *Gefaengnis* prison]. See <u>retirement</u>.

opprobrious (əp-prōb'bri-əs) adj. conveying reproach or scorn. 2. abusive, vituperative. [L, infamy, reproach < *opprobare* to reproach, taunt < *probrum* disgrace]. adv. **opprobriously**. n. **opprobriousness**. n. **opprobrium**. See <u>talk</u>.

oppugnant (op-pug'nənt) adj. opposing, antagonistic; contrary. [< L *oppugnare* to assault, assail, attack, storm; (fig.) to attack, assail]. n. **oppugnance**. n. **oppugnancy**. n. **oppugnation** (-pug-nay'shən) (all rare). vt. **oppugn** (op-pugn') = to controvert, call in question. n.

oppugner (-pugn'ur). See **mentality, mentation, behavior**. See **talk**. See **role**.

opsigamy (op-sig'gǝ-mee) n. marriage late in life. [< G *opsi* late + *gamos* marriage]. n. **opsigamist** (a man or woman marrying late in life). Cf. **anilojuvenogamy, anisonogamia, dysonogamia, isonogamia, nomogamosis, sororate**, q.v. See **marriage**. See **role**.

opsimath (op'si-math) n. one who learns late; a late bloomer. [< G *opsi* late + *manthanein* to learn]. n. **opsimathy**. (op-sim'ǝ-thee) = education, learning late in life. adj. **opsimathic** (-math'ik). Cf. **serotine**, q.v. See **role**.

opsimatria (op"si-may'tree-ǝ) n. the bearing of a child late in a woman's life. [< G *opsi* late + < L *mater* mother]. See **sex, love**. See **marriage**.

opsipatria (op"si-pat'tree-ǝ) n. the bearing of a child late in a man's life; becoming a father late in live. [< G *opsi* late + *pater* father]. See **sex, love**. See **marriage**.

opsiproligery (op"si-prō-lig'gǝ-ree) n. ability to have children late in life. [< G *opsi* late + < L *proles* offspring + *gerere* to bear]. See **sex, love**. See **marriage**.

opsomania (ops"sō-may'ni-ǝ) n. a longing, craving for a particular article of diet, or for highly seasoned food. [< G *opsos* seasoning + *mania* frenzy]. adj. **opsomaniacal** (-mǝ-nī'ǝ-kǝl). n. **opsomaniac**. See **manias**. See **drink, food**.

orthocrasia (awr-thō-kray'zi-ǝ, -kray-zhǝ) n. A condition in which there is a normal reaction to drugs, ingested proteins, etc., as distinguished from **idiosyncrasy**, q.v.

[ortho-, pref., straight, normal, correct < G *orthos* straight + *krasis* a mixing]. adj. **orthocrasic** (-kray'sik)/**orthocratic** (-kray'tik) (? -kra'tik). Cf. **dyscrasy, eucrasy, eucrasia**, q.v. See **health, illness**.

orthopnea (awr-thop'nee-ǝ or awr"thop-nee'ǝ) n. difficult breathing except in the upright position. [ortho-, pref., straight, normal, correct < G *orthos* straight + *pnoia* breath]. adj. **orthopneic**. Cf. **dyspnea, pursey**, q.v. See **breathing**.

orthoscopy (awr-thos'kō-pee) n. examination of the eye by means of an **orthoscope**. [ortho-, pref., straight, normal, correct, < G *orthos* straight + -scope, suff., denoting an instrument for examining or observing < *skopein* to view, examine]. n. **orthoscope** (awr'thō-skōp) = an apparatus which neutralizes the corneal refraction by means of a layer of water; it is used in examining the eye. adj. **orthoscopic** (-thos-kop'pik) = 1. pertaining to orthoscopy or an orthoscope. 2. having normal, undistorted vision. 3. pertaining to an optical system that produces undistorted images. 4. denoting an object correctly observed by the eye. See **eye**.

orthosis (awr-thō'siss) n.pl. **orthoses** (-seez), an orthopedic appliance or apparatus used to support, align, prevent, or correct deformities, or to improve the function of movable parts of the body. • The old **duffer**, q.v., nightly used a dental *orthosis* to prevent sleep apnea. [< G *orthosis* making straight]. n. **orthotics** (awr-thot'ikss) = the field of knowledge relating to orthoses and their use. n. **orthotist** (awr-thot'ist) = one skilled in **orthotics** and practicing its application in individual cases. See **orthotic**. See **role**. See **therapy**.

orthotic (awr-thot'ik) adj. serving to protect or to restore or improve function pertaining to the use or application of **orthoses**, q.v. The word, an adj., is incorrectly, but frequently, used as a noun in lieu of **orthosis**, q.v. [ortho-, pref., straight, normal, correct < G *orthos* straight + -ic, suff., pertaining to or characteristic of]. See **therapy**.

oscitancy (os'si-tən-seė) n. yawning; drowsiness; inattentiveness, being unfocused; lazy—a physical condition or a state of mind. • *Oscitancy* seems to increase exponentially with age. [< L *oscitans*, lit., yawning & fig., bored, pres.p. of *oscitare* to gape; to yawn < *os* mouth + *citare* to move, put into violent motion]. adj. **oscitant** = (also) woolgathering, oblivious; day-dreaming; dull; lazy; unmindful, neglectful. adv. **oscitantly**. n. **oscitation** (-tay'shən) = yawning; being drowsy; sleeping; being inattentive. vi. **oscitate**. See **sleep, wakefulness**. See **mentality, mentation, behavior**.

OSIF a chat- and text-message initialism = Oh s—t, I forgot. [NetLingo The Internet Dictionary: netlingo.com]. Cf. **CRAFT, CRAT, CRTLA, CRS, & SM**, q.v. See **memory**.

osmesis (oz-mees'siss) n. the act of smelling. • *Osmesis* is more pronounced in the elderly, which is an indication of diminished smell sense: **osmesthesia**, q.v. **Olfactory**, i.e., smelling function (See **olfaction**.) gradually declines with age, i.e., > age 50 years, and about 40% of the elderly have a diminished sense of smell, **hyposmia**, q.v.; a few also have an unpleasant taste in the mouth, **dysgeusia**, **dysosmia**, q.v. Gustatory function (taste) is divided into fine taste, which is an olfactory (smell) function, and crude taste—sweet, sour, bitter, salty—mediated by the tongue's taste buds. [G, smelling < *osme* odor]. adj. **osmatic** (oz-mat'tik). syn. **olfaction**, q.v. See **nose, smell**.

osmesthesia (oz"mes-theez'zha, -zee-ə) n. olfactory (smell) sensibility; the ability to perceive and distinguish odors. [< G *osmo-*, pref., < *osme* odor + *aesthesis* perception]. adj. **osmesthetic** (-the'tik). See **osmesis**. See **nose, smell**.

osophagist (ō-sof'fə-jist) n. a fastidious eater; one who picks and chooses. • *Osophagists* abound in retirement homes. [< G *oisophagos* gullet < *oisein* to carry + -phag, -phagia, -phagy, suff., < G *phagema* food < *phagein* to eat + -ist, suff., following a specific belief or school of thought]. n. **osophagia** (ō-sō-fay'ji-ə). See **drink, food**. See **role**.

ossify (os'si-fī) (-**fied**, -**fying**, -**fies**) vi.&vt. (1. to change or be changed from soft tissue, e.g., cartilage into bone, as a result of impregnation with calcium salts.) 2. to become or make somebody become rigidly set in a conventional pattern of behavior, beliefs, and attitudes. [< F *ossifier* turn into bone < L *os* bone]. n. **ossification** (os"si-fi-kay'shən). adj. **ossific** (os-sif'fik). See **past**. See **innovation, misoneism**.

oste(o) - (os'tee-ō) pref., denoting relationship to a bone or the bones < G *osteon* bone.

osteoarthritis (os"tee-ō-aarth rīt'tis) n. the most common joint disease, and a leading cause of disability in persons > 65 years of age, is a non-inflammatory degenerative disease occurring chiefly in the elderly; it is characterized by degeneration of the articular cartilage, hypertrophy of bone at the margins, and changes in the synovial membrane, i.e., the fluid-secreting joint membrane. It is accompanied by pain and stiffness, particularly after prolonged activity. Recent study shows that increasing physical activity, as measured by **walking speed**, q.v., can improve function in those with osteoarthritis of the knee. Those with a slow gait or walking speed of 4ft./sec. have the least physical activity; physical activity increases progressively as walking speed increases from 4.2 to 4.5ft./sec. [oste(o)-, pref., q.v., + < G *arthron* joint + -itis, suff., denoting inflammation of the part indicated by the word stem to which it is attached < G -*itis* a f. adjectival termination agreeing with G *nosos* disease (understood)]. adj. **osteoarthritic** (-rit'tik). syns. **degenerative arthritis, hypertrophic arthritis**, and **degenerative joint disease**. See <u>joint, extremities, back</u>.

osteoarthropathy (ost"tee-ō-aar-throp'pə-thee) n. any disease of the joints and bones. [oste(o)-, pref, q.v., + G *arthron* joint + *pathos* disease]. See <u>joint, extremities, back</u>.

osteoarthrosis (ost"tee-ō-aarth-rōs'siss) n. chronic arthritis of a non-inflammatory character. [oste(o)-, pref., q.v., + < G *arthron* joint + -osis, suff., denoting a process, especially a disease or morbid process, and sometimes conveying the meaning of abnormal increase]. See <u>joint, extremities, back</u>.

osteochondropathy (ost"tee-ō-kon-drop'pə-thee) n. any morbid condition affecting both bone and cartilage, or marked by abnormal endochondral (within cartilage) ossification. [oste(o)-, pref., q.v., + G *chondros* cartilage + *pathos* disease]. See <u>joint, extremities, back</u>.

osteopenia (ost"tee-ō-peen'ni-ə) n. low bone mass due either to not enough new bone formation (osteoid synthesis), or too much old bone reabsorption (osteoclasis or osteolysis), or both. [oste(o)-, pref, q.v., + G *penia* poverty]. adj. **osteopenic**. See **osteoporosis**. See <u>joint, extremities, back</u>.

osteoporosis (os"tee-ō-pō-rōs'siss) n. reduction in the amount of bone mass, leading to fractures after minimal trauma. It is diagnosed when bone density is at least 2.5 SD (standard deviations) below the young adult mean; when bone density lies between 1 and 2.5 SD below the young adult mean, the condition is termed **osteopenia**, q.v., (< G *penia* poverty). **Senescent**, q.v., bone loss is a constant feature of advancing age and is due to a decrease in formation of osteoblasts. (As many as half or all women and a quarter of men older than 50 years of age will break a bone due to osteoporosis. An average of 24% of hip-fracture patients who are 50 or more years of age die in the year following their fracture {Nat'l. Osteoporosis Foundation data} A daily calcium supplement improves bone density, but a recent study reported in the British Medical Journal raised concern, i.e., a 30% higher risk of heart attack in healthy older women who took calcium supplements.) [oste(o)-, pref., q.v., + < G *osteon* bone + *poros* passage + -osis, suff., indicating a process, condition, or state, usually abnormal]. adj. **osteoporotic**. See **joint, extremities, back**.

otacoustic (ō-tə-koos'tik) adj. helping to hear, aiding the sense of hearing. [ot-, pref., relating to the ear < G *ous* ear + *akoustikos* relating to hearing < *acouein* to hear]. n. **otacoustic** = a hearing device, aid. See **ear, hearing**.

otalgia (ō-tal'ji-ə or -tal'jə) n. pain in the ear, earache. [G, *otalgia* earache]. adj. **otalgic**. See **ear, hearing**.

otiant (ō'shi-ənt, -ti-ənt) adj. dormant; unemployed, idle, resting. • The retirement home had many *otiant* members (**otiants**) lounging about. [< L *otium* leisure, free time, relaxation; freedom from public affairs, retirement; peace, quiet, ease, idleness, inactivity < *otiari* to take it easy]. n. **otiant** = one who is dormant; unemployed, idle. See **role**. See **work, activity**.

otiatrus (ōt"ti-at'rəs/ō-tī'ə-trəs) n. an ear specialist. [ot(o)-, pref., relating to the ear < G *ous* ear + *iatros* physician]. n. **otiatria/otiatrics** (ōt"ti-at'ri-ə/ō-tī'ə-triks) = the treatment of diseases of the ear. adj. **otiatric** (ōt"ti-at'rik/ō-tī'ə-trik). syns. = **aurist**, qv., audiologist. See **ear, hearing**. See **role**.

otic (ō'tik) adj. relating to the ear. [< G *otikos* < *ous* ear]. See **ear, hearing**.

otiose (ō'shee-ōz) adj. 1. ineffective, having no useful result or practical purpose. 2. having little or no value, worthless. 3. unwilling or uninterested in being active, working, lazy (archaic). n. **otiosity**(-os'sə-tee). adv. **otiosely**. [< L *otiosus* at leisure, idle < *otium* leisure]. See **work, activity**.

ot(o)-, pref., relating to the ear. [< G *ous*, genitive of *otos*, ear].

otocleisis (ō-tō-klī'siss) n. 1. closure of the Eustachian tube (which can occur during airplane descent and sometimes can result in **otalgia**, q.v., and hearing loss). 2. closure of the external auditory meatus by accumulation of cerumen (ear wax) or a new growth (both of which can result in hearing loss, deafness). • Earwax accumulation occurs more frequently in the elderly and can not infrequently result in *otocleisis*. [ot(o)-, pref., q.v., < G *ous* ear + *kleisis* closure]. See **ear, hearing**.

otology (ō-tol′lə-jee) n. the study of the ear and its diseases. [ot(o)-, pref., q.v., + *logos* study]. adj. **otic**. n. **otologist** = **otiatrist**, q.v. syn. **auricular**, q.v. Cf. audiologist. Cf. audiology. See **ear, hearing**.

otorhinolaryngologist (ōt″tō-rīn″nō-lar″ən-gol′lə-jist) n. a physician specializing in diseases of the ear, nose, and throat, an ENT specialist. [ot(o)-, pref., q.v., + < G *rhis* nose + *larynx* + *logos* study]. n. **otorhinolaryngology**. adj. **otorhinolaryngological** (-gō-loj′ji-kəl). See **role**. See **ear, hearing**. See **nose, smell**.

otosclerosis (ō″tō-sklair-rō′sis) n. a conductive type of hearing loss in the aged in which inner ear bones, especially the stapes, become **ankylosed**, q.v. [< ot(o)-, pref., q.v., + *sklerosis* hardening]. See **ear, hearing**.

otosis (ō-tōs′siss) n. a hearing malfunction; not hearing correctly; the misunderstanding of spoken sounds or an alteration of words because of such misunderstanding. [ot(o)-, pref., q.v., + -osis, suff., (properly added only to words formed from Greek roots) a process, condition, or state usually abnormal or diseased]. See **ear, hearing**.

ototoxic (ō-tō-tox′ik) adj. having a deleterious upon the eighth nerve, or upon the organs of hearing (hearing loss) and balance, e.g., prolonged exposure to very loud music or noise—an estimated half of all hearing loss cases in the U.S.—to certain drugs, e.g., aspirin, quinine, gentamycin, etc. [< ot(o)-, pref., q.v., + G *toxikon* poison]. n. **ototoxicity**. See **ear**.

outrance (utrãs) n. utmost; excess. [F]. *à outrance* (a utrãs) (adv.) = to the bitter end (a pun on a senior's life's end); excessively. (*guerre à outrance* (or *guerre à mort*) war to the knife.) See **end-of-life, death**.

outré (utre) adj. outside the bounds of what is considered usual, correct, proper, or generally acceptable; exaggerated, strained, undue, excessive. (Beyond the tomb = *outre-tombe*.) [F < OF pp. of *outrer* exceed < L *ultra* beyond]. See **mentality, mentation, behavior**.

overslaugh (ōv'vur-slaw) vt. 1. To pass over someone in favor of another, as in selecting one over another. 2. To bar or to hinder. ● The grandame thought that the retirement home's social worker had *overslaughed* her in assigning the home's best room. [< Du *overslaan* to pass over, omit, < *over* over + *slaan* to strike]. See **mentality, mentation, behavior**.

oxter (oks'tər) vi.&vt. to lead or support with one's arm; to walk arm in arm; to put one's arm around; to embrace; to support by the elbow; to take and carry under the arm. ● The centenarian could not manage alone, but had to be *oxtered* to the dining table. [OE *oxta*, *ohsta*, Du *oksel*, Ger. *achsel*, L *axilla*, dim. of *axula*, all in the same sense: armpit]. n. **oxter** = the armpit. See **standing, walking, wandering**.

ozostomia (ōz"zō-stōm'mi-ə) n. foulness of breath. [< G *oze* stench + *stoma* mouth + -ia, suff.]. See **nose, smell**.

P

"Peu de gens savant être vieux."
(Few people know how to be old.) [Fr].

"Grow old along with me!/ The best is yet to be,/ The last of life for which the first was made./ Our times are in his hand." Robert Browning: *Rabbi Ben Ezra* (1864), st. 1.

padnag (pad'nag) n. lit., an old, slow, worn out horse; fig. an old person or thing. [E pad, a piece of soft material; fleshy cushion of an animal's paw + nag, a horse]. See **old person(s)**.

paedomorphism/pedomorphism (peed'dō-mawr'fiz-əm) n. description of adult behavior in terms of child behavior. [< G *pais* (*paid*) child + *morphe* form]. adj. **pedomorphic**. adv. **pedomorphically**. n. **pedomorph** (peed'ō-mawrf) = an adult who behaves like a child. See **mentality, mentation, behavior**. See **role**.

pain: **algophobia, angina, charlie horse, claudicant, claudication, dyspragia, dyspraxia, odynophobia, ombrosalgia, podagra, podalgia, pododynia, sciatica, spinal stenosis, suralgia, surbate, tarsalgia,**

pain: Subcategories

I. Cardiac:
 1. Pain in the left chest (heart), throat, or jaw: **angina**
II. Fear of pain:
 1. General fear of pain: **algophobia, odynophobia**
III. General:
 1. Impaired or painful functioning of any organ: **dyspraxia**
IV. Leg, foot, toe:
 1. A cause of sciatica: **spinal stenosis**
 2. Calf pain: **suralgia, charlie (or charley) horse**
 3. Foot pain: **podalgia, pododynia, tarsalgia**
 4. Gouty pain in the great toe: **podagra**
 5. Leg pain on walking: **claudication (& intermittent claudication)**
 6. Relating to leg pain on walking: **claudicant**
 7. Thigh, buttock, outer leg pain: **sciatica**
 8. To make or become footsore (vt.): **surbate**
 9. Upper anterior leg pain: **charlie horse**
V. Performance-related: **dyspraxia**
VI. Rainy weather pain: **ombrosalgia**

paleoanthropic (pay"lee-ō-an-throp'pik) adj. pertaining to the earliest (oldest) types of human beings. [paleo-, pref., ancient, prehistoric; primitive, early < G *palaios* < *palai* long ago + *anthropos* man]. See **old**.

paleography (pay'lee-og'grə-fee) n. 1. the study of ancient manuscripts and handwriting. 2. an ancient manuscript or piece of handwriting. [< paleo-, pref., ancient, prehistoric; primitive, early < G *palaios* < *palai* long ago + -graphy, suff., writing about or study of a particular subject < L -*graphia* < G *graphein* write]. adj. **paleographic** (pay"lee-ə-graf'fik) adv. **paleographical**. n. **paleographer** (pay"lee-og'grə-fər). See **role**. See **old**.

paleomnesia (pay"lee-om-neez'zi-ə) n. a good memory for events of the far past. [paleo-, pref., ancient, prehistoric, primitive, early < G *palaios* < *palai* long ago + *mneme* memory]. See **memory**.

palikinesia (pal"li-kin-eez'zi-ə)/**palicinesia** (-sin-) n. involuntary repetition of movements. [paleo-, pref., ancient, prehistoric; primitive, early < G *palaios* < *palai* long ago + *kinesis* movement]. See **nerve, muscle, movement, touch**.

palliative (pal'lee-ə-tiv, pal"lee-ayt'tiv) adj. 1. reducing the bad effects of something, e.g. soothing anxiety. 2. treating symptoms only, without eliminating the cause. [< L *palliate*- pp. of *palliare* cover or hide < *pallium* covering]. n. **palliative** (pal'lee-ə-tiv) = something that is palliative, especially a medicine that treats symptoms only. adv. **palliatively** (pal"lee-ayt'tiv-lee). See **therapy**.

pallid (pal'lid) adj. 1. having an unhealthy paleness, pallor. 2. lacking color, spirit, or intensity. [< L *pallidus* < *pallere* to be pale]. n. **pallidity** (pal-lid'ə-tee). adv. **pallidly**. See **color**. **mentality, mentation, behavior**. See **talk**.

palinoia (pal-i-noy'yə) n. compulsive repetition of an act until it is performed perfectly. It can be a sign, but not necessarily so, of mental derangement. [< G *palin* back again, over again + *noeo* to think]. (A closely related word is **palinode**, an ode recanting something said in a former ode. [< L *palinodia* < G *palinodia* singing over again, repetition, esp. recantation < *palin* + *ode* song, a name first given to an ode by Stesichorus in which he recants his attack upon Helen of Homer's Iliad]). **See mentality, mentation, behavior**.

palter (pawl'tər) vi. 1. to mumble or babble. (2. to act insincerely. 3. to bargain, haggle.) [?]. n. **palterer**. See **talk**. See **role**.

palsy (pawl'zee) n. (archaic) paralysis: muscular inability to move part or all of the body, e.g., Bell's (facial) palsy, due to paralysis of the facial (7th cranial) nerve. [13th C. < OF *paralisie* < L *paralysis* < G *paralusis* < *paraluesthai* be unable ot move < *para*- on one side + *luein* release]. adj. **palsied**. See **nerve, muscle, movement, touch**.

panacea (pan-ə-see'ə) n. a remedy or supposed cure for all diseases, or troubles. [< G *panakeia* < *panakes* all healing < *akos* remedy]. adj. **panacean**. syn. **holagogue**, q.v. Cf. **panpharmacon, catholicon**. See **therapy**.

pandiculation (pan"dik-yoo-lay'shən) n. the act of stretching and yawning in which there is a stretching and stiffening of the skeletal muscles. [< L *pandiculari* to stretch oneself]. See **nerve, muscle, movement, touch**. See **sleep, wakefulness**.

panmnesia (pan-neez'zi-ə) n. retention of all mental impressions, memories that remain in the memory; some psychologists believe they are retained lifelong. (There is a recently discovered "superior autobiographical memory" that a certain extremely few people have; it allows them to remember every day of their lives since some time in childhood. Only about six persons so far have been credited with this ability. They can remember in detail what happened on a specific date many years ago as if it were yesterday, including the day, date, day of the week, and year of an event. None found so far are old enough to know what happens to this power with age. Brain scans show the temporal lobes and second caudate nucleus are 6-7 standard deviations larger than normal—the caudate nucleus is involved in obsessive-compulsive disorders.) [pan-, pref., all, any, everyone < G, a form of *pas* all + *mneme* memory]. See **memory**.

panpharmacon (pan-for'mə-kon) n. an all-purpose medicine. • That **beldam**, q.v., aggravated by the tedium of taking so many medicines, eagerly sought a *panpharmacon*. [pan-, pref., all < G *pan* all + *pharmakon* a drug, medication, poison]. See **therapy**.

par(a)- (par, par'a) pref. beside; beyond; denoting a departure from the normal. [< G *para*- beside, along side of; near; amiss].

paracme (par-ak'mee) n. the stage after one's peak, i.e., the highest point of perfection or achievement; when decline and senescence set in. [par(a)-, pref., q.v., + *akme* highest point]. Cf. **presenium**, q.v. See **old age**.

paracusis (par-ə-kyoo'siss) n. disordered hearing. [par(a)-, pref., q.v., + *akousis* hearing]. See **ear, hearing**.

parahypnosis (par"rə-hip-nōs'siss) n. any type of abnormal or disordered sleep, e.g. nightmare, sleep apnea, somnambulism, **PLMD** q.v., restless leg syndrome (RLS), leg movement disorder, etc. [par(a)-, pref., q.v., + *hypnos* sleep + -osis, suff., meaning a process, condition, or state, usually abnormal or diseased]. syn. **parasomnia**, **somnipathy**, q.v. See **sleep, wakefulness**.

paralipophobia (par'rə-līp"pŏ-fŏb'bi-ə) n. morbid fear of responsibility, or of neglecting a duty. [< G *paraleipein* to leave to one side, to omit + *phobos* fear]. adj. **paralipophobic**. n. **paralipophobe**. syn. **hypengyophobia**, q.v. See **phobias**.

paralogize (pə-ral'lə-jīz, -lō-jīz) vi. unintentionally to comment or argue illogically, or draw illogical conclusions from a series of facts [via L *paralogismus* < G *paralogos* contrary to reason < par(a)-, pref., q.v., + *logos* reason]. n. **paralogism** (par"rə-lōj'jiz-əm). n. **paralogist** (pə-ral'-lə-jist, lō-jist). adj. **paralogistic** (par"rə-lō-jis'tik). adv. **paralogistically** (par"rə-lō-jis'ti-kə-lee). See talk. See role.

paralysis agitans (pə-ral'lə-siss aj'ji-tanss) n.phr. a form of parkinsonism of unknown etiology usually occurring late in life, although a juvenile form has been described. It's slowly progressive, characterized by mask-like facies, a characteristic tremor of resting muscles, a slowing of voluntary movements, a **festinating**—peculiar accelerating—gait, peculiar posture (**kyphosis**, q.v.), weakness of the muscles, and sometimes excessive sweating and feelings of heat. Alternative names are **Parkinson's disease**, q.v., and **shaking palsy**. [par(a)-, pref., q.v., + *lyein* to loosen + < L *agitatio* agitation, motion, movement; activity < *agitare* to hurry]. syn. **parkinsonism**, q.v. See nerve, muscle, movement, touch.

paramnesia (par-am-neez'zhə, -zee-ə) n. 1. inability to recall the meaning of some familiar words, e.g., as in forgetting whether the benediction comes first or last in a mass. 2. a feeling that one has previously visited a place or has had an experience that is actually happening for the first time. 3. a disorder in which one claims to remember events that didn't happen; also known as **pseudomnesia**, q.v. [par(a)-, pref., q.v., + < G *mneme* memory]. adj. **paramnestic** (-nes'tik). n. **paramnesiac** (-zee-ak). See memory. See role.

paraphasia (par"raa-fay'zhə, -zee-ə)/ **paraphrasia** (par" raa-fray'shə, -zee-ə) n. partial aphasia in which wrong words are used in wrong or/and senseless combinations. A brain lesion causes the *central* type. No specific lesion causes the *literal* type in which one or more sounds are replaced in otherwise correct words, e.g., "far" for "of", "**paraphasia**" for "**paraphrasia**". In the *verbal* type of paraphasia, one correct word or phrase is substituted for another, sometimes related in meaning and sometimes completely unrelated. [par(a)-, pref., q.v., + G *aphasia*, q.v., speechlessness/*phrasis* utterance]. See talk.

parapraxis (par"-rə-praks'siss) n. a sudden blank in memory; a slip of the tongue; a lapse; an error; something unconventional. [par(a)-, pref., q.v., + G *praxis* custom, behavior, action, deed < *prattein* to do]. adj. **parapraxic**. adv. **parapraxically**. n. **parapraxia** = erroneous, faulty blundering action in general. See **memory**. See **mentality, mentation, behavior**.

paraprosexia (par"rə-prŏ-seks'si-ə) n. heightened sexuality, over sexed. [par(a)-, pref., q.v., in medicine, para- = functionally disordered + pro-, a comb. form < G *pro*, in front of, for, on behalf of + < L *sesus*, -*us* sex + -ia, suff.]. syns. **acolasia, aidoi(o)mania, concupiscence, edeomania, erotomania, hyperprosexia, satyriasis**, q.v. See **mentality, mentation, behavior**. See **sex, love**.

parasomnia (par"rə-som'ni-ə) n. disturbed sleep; any sleep disorder, e.g. snacking on high-caloric foods during the night while sleepwalking. Parasomnias occur more frequently in the elderly; they include restless leg syndrome (RLS), periodic limb movement disorder (**PLMD**, q.v.) of sleep (nocturnal myoclonus), and REM (rapid eye movement), a sleep-behavior disorder that is much more frequent in men. [par(a)-, pref., q.v., + < G *somnos* sleep]. syn. **parahypnosis**. See **sleep, wakefulness**.

parcener (paar'sə-nər) n. a coheir or joint heir. [< L *parti(ti) onarius* < *partitionem* < *partiri* to part + -er, suff.]. n. **parcenary** (-air-ee)/**-ery** (-ə-ree) = joint heirship. syn. **coparcener**, q.v. See **finance**. See **role**.

parergon (par-er'gon) n. secondary work or business separate from one's main or ordinary work. • After retiring as an accountant, she continued her former *parergon*, a small ceramics shop. [par(a)-, pref., q.v., + G *ergon* work]. See **work, activity**.

pareschatology (par-esk"kə-tol'lə-gee) n. the name given to theories about life after physical death, but before the final (Christian) resurrection. [< par(a)-, pref., q.v., + G *eskhatos* last + -ology, suff., study, i.e., study of next-to-last things]. See **end-of-life, death**.

paresis (pa-rees'siss, par'ree-siss) n. slight or incomplete paralysis. [G, relaxation]. adj. **paretic** (pa-ret'tik) = pertaining to or affected with paresis. See **nerve, muscle, movement, touch**.

paresthesia (par-es-theez'zee-ə, -theez-zhə) n. morbid or perverted sensation; an abnormal sensation, such as burning, prickling, formication, etc. [par(a)-, pref., q.v., + < G *aesthesis* perception]. adj.

paresthetic (par-es-thet'tik) = pertaining to or marked by paresthesia. See **nerve, muscle, movement, touch**.

Parkinson's facies (paark'kin-sən fay'shee-eez, fay'seez, faysh'ee-eez), pl. **facies**, n.phr. the expressionless or mask-like countenance characteristic of parkinsonism. [L *fascies* face, countenance]. syn. **Parkinsonian facies**. See **physique, appearance**.

parkinsonism (paark'kin-sən-iz"zəm) n. Parkinson's (paar'kin-sənz) disease, or simply Parkinson's, which is a form of **paralysis agitans**, q.v., a nervous disorder of unknown etiology marked by symptoms of trembling hands—an involuntary tremor—lifeless face (**Parkinson's facies**, q.v.), monotone voice, slow movement, muscular rigidity, and a slow, shuffling, small-stride gait. Recently, Parkinson's is found to alter the brain's cognitive function, particularly that of the hippocampus, the key to memory. There is some loss of "executive function": planning, decision-making, and emotional control. There is some shrinkage of cells in the brain's substantia nigra, the site of dopamine production; low dopamine levels are associated with Parkinson's. Lewy bodies, which are clusters of alpha-synuclein protein, accumulate in Parkinson's. [< James Parkinson, English physician, 1755-1824. (Parkinson's law, < C. Northcote Parkinson, 1909-'93, is unrelated; he observed that work always expands to fill the time allotted for it.)]. adj. **Parkinsonian** (-sōn'ni-ən). See **nerve, muscle, movement, touch**. See **intelligence**.

Paro (paa'rō) n. a robo-seal, i.e., a $6,000 white-furred computerized device built to resemble a baby harp seal. It is a pet substitute for the elderly, particularly those who are demented, and it provides "pet therapy" visits for emotional support. Paro was built in 2005 in Japan, has an antibacterial plush white coat, weighs about six pounds, makes a few sounds when stimulated, has twelve tactile sensors, touch sensitive whiskers, can move its parts, sucks on a pacifier, can recognize voices, track motion, and "remember" behaviors that elicit positive responses from patients. It's a "hassle-free" pet. When stroked, it can bat its eyelashes and track movement with its head and eyes. A study has found that the faux relationship with Paro soothes dementia patients and helps them to communicate. [? < Japanese. Perhaps the first two letters in the name are < G *para*-, pref., meaning beside, alongside of, near, along with + the last two letteres in the name are < the initial two letters of robot]. See **therapy**.

parorexia (par-ō-reks'si-ə) n. perverted appetite; demanding strange foods. [< para- pref., q.v., + G *orexis* appetite]. See **drink, food**.

parsimony (paar'si-mō-nee) n. 1. carefulness in use of money, etc., especially excessive carefulness with money; lack of generosity, stinginess; frugality. 2. economy in the use or means to achieve something, especially the principle of endorsing the simplest explanation that covers a case. Cf. **Occam's razor**. [< L *parsimonia* < *pars*-, pp. of *parcere* to spare]. adj. **parsimonious** (paar"-sə-mō'nee-əss). See **finance**. See **mentality, mentation, behavior**.

passé **-e,** (pɑse -ə) adj. past, gone; outdated, outmoded, unfashionable; faded; vanished. [F]. See **past, time**. See **old**.

passulation (pas-yoo-lay'shən) n. the act or process of drying up and turning into a raisin; fig., to dry up, wrinkle up. • "Wrinkle, wrinkle, every day,/We *passulate*, then pass away."—Prunella Croon—cited by C. H. Elster: "There's A Word For It!". [< L *passulatus* dried in the sun—L *uva passa* = raisin < uva grape & *passum* raisin-wine made from dried grapes, neuter of *passus* spread out, (of fruit) spread out to dry, dried, pp. of *pandere* to spread]. adj. **passulate** = dried up, wrinkled, shrunken. vi. **passulate** = to make or turn (a grape) into a raisin; fig., to dry up, shrink, wrinkle. See **skin**. See **physique, appearance**.

past, time: consuetude, diuturnal, erstwhile, filiopietistic, fusty, hesternal, moss-grown, omniana, ontogeny, ossify, *passé*, prelapsarian, prepresbyophrenia, preterist, quondam, *retardataire*, retrospective, skeuomorph, tralatitious, whilom, yesterfang.

past, time: Subcategories

I   Ancient past:
     1. Before the fall: **prelapsarian**
II.   Former:
     1. In the past was something that no longer is, a time in the past: **erstwhile, quondam, whilom**
     2. Of yesterday: **hesternal**
III. Great reverence for the past:
     1. For ancestors, tradition: **filiopietistic**

IV. History:
1. Life history of an individual organism (a person): **ontogeny**
2. Representative of an artist's lifework; past and present happenings: **retrospective**
3. Something taken at some past time (poetic): **yesterfang**
4. Traditional, handed down from one generation to the next: **tralatitious, consuetude**
V. One who lives in the past: **preterist**
VI. Outdated:
1. Characteristic of an earlier period, behind the times: **retardataire**
2. Currently functionless item replicating an item that previously was functional: **skeuomorph**
3. Old-fashioned, out-of-date: **démodé**
4. Old fashioned, out-of-date, conservative: **moss-grown, fusty**
5. Outmoded, past: **passé**
VII. Time:
1. Before the onset of senile dementia: **prepresbyophrenia**
2. Daily: **diurnal**
2. Re: long duration: **diuturnal**
VII. To rigidly set in a pattern of belief, behavior, attitudes: **ossify**
VIII. Writings:
1. Notes, jottings, scraps of information, etc.: **omniana**

path(o)-, -pathy, combining forms meaning disease, < G *pathos* suffering, disease.

patharmosis (path"aar-mōs'siss) n. mental adjustment to one's disease. [path-, pref., q.v., + L & G *harmonia* a joining; agreement, accord; harmony]. See **health, illness**. See **mentality, mentation, behavior**.

pathocryptia (path"ō-krip'ti-ə) n. unwillingness to talk about or believe in one's illness. [patho-, pref., q.v., + *kryptos* hidden, concealed; without apparent cause]. n. **pathocryptic** = one who is unwilling to talk about or believe in one's illness. adj. **pathocryptic**. See **health, illness**. See **talk**. See **mentality, mentation, behavior**. See **role**.

pathomimetic (path"ō-mi-met'tik) n. someone who feigns illness, a malingerer. [patho-, pref., q.v., + *mimesis* imitation]. n. **pathomimesis** (-mees"siss) = **pathomimicry** (-mim'mik-ree). adj. **pathomimetic.** adv. **pathomimetically.** Cf. **Munchausenism**, q.v. See **health, illness**. See **role**.

pathomiosis (path"ō-mī-ōs'siss) n. the attitude of a patient leading him/her to minimize his/her disease. [patho-, pref., q.v., + G *meiosis* a lessening]. See **health, illness**.

pathoneurosis (path"ō-noo-rō'siss) n. a neurotic or hysterical preoccupation with real illness. [patho-, pref., q.v., + G *neuron* nerve + -*osis* condition]. adj. **pathoneurotic.** n. **pathoneurotic** = one who is neurotically preoccupied with real illness. See **health, illness**. See **role**.

pathophobia (path"ō-fōb'bi-ə) n. fear of disease or of becoming ill. [patho-, pref., q.v., + -phobia, suff., fearing < G -*phobia* < *phobos* fear]. adj. **pathophobic.** n. **pathophobe.** syn. **nosophobia**, q.v. See **phobias**. See **health, illness**.

patriarch (pay'tree-aark) n. family head; respected senior; biblical ancestor; Hebrew leader; oldest member; founder; Eastern Orthodox bishop; senior Roman catholic bishop; Latter-Day-Saints dignitary. [< G *patriarkhes* head of a family < *patria* family]. adj. **patriarchal** (-aark'kəl), **patriarchic** (-aark'kik). n. **patriarchy.** See **role**. See **old man**.

patriarchalism (pay"tree-aark'kəl-iz-əm) n. institutionalized domination by men, with women being regarded as socially or constitutionally inferior. [< G *patriarkhes* head of a family < *patria* family + -ism, suff., doctrine, system of beliefs < L –*ismus* < G -*ismos*].

patrimony (pat'tri-mōn"nee, pat'-trə-), pl. **patrimonies** (-mon"nees) n. 1. an inheritance or legacy from an ancestor, especially a father, or male ancestor. 2. the objects, traditions, or values that one generation has inherited from its ancestors. (3. estate(s) belonging to a church.) [L < *patrimonium* < *pater* father]. adj. **patrimonial** (pat"tri-mōn'nee-əl, pat"-trə-). adv. **patrimonially** (-mōn'nee-əl-lee). See **finance**. See **end-of-life, death**.

patroiophobia (pa-troy"ō-fōb'bi-ə) n. morbid fear of hereditary disease. [< L *pater* + father (? + G *oidium*, diminutive of *oon* egg) + -phobia, suff., fearing < G -*phobia* < *phobos* fear]. adj. **patroiophobic.** n. **patroiophobe** (pa-troy'-ō-). See **phobias**. See **health, illness**.

pauciloquent (paw-sil'lŏk-kwent) adj. using the fewest possible words to make the point. [< L *paucitas* < *paucus* few, little + < L *loqui* speak, talk, say, speak about, tell]. adv. **pauciloquently.** n. **pauciloquence.** ant. **logomania**, q.v. Cf. **breviloquent, omniloquent, polyloquent,** q.v. See **talk**.

peccatiphobia/peccatophobia (pek"kə-ti-fōb'bi-ə/pek"kə-tō-fōb'bi-ə) n. morbid fear of sin or sinning. [< L *pecco* to sin + < G *phobos* fear]. adj. **peccatiphobic/peccatofobic.** n. **peccatiphobe/peccatofobe** (pek-kat'ti-fōb, -tō-fōb). syn. **hamartophobia**, q.v. Cf. **enissophobia, enosi(o)phobia**, q.v. See **phobias**. See **religion, theology, morality**.

peccavi (pek-kaav'vee) n. an admission of guilt or sin. [L, *peccavi* I have sinned < *peccare* to err. (An apocryphal story is that British General Sir Charles Napier, upon annexing Sind, an Indian province, in battle, telegraphed home his victory with a single word, "Peccavi.", i.e., "I have Sind.")]. See **talk**. See **religion, theology, morality**.

Pecksniff (pek'snif) n. unctuous hypocritical prating of benevolence and making a show of high moral principles. [< Pecksniff, a character in Charles Dickens's *Martin Chuzzlewit* (*1844*)]. adj. **Pecksniffian.** See: **role**. See **mentality, mentation, behavior**. See **talk**.

pediculosis (pe-dik'kyoo-lōs'siss) n. lousiness, **phthiriasis** (thir-rī'ə-siss)—< G *phtheiriasis* < *phtheir* louse—the state of being infested with pediculi, lice. One form, *phthirus pubis* or *pediculosis pubis* is usually spread by sexual contact, but possibly is transmitted by clothing, towels. That infestation produces intense itching (**pruritus**, q.v.) in the genital area. *Pediculosis humanus capitis* (head) and *p. corporis* (body) are the other two common forms; *p. palpebrarum* involves the eyelashes. Scabies (*sarcoptes scabiei*) is one other common parasitic skin disease found in the elderly, and spread by contact between residents of the same household, nursing home, or other institution. • Nursing homes are sometimes *pediculous*. [< L *pediculus* louse + G suff. −*osis* condition]. adj. **pediculous** (pe-dik'kyoo-ləs). syn. **pediculation, phthiriasis**. See **hair**. See **genitourinary**. See **skin**.

peladophobia (pe-lad"dō-fōb'bi-ə) n. 1. fear of baldness or of bald people. 2. fear of becoming bald. [< F *peler* to remove hair from a hide + < G *phobos* fear]. n. **peladophobe**. adj. **peladophobic**. syn. **alopeciaphobia, phalacrophobia**, q.v. See **phobias**. See **hair**.

Pelmanism (pel'mən-izm) n. 1. a memory-training system developed by W. J. Ennever, founder of the Pelman Institute, established c. 1900. (2. the name of a children's card game dependent on mental concentration and memory.) [The name, Pelman, was selected arbitrarily on the basis that it would be easy to remember]. vi.&vt. **Pelmanize** = to get good results through memory training. See **memory**.

pelvic-support disorders n.phr. comprise: 1. hernia-like protrusions into the vagina by a.) the bladder, a **cystocele**, b.) the rectum, a **rectocele**, or c.) the uterus, a **uterine prolapse**. 2. a true **herniation of the peritoneum** (a membranous covering of the abdominal contents) and small bowel usually down into the space between the uterosacral ligaments and the rectovaginal space, an **enterocele**. 3. **procidentia**—a falling forward < L *procido* to fall forward—i.e., prolapse of the uterus and vagina (called total vaginal vault prolapse), an eversion (turning inside-out) of the entire vagina, **procidentia uteri**, which can occur after hysterectomy. • *Pelvic support disorders* occur with increasing frequency in older women as they age. syn.= pelvic organ prolapse. See **colporraphy** for treatment. See **genitourinary**.

pendulous (pen'dyoo-ləs, pen'jə-, pen'dyə-) adj. 1. hanging. (2. undecided.) • *Pendulous* parts are part and parcel of **presbyatrics**, q.v. [< L *pendulus* < *pendere* to hang]. See **physique, appearance**.

pensioner (pen'shən-ur) n. 1. a retired, usually older, person receiving a stipend for work done over a number of years. (2. as defined by Dr. Samuel Johnson, "A slave of state hired by a stipend to obey his master. In England it is generally understood to mean pay given to a state hireling for treason to his country." Dr. Johnson's definition became a sharp weapon in the hands of his enemies when he himself accepted a pension from George III. (3.{archaic or literary} somebody whose services are bought, especially somebody paid to do menial or unpleasant work.) [via F < L *pension*- payment < pens- pp. of *pendere* hang, hang down; be suspended; hover]. See **old man**. See **old woman**. See **retirement**. See **role**.

percipient (pər-sip'pee-ənt) adj. perceptive, observant, or discerning.
• The often touted wisdom of old age was confirmed by that *percipient*
oldster, q.v. [< L *percipere* to seize completely < *capere* seize]. n.
percipience. n. **percipiency**. adv. **percipiently**. Cf. **perspicacious**.
See **intelligence**.

perdition (pur-dish'ən) n. the state, in some religions, of ultimate and
everlasting punishment for mortal sin in hell; hell itself. [< L *perdere*
put to destruction < *per* (prep.) through + *dare* put]. See **religion,
theology, morality**.

perennate (per'rə-nayt) vi. to persist from season to season, to
be perennial. • Despite her advanced age the old girl continues to
perennate beautifully. [< L *perennare* to last]. See **old age**.

peripheral atherosclerosis (pər-if'fər-əl ath"hər-ōs"sklə-rōs'siss)
n.phr. the major cause of peripheral (vs. central, i.e., chest and
brain) arterial disease (PAD), is age-related and found mainly in the
elderly; it's exacerbated by diabetes, cigarette smoking, obesity,
hyperlipidemia ("bad" cholesterol), polycythemia (high red-blood-cell
count), and hypertension. Atheroma formation that occurs in the inside
layer (intima) of the peripheral arteries leads to curtailment of blood
flow that causes intermittent **claudication**, q.v.—pain on muscular
exercise, i.e., walking—and numbness, paresthesias, coldness.
[athero-, pref., denoting fatty degeneration or relationship to an
atheroma < G *athere* gruel + sclerosis < *sklerosis* hardness]. See
atherosclerosis, arteriosclerosis. See **blood, circulation, glands**.

periphrasis (per-if'rə-siss)/**periphrase** (per'ri-frayz) n. circumlocution,
a roundabout way of expressing oneself: using longer expressions
when shorter ones are adequate, introducing double negatives,
passives, superfluous description, using abstract generalities, etc.
[peri-, pref., around, surrounding; near < G *peri-*, pref., around +
phrasis speech < *phrazein* to speak]. adj. **periphrastic** (-fras'tik). adv.
periphrastically (-fras'tik-kal-). See **talk**.

perissology (per-is-sol'lə-jee) n. verbiage, excessive talk. [< G
perissologia, *perissos* excessive + *logos* speech, discourse]. syn.
periphrasis, pleonasm, q.v. See **talk**.

peritoneoscopy (per"i-tō-nee-os'kō-pee) n. examination of the
peritoneal cavity by an instrument inserted through the abdominal

wall. [< G *peritonaion* peritoneum < *per* around + *teinein* to stretch + *skopein* to examine]. n. **peritoneoscope** (-nee'-os-kōp) = an instrument for performing peritoneoscopy. n. **peritoneoscopist** = a physician performing the procedure. See <u>gastrointestinal</u>. See <u>role</u>.

pernoctation (pur-nok-tay'shən) n. passing the night; (ecclesiastical) an all-night vigil. [< L *pernoctatio* < per-, pref., through < *per* through + *noctare* < *nox* night + -ation, suff., an action or process or the result of it < -*ationem*, an instance of this, resulting state]. Cf. **insomnia**, q.v. See <u>sleep, waking</u>.

perseverate (pur-sev'və-rayt) vi. 1. to continue action, etc., for an unusually or excessively long time. 2. in psychology, to tend to prolong or repeat a response after the original stimulus has ceased. [< L *perseverare* to persist < *perseverus* very strict (as per-, pref., through, all over; completely < L by means of, by; through + *severus* severe]. n. **perseveration** (-sev"və-ray'shən). n. **perseverance** (pur"sə-veer'ənss). adj. **perseverant** (-sev'ər-ənt). adv. **perseverantly**. See <u>talk</u>. See <u>work, activity</u>.

persiflage (pur'sə-flaaj) n. 1. light or teasing good-natured talk, banter. 2. light-heartedness, flippancy, or frivolity in the treatment of a subject. [< F *persifler* to banter < *siffler* to whistle via OF < L *sibilare* to hiss (onomatopoeic)]. Cf. **badinage**, q.v. See <u>talk</u>.

perspicacious (pur"spi-kay'shəs) adj. having or showing great insight, astuteness; penetratingly discerning. • His *perspicacious* insight belied his very advanced years. [< L *perspicac-*, stem of *perspicax* < *perspicere* look closely < *specere* to look at]. n. **perspicacity** (-kas'-). n. **perspicaciousness**. adv. **perspicaciously**. Cf. **percipient**, q.v. See <u>intelligence</u>.

pertinacious (pur-tin-ay'shəss) adj. 1. determinedly resolute in purpose, belief, or action. 2. highly persistent, stubbornly unyielding. adv. **pertinaciously**. n. **pertinaciousness**. n. **pertinacity** (-nas'si-). [L *pertinac-* stem of *pertinax* very tenacious < *per-* thoroughly + *tenax* holding fast, tenacious < *tenere* to hold]. See <u>mentality, mentation, behavior</u>.

pervicacious (pur-vi-kay'shəss) adj. extremely obstinate; willful. [< L *pervicacia* persistence, stubbornness]. See <u>mentality, mentation, behavior</u>.

petechia (pee-teek'kee-ə), pl. **petechiae** (-kee-ī) n. minute intradermal or submucosal hemorrhagic spots of pinpoint-to-pinhead size. [modern L < It *petecchie*]. adj. **petechial**. Cf. **ecchymosis**. See **blood, circulation, glands**. See **skin**.

pettifogger (pet-tee-fog'gər) n. 1. a person overly concerned with, or who argues about, small details; someone who nitpicks, a niggler, a quibbler. (2. a lawyer whose practice is small or insignificant.) vi. **pettifog** (pet'tee-). n. **pettifoggery**. adj. **pettifogging**. [< petty < OF *peti*, a variant of *petit* small + fogger <?]. See **mentality, mentation, behavior**. See **role**.

phalacrophobia (fal"lak-rō-fōb'bi-ə) n. fear of baldness, going bald. [< G *phalakrosis* shining, white < *phao* to shine + *phobos* fear]. adj. **phalacrophobic**. n. **phalacrophobe**. syn. **alopeciaphobia**, **peladophobia**, q.v. See **phobias**. See **hair**.

phalacrosis (fal'ə-krōs'siss) n. (obs.) baldness. [< G *phalakrosis* shining, white < *phao* to shine]. syns. **acomia, alopecia, atrichia, calvites, canescent, canities, depilous, pilgarlic, poliosis, psilosis** (10 baldness syns.!), q.v. See **hair**.

phaneromania (fan"nər-ō-may'nee-ə) n. the compulsive habit of picking at scabs or growths on the skin. [phaner(o)-, pref., denoting visible or apparent < G *phaneros* visible + *mania* madness]. adj. **phaneromaniacal** (-mə-nī'ə-kəl). n. **phaneromaniac**. See **manias**.

Pharisaic/Pharisaical (far"ri-say'ik/ -say'i-kəl, -rə-sī'ik/-rə-sī'ə-kəl) adj. hypocritically self-righteous; emphasizing strict adherence to the superficiality of law or ritual rather than the spirit of an observance or ceremony. [< the Pharisees, a Hebrew sect during the time of Christ; its members were noted for their strict observance of Hebraic rites, rituals, and laws, and their self-righteousness, because of it. Derivation is via L, G, & ultimately Aramaic *prishayya*, pl. of *prish* or *parush* separated]. n. **Pharisee** = one with pharisaical characteristics of some of the ancient Jews. n. **Pharisaism**. adv. **Pharisaically**. See **mentality, mentation, behavior**. See **role**.

pharmacomania (faar"mə-kō-may'ni-ə) n. Uncontrollable desire to take or administer medicines. [pharmaco-, pref., denoting drugs, medicine < G *pharmakon* drug, poison + *mania* frenzy]. adj.

pharmacomaniacal (-mə-nī'ə-kəl). n. **pharmacomaniac**. See **manias**. See therapy.

pharmacophobia (farm"mə-kō-fōb'bi-ə) n. the morbid fear of medicine or drugs. [pharmaco-, pref., relating to drugs < G *pharmakon* drug, medicine + *phobos* fear]. adj. **pharmacophobic**. n. **pharmacophobic**. Cf. **neopharmacophobia**, q.v. See phobias. See therapy.

phatic (fa'tik) adj. emotional language that conveys friendship, shared feelings, or sociability, and creates good will rather than providing information. • Discussion was mainly *phatic* rather than logical at the **oldsters'**, q.v., reunion. [< G *phasis* utterance < *phatos* spoken < *phanai* to say]. adv. **phaticly**. See talk. See emotion.

phengophobia (fen"gō-fōb'bi-ə) n. morbid fear of the daylight, sunlight. • Concern about **actinic keratosis**, q.v., renders the aged *phengophobic*. [< G *phengos* daylight + *phobos* fear]. adj. **phengophobic**. n. **phengophobe**. syn. **heliophobia**, q.v. See phobias.

phil(a)-, **philo-**, prefs., denoting a love, fondness, affinity or craving for. [< G *philos* fond, loving < *phileo* to love].

philalethe (fil'ə-leth) n. one who loves to forget—not a **philalethist**, one who loves the truth, or a **philatelist**, one who loves to collect and study postage stamps. [< phila-, pref., q.v., + < G *lethe* forgetfulness]. See memory. See role.

philobat (fil'lō-bat) n. someone who loves to travel widely. [philo-, pref., q.v., + bat? (an animal that travels widely)]. See role. See work, activity.

philodox (fil'lō-doks) n. one who loves his/her own opinions; a dogmatist. [philo-, pref., q.v., + *doxa* opinion]. adj. **philodoxical** (fil"lō-doks'si-). adv. **philodoxically** (fil"lō-doks'si-). See role.

philopatrodomania (fil"lō-pat"trō-dō-may'ni-ə) n. homesickness. [philo-, pref., q.v., + < L *pater* father + < F *domaine*, alteration of *demeine* (land), belonging to a lord < L *dominicus* < *dominus* lord]. adj. **philopatrodomaniacal** (-may-nī'ə-kəl). n. **philopatrodomaniac** (-may'ni-ak). Cf. **nostomania**, **oikomania**, **ecomania**, q.v. See manias.

philopolemist (fil"lō-pō-lem'mist) n. a lover of argument, controversy, or of otherwise verbally contending. [philo-, pref., q.v., + < G *polemikos* < *polemos* war]. adjs. **philopolemic, philopolemical.** adv. **philopolemically.** See role. See talk.

philosophastering (fil-os"sō-fas'tər-ing) adj. pseudo-philosophizing. [< G *philosophos* love of knowledge < *philos* loving + *sophia* learning, wisdom + *phases* utterance < *phanai* to say]. n. **philosophaster** (-os'sō-fas"tər) = a pseudophilosopher. See talk. See role.

phlegmatic (fleg-mat'tik) adj. having a sluggish temperament, apathetic. 2. calm or composed. [< G *phlegmatikos* < *phlegm* that one of the four humors identified with those (phlegmatic) qualities < *phlegein* to burn]. adv. **phlegmaticly.** See mentality, mentation, behavior.

phobias (fōb'bi-əs) pl.n. fears. [G -*phobia*, suff. < *phobos* fear]. An alphabetical list of phobias, q.v., associated with the aged follows: **algophobia, ambulophobia, amnesiophobia, anemophobia, anginophobia, asthenophobia, autophobia, bacillophobia, bacteriophobia, basiphobia/basophobia, basistasiphobia, basostasophobia, caino(to)phobia, cancerophobia, carcinophobia, carcinomatophobia, cardiophobia, centophobia, chronophobia, cleptophobia, climacophobia, coimetrophobia, compuphobia, coprostasophobia, cyberphobia, deisidaimonia, dentophobia, dextrophobia, dysmorphobia, enissophobia, enosi(o)phobia, erem(l)ophobia, ermitophobia, geniophobia, gerascophobia, gerontophobia, hamartophobia, harpaxophobia, heliophobia, heresyphobia, hierophobia, homophobia, hypegiaphobia, hypengyophobia, hypnophobia, iatrophobia, isolophobia, kaino(to)phobia, kilobytophobia, kleptophobia** (or **cleptophobia**), **kopophobia, levophobia, medomalacophobia, microbiophobia, molys(o)mophobia, monophobia, my** (or **i**) **sophobia, neopharmaphobia, nosocomephobia, nosophobia, odontophobia, odynophobia, paralipophobia, pathophobia, patroiophobia, peccatiphobia, peccatophobia, peladophobia, phalacrophobia, pharmacophobia, phengophobia, ponophobia, prosophobia, rhytiphobia, satanophobia, sinistrophobia, solophobia, stasibasiphobia, stasobasiphobia, stasiphobia, stasophobia, stygiophobia, tachophobia, taphephobia/ taphophobia, taxophobia, technophobia, thanatophobia,**

theophobia, tomophobia, tropophobia, trypanophobia, xeniatrophobia, xenophobia.

Alphabetic listing of things feared: baldness or bald people; being buried alive; being reproached; cancer; cemeteries; change, making changes; chins, double chins; climbing up (or falling down) stairs; computers, informational technology, high technology; constipation; contamination; daylight, sunlight; death; deformity; dentists; devils, Satan; doctors; drugs, medicine; error; falling down (or climbing up) stairs; foreign doctors; foreigners; forgetting, amnesia; germs, bacteria; God, gods, God's wrath; growing old; having a heart attack; having committed an unpardonable sin; heart disease; hell; hereditary, genetically transmitted disease; hospitals; illness, disease; infection; injections, inoculation; heresy; homosexuals, homosexuality; (the) left, or of things located there; loneliness, being alone, solitude; losing an erection during sexual intercourse; new drugs; novelty, newness; old age; old people; oneself, being alone, loneliness; overwork, fatigue, exhaustion; passage of time; progress; religious or sacred objects; responsibility; neglected duty; (the) right, or of things located there; sameness, monotony; sinning; sleep & not waking; speed; standing & walking; strangers; sunlight; supernatural powers; surgery; taxes; thieves; walking; weakness; wind; wrinkling.

phobias: Subcategories

Morbid Fear Of:

I. Age:
    1. Growing old: **gerascophobia, gerontophobia**
    2. Old age: **gerascophobia**
    3. Old persons: **gerontophobia**
II. Appearance:
    1. baldness or bald people: **peladophobia, phalacrophobia**
    2. chins, double chins: **geniophobia**
    3. deformity: **dysmorphobia**
    4. wrinkling, getting wrinkles: **rhytiphobia**
III. Balance, locomotion, stability:
    1. Climbing up stairs: **climacophobia**
    2. Falling down stairs: **climacophobia**

IV. Change, innovation, newness, novelty, progress:
1. Change, making changes: **centophobia, tropophobia**
2. New drugs: **neopharmaphobia**
3. Novelty, newness: **caino(to)phobia, kaino(to) phobia, centophobia**
4. Progress: **prosophobia**
5. Strangers, foreigners: **xenophobia**.

V. Criticism:
1. Being reproached: **enissophobia**

VI. Computers, Internet, technology, Web:
1. Computers, informational technology, high technology: **compuphobia, cyberphobia, kilobytophobia, technophobia**

VII. Death:
1. Being buried alive: **taphephobia/ taphophobia**
2. Cemeteries: **taphephobia/ taphophobia, coimetrophobia**
3. Death: **thanatophobia**

VIII. Dirt, contamination, uncleanness:
1. Contamination: **my(or i)sophobia**
2. Germs, bacteria: **bacillophobia, bacteriophobia, microbiophobia**

IX. Light, daylight, sunlight:
1. Daylight, sunlight: **phengophobia**
6. Sunlight: **heliophobia**

X. Medical, physical, dental:
1. Cancer: **cancerophobia, carcinophobia, carcinomatophobia**
2. Constipation: **coprostasophobia**
3. Deformity: **dysmorphobia**
4. Dentists: **dentophobia, odontophobia**
5. Doctors: **iatrophobia**
6. Drugs, medicine: **pharmacophobia**
7. Foreign doctor: **xeniatrophobia**
8. Germs, bacteria: **bacillophobia, bacteriophobia, microbiophobia**
9. Having a heart attack: **anginophobia**
10. Heart disease: **cardiophobia**
11. Hereditary, genetically transmitted disease: **patroiophobia**
12. Hospitals: **nosocomephobia**
13. Illness, disease: **nosophobia, pathophobia**.

        14. Infection: **molys(o)mophobia**.
        15. Injections, inoculation: **trypanophobia**
        16. New drugs: **neopharmaphobia**
        17. Pain: **algophobia, odynophobia**
        18. Surgery: **tomophobia**
        19. Weakness: **asthenophobia**

XI. Mental, mind, intellect:
        1. Forgetting, amnesia: **amnesiophobia**

XII. Mistake, error:
        1. Error: **hamartophobia**

XIII. Pain:
        1. Pain: **algophobia**

XIV. Religion:
        1. Devil, Satan: **satanophobia**
        2. God, gods, God's wrath: **theophobia**
        3. Having committed an unpardonable sin: **enosi(o) phobia**
        4. Hell: **stygiophobia**
        5. Heresy: **heresyphobia**
        6. Religious or sacred objects: **hierophobia**
        7. Sinning: **hamartophobia, peccatiphobia**

XV. Responsibility:
        1. Responsibility, neglect of duty: **hypegiaphobia, hypengyophobia, paralipophobia**

XVI. Sameness, monotony: **homophobia**

XVII. Sex:
        1. Homosexuals, homosexuality: **homophobia**
        2. Losing an erection during sexual intercourse: **medomalacophobia**

XVIII.Sleep:
        1. Sleep and not waking: **hypnophobia**

XVIX.Solitude, aloneness, loneliness:
        1. Loneliness, being alone, solitude: **autophobia, erem(i)ophobia, ermitophobia, isolophobia, monophobia, solophobia**
        2. Oneself; being alone; loneliness: **autophobia**

XX. Speed: **tachophobia**

XXI. Standing, walking:
        1. Standing and walking: **basistasiphobia, basostasophobia, stasibasiphobia, stasobasiphobia, stasiphobia, stasophobia**
        2. Walking: **ambulophobia, basiphobia, basophobia**

XXII. Superstition, clairvoyance, magic, supernatural:
    1. Left or things located there: **levophobia,**
       sinistrophobia
    2. Right or things located there: **dextrophobia**
    3. Supernatural powers: **deisidaimonia**
XXIII. Taxes: **taxophobia**
XIV. Theft:
    1. Thieves: **cleptophobia, kleptophobia, harpaxopho-**
       bia
XXV. Time:
    1. Passage of time: **chronophobia**
XXVI. Wind: **anemophobia**
XXVII. Work:
    1. Overwork, fatigue, exhaustion: **kopophobia, pono-**
       phobia

phonasthenia (fōn"nas-theen'ni-ə) n. a weak or hoarse voice; difficult or abnormal voice production with enunciation being too high, too loud, or too hard; functional voice fatigue. [phon(o)-, pref., < G *phone* sound, voice + *asthenia* < a- priv. + *sthenos* strength]. adj. **phonasthenic.** adv. **phonasthenicly.** See **talk**.

phrontifugic (fron"ti'fyooj'jik) adj. helping to escape one's thoughts or cares. [< G *phronema* mind (that portion of the cortex of the brain which is occupied by thought or association centers) + -fuge, suff., denoting an agent that drives away or banishes < L *fugare* to put to flight]. • *Phrontifugic* relief is sought due to the duress of old age. n. **phrontifuge.** See **therapy**.

phrontistery (fron-tis'tər-ee) n. a place for thinking, or where a deep thinker, an intellectual, reads, studies, or meditates. [< G *phrontisterion* < *phrontizo* to think < *phrontis* thought]. n. **phrontistes** [G] = a deep thinker. See **intelligence**. See **role**.

physagogue (fiz'zə-gog) n. & adj. a **carminative**, q.v., or medicine that induces farting, **crepitus**, q.v. [< G *physikos* natural, physical + -agogue, -agog, suff., indicating a promoter or stimulant of < G *agogos* leading forth]. See **therapy**. See **gastrointestinal**.

physique, appearance: **abdominous, adipose, aesthetics/ esthetics, agerasia, allochrous,** *arcus corneae/arcus cornealis, arcus senilis,* **atrophy, attenuate, bariatrics, buccula, cachexia,**

caducity, caducous (adj.), canities, cereous, cernuous, compursion, contabescent, crine, decrepit, decrepitude, desiccated, dewlap, discalceate, discinct, draconic, dropsy, dyspnea, *éboulement*, edema, elflock, enophthalmos/ enophthalmus, exility, exsuccous, *feuillemorte*, frowzy, fubsy, fuliginous, fusty, geromarasmus, geromorphism, glabrous, gleet, gnarled, graybeard, grisard/grizard, heteromorphic, hirsutulous, hoary, irrugate, jollop, juvenescent, kyphosis, lardy, leptorrhine, leptosomatic, macilent, marasmus, marcescent, marcescible, myxedematous, neanimorphism, onychauxis, onychogryphosis/onychogryposis, paedomorphism, Parkinson's facies, passulation, pendulous, pinguid, prolapse, rigescent, senescent, *shibui*, slaver, snurp/snerp/snirp, steatopygous, tabes, tabescence/tabetic/tabic/tabid, tabefaction, tabefy, trumpery, urceolate, ventricous, vibrissa, wan, wanze, waspish, wattle, withered, wizened/wizen/weazen.

physique, appearance: Subcategories

I. Age:
  1. Approaching an advanced age: **senescent**
  2. Beauty revealed by time, old age: *shibui*
II. Attitude:
  1. Appearing conservative, old fashioned: **fusty**
  2. Darkly mysterious: **fuliginous**
  3. Subtlety: **exility**
III. Back:
  1. Hunchback: **kyphosis**
IV. Discharge:
  1. Viscous transparent discharge from a mucous surface: **gleet**
V. Dress:
  1. Barefooted: **discalceate**
  2. Beltless, loosely dressed: **discinct**
  3. Dirty, untidy, unkempt: **frowzy**
  4. showy, trashy, worthless: **trumpery**
VI. Face:
  1. Double chin, loose skin under the chin: **buccula**, **dewlap**, **jollop**, **wattle** (Strictly, all except the first refer to animals, birds.)
  2. Dried out: **desiccated**
  3. Long, narrow nose: **leptorrhine**

4. Mask-like, lifeless countenance: **Parkinson's facies**
5. Plastic surgery: **aesthetics/esthetics**
6. Sunken eyes: **enophthalmos/enophthalmus**
7. To become shriveled, wrinkled: **snurp/snerp/snirp**
8. To dribble, drool saliva: **slaver**
9. To wrinkle (vt.), e.g., one's face: **irrugate**
10. White or gray ring in the eye's corneal margin: *arcus corneae/arcus cornealis, arcus senilis*
11. Wrinkling one's face (n.): **compursion**.

VII. General physical appearance:
1. Appearing older than one's age or prematurely senile: **geromorphism**
2. Atrophy, wasting of old age: *éboulement*, **geromarasmus**
3. Dried up, wrinkled up (n.); (adj.): **passulation**; **desiccated**
4. Drooping, hanging down: **cernuous, pendulous, caducity**
5. Dropping off, unenduring: **caducity**
6. Dry, sapless, dried up: **exsuccous**
7. Edematous (swollen): **myxedematous**
8. Growing rigid, stiff, or numb: **rigescent**
9. Having a stale smell, musty: **frowzy**
10. Ill-smelling or musty: **fusty**
11. Knobby, twisted, rugged: **gnarled**
12. Of or like a dragon: **draconic**
13. Pale, sickly; feeble; bland: **wan**
14. Short of breath (n.): **dyspnea**
15. Shrink, shrivel up: **crine**
16. Smokey, sooty, dark: **fuliginous**
17. Swelling of body tissues: **dropsy, edema**
18. Tending to wither, fade (adj.): **marcescible**
19. Thin, lean: **macilent, leptosomatic**
20. Thinness: **exility**
21. To become wrinkled, shriveled: **snurp/snerp/snirp**
22. Wasp-like: **waspish**
23. Wasting away of the body: **marasmus**
24. Waxen: **cereous**
25. Yellow, yellowish brown appearance: *feuillemorte*

VIII. Loss of function:
1. Being old and worn out (n.): **decrepitude**
2. Especially old, malfunctioning: **decrepit, caducous**

3. Make thin, weaken: **attenuate**

IX. Obesity; fat, pot-bellied:
1. Branch of medicine re: treatment of obesity: **bariatrics**
2. Fat (adj.): **adipose, lardy, fubsy, pinguid**
3. Fat and with a large abdomen; large abdomen: **abdominous; ventricous**
4. Fat with protuberant, large buttocks: **steatopygous**
5. Pitcher-shaped: **urceolate**

X. Overgrown fingernails and toenails:
1. Gross hypertrophy, thickening of nails: **onychogryphosis/onychogryposis**
2. Simply long finger and/or toenails: **onychauxis**

XI. Size:
1. Squat: **fubsy**
2. Varied lifecycle forms: **heteromorphic**

XII. Skin & Hair:
1. Become shriveled, wrinkled (vi.); (adj.): **snurp/snerp/ snirp; wizeńed/wizen/weazen**
2. A bristle, hair, especially in the nose: **vibrissa**
3. Changing color: **allochroous**
4. Dry, sapless: **exsuccous**
5. Gray-haired person: **canities, graybeard** (man only), **grisard/grizard**
6. Having gray, white, gray-white hair; venerable: **hoary**
7. Minutely hairy: **hirsutulous**
8. Smooth & hairless: **glabrous**
9. Tangled hair: **elflock**
10. Yellowish, yellowish brown color: *feuillemorte*

XIII. Stability:
1. Falling down, slipping of a body part, viscus (pl. = viscera): **prolapse**

XIV. Wasting:
1. Atrophy, wasting of old age: **geromarasmus**
2. Shrink, shrivel up: **crine**
3. Shriveled, dried up, shrunken, having lost vitality: **withered**
4. Tending to wither, fade (adj.): **marcescible**
5. Wasting away (adj.): **tabescent/tabetic/tabic/tabid**
6. Wasting away; wasting away due to inadequate nutrition; wasting away due to disease; withering: **tabes** (n.), **wanze** (vi); **atrophy** (n), **cachexia** (n.),

contabescent (adj.); tabefaction (n.), tabefy (vt., vi.); marcescent (adj.)
XV.Youthful:
  1. Appearing younger than one's years: agerasia, neanimorphism, paedomorphism
  2. Becoming youthful (ant.): juvenescent

PICALM n. is the name of a recently discovered Alzheimer's disease gene. It appears "to play a role in maintaining healthy synapses (neural connections) in the brain." Other Alzheimer-related genes are: ApoE4, CLU, and TOMM40, q.v., and also CALHM1 and TREM2. See Alzheimer's disease. See intelligence.

picaresque (pik-ə-resk') adj. 1. relating to or typical of rogues or scoundrels. • Don Quixote—Alonso Quijano, his true name, was nearly 50 years of age and an aging rogue—was the original picaresque character: quixotic. (2. belonging to or characteristic of a type of prose fiction featuring a rogue.) [via F < Sp picaresco < picaro rogue < assumed vulgar L piccare to prick]. See mentality, mentation, behavior.

pickmote (pik'mōt) n. one who habitually points out and dwells on petty faults. [E, pick, to find fault, be petty, or fault finding < assumed OE pickian to prick, Old Icelandic pikka + E mote, a tiny speck or particle < OE mot <?]. See role. See mentality, mentation, behavior.

Pickwickian (pik-wik'kee-ən) adj. 1. said of words used in a Pickwickian sense, i. e., in a technical, constructive, or esoteric sense; meaningless; not typical or literal in usage or meaning, as in the Pickwick Papers. (Pickwickian words or epithets are usually of a derogatory or insulting type, but should not be taken that way. In the Pickwick Papers Samuel Pickwick accused Mr. Blotton of "acting in a vile and calumnious manner", but did not mean it literally.) 2. generous, naïve, or benevolent. • "It were better," said the old gnoff (q.v.), "had you called him a humbug in strictly a Pickwickian sense." [< Pickwick Papers, Chapter 1., Charles Dickens, 1837]. See mentality, mentation, behavior. See talk.

piddle (pid'əl) vi. (arch.) 1. to pick at one's food, "eat like a bird". 2. work, act in a trifling way. 3. (colloquial or childish) to urinate, make water. [< Swedish dialect; ? imitative;?]. adj. piddling. n. piddling. See drink, food. See work, activity. See genitourinary.

piffle (pif'fəl). n (dated informal) silly talk or ideas. vi. to behave in a silly or ineffective way. ● Such *piffle* is not unusual in those with dementia. syns. **balderdash, blather, glossolalia, prate, prattle,** etc., q.v. See **talk**. See **mentality, mentation, behavior**.

pilgarlic (pil-gaar'lik) n. 1. (arch.) a bald head that looks like a smooth peeled garlic bulb; bald-headed man; poor creature. 2. (arch.) a facetious term of contempt or pity to describe a person as a poor wretch or a sad sack, especially one abandoned by his friends, and was used of oneself as a term of self-pity. (". . . we jogged off to bed for the night; but never a bit could poor *pilgarlic* sleep one wink, for the everlasting jingle of bells." < Rabelais's "Pantagruel". {N. W. Schur}). [E < pilled, obs., to make or become hairless, or like peeled garlic]. syns. **acomia, alopecia, atrichia, calvities, depilous, phalacrosis, poliosis, psilosis,** q.v. See **hair**.

pingle (pin'gəl) vi. to fiddle or trifle with one's food, showing little interest or appetite. [< E & Sc dialect <?]. Cf. **piddle,** q.v. See **drink, food**.

pinguecula (pin-gwek'kyoo-laa, -lə)/**pinguicula** (-gwik'), pl. **pingueculae/pinguiculae** (-ee, -ī). n. a yellowish spot sometimes seen on either side of the cornea in the aged; it is a connective tissue (non-fatty) thickening of the conjunctiva (the outermost delicate, clear, thin-tissue covering of the eyeball—except for the lens—and the inner eyelids). By growth and vascularization a pinguecula can invade the cornea and become a **pterygium,** q.v. ● The elderly are more subject to *pingueculae*, especially those who have spent a lot of time outdoors in sun, dust, wind. [< L *pinguiculus* fattish, somewhat fatty < *pinguis* fat]. Cf. **pterygium,** q.v. See **eye**.

pinguid (pin'gwid) adj. fat; containing a lot of fat, oil, grease. [< L *pinguis* fat]. n. **pinguidity** (pin-guid'di-tee). syns. **adipose, lardy,** q.v. Cf. **fubsy; abdominous, ventricous; pursy,** q.v. See **physique, appearance**.

pinna (pin'aa or -ə) pl. **pinnae** (pin'nī, -nee,-nas) n. the projecting part of the ear lying outside of the head. ● The elderly seem to have large *pinnae*, which is actually due to normal enlargement of the *pinnae* with age. [L, wing]. adj. **pinnal** = pertaining to the pinna. syn. **auricula,** q.v. See **ear, hearing**.

piss-proud (piss'prowd) adj. having a somewhat incomplete, i.e., faltering, erection. This may be said of an old man with a young wife—a situation of **alphamegamia** or **anisonogamia**, q.v. The penis or *membrum virile* (L, penis) is not fully **rigescent**, q.v., lacks complete obtumescence (swelling up). The term currently can also refer to someone with a false ego. [The phrase first appeared in 1788 in ed. 2 of the" Vulgar Tongue" by Francis Grose (British), and originally referred to some degree of penile erection, thus swollen and prideful, present on awakening after a night's sleep, and due to pressure by a full urinary bladder on the prostate. < www.Everything2.com]. See **sex, love**. See **genitourinary**.

pixilated (piks'i-layt'ted) adj. 1. mentally unbalanced, slightly crazy; eccentric. 2. whimsical. [< pixie, a 17ᵗʰ C. mischievous fairylike creature; origin unk.]. See **intelligence**.

planeticose (plə-neet'ti-kōss) adj. liking to wander—on foot or (fig.) in talking. [G, wander]. • The elderly raconteur was invariably *planeticose*. See **standing, walking, wandering**. See **talk**.

platitudinarian (plat"ti-tood-in-air'ri-ən) adj. & n. a dealer in platitudes; full of platitudes; speaking platitudes. [< L *plattus* broad < G *platus* flat + -tude, comb. form, suff., for forming abstract nouns < adjs., pps., or v. stems, in E direct < L, e.g., altitude < F, e.g., solitude, or on L analogy, e.g., exactitude, + -ian, suff.]. See **talk**. See **role**.

pleniloquence (plen-il'lō-kwəns) n. excessive talking, loquacity. [< L *plenus* full + *loquitari* to chatter away < *loqui* to speak + -ence, suff., forming nouns of quality or action < *-entia* < pres. p. in *-ent-* (nom. *-ens*)]. adj. **pleniloquent**. adv. **pleniloquently**. syn. **longiloquence**, **multiloquence**, q.v. Cf. **logomania**. See **talk**.

pleonastic (plee-ō-nas'tik) adj. pertaining to oral or written repetitiousness, redundancy of expression. n. **pleonasm**. adv. **pleonastically**. [< G *pleonasmos* (*pleonazo* add superfluously < *pleon* more]. syn. **tautologic**, q.v. See **talk**.

plica polonica (plīk'kə pō-lon'ni-kə) n.phr. a twisted, matted, and crusted condition of the hair usually as a result of neglect, filth, or parasitic infestation. (Apparently the term originated in Poland and was associated with an inflammation of the scalp due to lice {**pediculosis**, q.v., **capitis**} infestation.) [L, a fold or plait & *polonica* Polish]. See **hair**.

PLMD an initialism: Periodic Limb Movement Disorder, which occurs frequently in the elderly: some 45% of community-dwelling elders older than 65 years of age have PLMD. Movement of the big toe, ankle, and partial flexion of the knees and hip occur during NREM (non-rapid-eye-movement) sleep; movements last 2-4 sec., and occur throughout the night. Usually patients are not aroused and are unaware of the movements. PLMD causes disordered, inefficient sleep. Daytime drowsiness can be a prominent symptom, but sometime the disorder is asymptomatic. The condition responds usually to dopamine antagonists, or to benzodiazepines such as clonazepam. PMLD's cause is unknown, but age-related decrease in dopamine receptors may be etiologic. See **parahypnosis**, **parasomnia**, and **somnipathy**. See **sleep, wakefulness**. See **joint, extremities, back**.

pneuma (noo'maa) n. 1. air. 2. intelligence; breath; soul, psyche. (In ancient G philosophy and medicine, air, or a pervasive fiery essence therein, which was the creative and animating spirit of the universe, was drawn into the body via the lungs where it generated or sustained the innate heat in the heart's left ventricle and was thereby circulated to all parts of the body.) [G, air, breath]. See **intelligence**.

pococurante (pōk"kō-koo-raan'tay, -kyoo-) adj. indifferent, apathetic, nonchalant, devil-may-care. [< It *poco* little + *curante* pres.p. of *curare* to care < L *curare*, *cure* care]. n. **pococurante** = a careless or indifferent person. See **mentality, mentation, behavior**. See **role**.

pod(o)-, pref., meaning foot or foot-shaped, or relationship to the foot. [< G *pous*, *podos* foot].

podagra (pō-dag'grə) n. gouty pain in the great toe. • Famous *podagra* sufferers include Leonardo da Vinci, Galileo, Martin Luther, Ben Franklin, Thomas Jefferson, Benjamin Disraeli, and Karl Marx. [pod(o)-, pref., q.v., + *agra* seizure]. adj. **podagral**. adj. **podagric**. adj. **podagrous**. See **pain**. See **joint, extremities, back**.

podalgia (pō-dal'jee-ə, -ji-ə, -jhə) n. pain in the foot. [pod(o)-, pref., q.v., + -algia, suff., denoting a painful condition < G *algos* pain].

syns. **pododynia**, **tarsalgia**, q.v. Cf. **lassipedes**, q.v. See **standing, walking, wandering**. See **pain**. See **joint, extremities, back**.

podarthritis (pod-arth-rīt'tis) n. inflammation of any of the tarsal or metatarsal joints of the foot. [pod(o)-, pref., q.v., + G *arthron* joint + -itis, suff. inflammation]. See **joint, extremities, back**.

podiatrist (pō-dī'ə-trist) n. a practitioner of **podiatry**, q.v. • Due to near vision and **osteoarthritic**, q.v., difficulties the elderly often cannot trim their toenails themselves, but require a *podiatrist*. [pod(o)-, pref., q.v., + *iatros* physician]. syn. **chiropodist**, q.v. See **role**. See **joint, extremities, back**. See **role**.

podiatry (pō-dī'ə-tree) n. the specialty that includes the diagnosis and/ or medical, surgical, mechanical, physical, and adjunctive treatment of the diseases, injuries, and defects of the human foot. [pod(o)-, pref., q.v., + G *iatreia* medical treatment]. adj. **podiatric** (pō-di-at'rik). adj. **podalic** (pō-dal'lik) = relating to the foot. syn. **chiropody**, q.v. See **joint, extremities, back**.

pododynia (pod"dō-din'ni-ə, -ee-ə) n. pain in the foot. [pod(o)-, pref., q.v., + G *odyne* pain + -ia, suff.]. syn., **podalgia**, q.v. See **joint, extremities, back**. See **pain**. See **standing, walking, wandering**.

poliosis (pō-lee-ōs'siss) n. the loss of hair color, particularly of the scalp hair, and often as the result of various pathologic conditions; premature graying of the hair. [< G *polios* gray]. See **color**. See **hair**.

poltophagy (pōl-tof'fə-jee) n. thorough chewing of food so that it becomes reduced to a porridge-like, semiliquid mass: extended mastication. [< G *poltos* porridge + *phagein* to eat]. adj. **poltophagic** (-tō-fay'jik). See **drink, food**.

polyhistor (pol-ee-his'tawr) n. a universal scholar, one remarkably learned in many subjects. [< G, *poluistor* < *polus* much (poly-, pref., more than one) + *histor* < L *historia* history + -or, suff.]. adj. **polyhistoric** (-stawr'rik) n. **polyhistorian** (-tawr'ri-ən). n. **polyhistory** (-his'-). syn. **polymath**, q.v. See **role**.

polylogy (pō-lil'lə-jee) n. wordiness. [poly-, pref., more than one or normal < G *polus* much + -logy, suff., speech, expression; science, study < -*logia*, suff., < *logos* word, reason & < -*logos*, suff., speaking]. See **talk**.

polyloquent (pō-lil'lō kwent). adj. talking about many things. [poly-, pref., meaning many or much, < G *polys* many + L *loqui* speak, talk, say, speak about, tell]. n. **polyloquence**. adv. **polyloquently**. syn. **omniloquent**, q.v. ant. **pauciloquent**, q.v. See **talk**.

polymath (pol'lee-math") n. a person with extraordinarily broad and comprehensive knowledge. • It goes without saying that one must be old in order to have acquired the extraordinarily broad and comprehensive knowledge of a *polymath*. [< G *polumathes* somebody with much learning < *polys* many + *manthanein* to learn]. adj. **polymathic** (-math'hik). n. **polymathy** (pol-lim'ə-thee, pə-lim'ə-thee). syn. **polyhistor**, q.v. See **role**.

polypharmacy (pol"ee-faar'mə-see) n. 1. the use of two or more drugs together, usually to treat a single condition or disease. 2. the use or prescription of too many drugs together, especially when they are used to treat one condition, i.e. the use of excessive medication. Increased drug reactions may result from polypharmacy. The term "pill burden" refers to the number of medications—pills, tablets, liquid doses, etc.—taken on a regular basis. [poly-, pref., meaning many or much, < G *polys* many + *pharmakeia* medication or drugs]. See **therapy**.

polysomnography (pol"lee-som-nog'grə-fee) n. registration, typically in a sleep laboratory, of a patient's electroencephalogram (EEG), respiration, pulse, blood pressure, oxygenation, etc., during sleep in order to detect sleep disorders, such as **sleep apnea**, q.v., which are most frequent in the elderly. (An objective definition of sleep apnea is the "apnea-hypopnea index", which is defined as the number of hours slept divided into the number of airflow interruptions {apneas} and airflow reductions {hypopneas} that occurred during sleep. Greater than 5 apneas &/or hypopneas per hour indicate sleep apnea.) [poly-, pref., meaning many or much < G *polys* many + < L *somnus* sleep + -graphy, suff, meaning the process of writing or recording or a method of recording < G -*graphia* < *graphein* to write]. See **PMLD**. See **sleep, wakefulness**.

ponophobia (pōn"nō-fōb'bi-ə) n. morbid fear of becoming overworked or of becoming fatigued. [pono-, pref., denoting bodily exertion, fatigue, overwork, pain < G *ponos* toil, fatigue, pain + < G *phobos* fear]. adj. **ponophobic**. n. **ponophobe**. syn. **kopophobia**. See **phobia**. See **work, activity**.

poriomania (pawr"ri-ō-may'ni-ə) n. wanderlust. "A disease of cats, teenagers, and elderly ladies." (Peter Bowler). [? < G *poros* pore, a passage < *peran* to pierce + -mania, suff., q.v.]. adj. **poriomaniacal** (-mə-nī'ə-kəl). n. **poriomaniac**. See **manias**. See **standing, walking, wandering**.

porlockian (pawr-lok'-ki-ən) adj. intrusive, interrupting. [< a man from Porlock, a coastal village and civil parish in Somerset, England, who wrecked Coleridge's train of thought by intruding during his writing of *Kubla Khan*]. See **mentality, mentation, behavior**.

pornogenarian (pawr'nō-gen-air'ree-ən) n. a "dirty old man", an elderly lecher, a libidinous duffer, a skuzzy-duddy, a sexagenarian (pun by David Grambs). [< G *porne* prostitute + < -gen, suff., something that produces < G *−genes* born + -ian, suff., belonging to, coming from, being involved in, or being like something < L *-ianus*, suff.]. syns. & Cf. **aidoi(o)maniac, capripede, cretomaniac, edeomaniac, erotomaniac, gynecomaniac, lewdster, lovertine, satyr**, q.v., **nymphomaniac**. See **old man**. See **role**. See **sex, love**.

poroma (por-ōm'mə) n. a corn. [G, < *poros* stone]. Syn. **clavus**, q.v. See **skin**. See: **joint, extremities, back**.

posiomania (pōs"si-ō-may'ni-ə) n. alcoholism, dipsomania. [< G *posis* drinking + *mania* frenzy, madness]. adj. **posiomaniacal** (-mə-nī'ə-kəl). n. **posiomaniac**. syns. **alcoholomania, dipsomania, methomania**, q.v. Cf. **oenomania**, q.v. See **manias**. See **drink, food**. See **role**.

potatory (pōt'tə-tawr-ee) adj. pertaining to or given to drinking. [< L *potatorius* < *potatus*, pp. of *potare* to drink]. See **drink, food**.

prate (prayt) vi. talk too much in a silly way about nothing important, with little or no purpose; chatter; talk idly. [< MD *praten*]. n. **prate**. n. **prater**. adv. **pratingly**. See **talk**. See **role**.

prattle (prat'təl) vi.&vt. to talk in a silly, idle, childish way. [mid-16th C. < MLG <?]. n. **prattle** = childish chatter, small talk. n. **prattler.** adv. **prattlingly.** syn. **prate**, q.v. See **talk**. See **role**.

pre- (pree), pref., before, earlier; in advance; in front of. [< L *prae* in front, before].

preagonal (pree-ag'gən-əl) adj. a period of suffering or struggle immediately preceding death. [pre-, pref., q.v., + < L *agonia* < G *agonia* (mental) struggle, anguish < *agon* contest]. See **end-of-life, death**.

precant (preek'kənt) n. one who prays. [< L *precari, precorare* to pray]. See **role**.

prefrontal cortex (pree-fron'tal kawr'teks") n.phr. a brain area involved in concentration and "working memory", e.g., remembering a phone number long enough to "dial" it. [pre-, pref., q.v., + < L *front-*, stem of *frons* forehead, front + L, *cortex* bark, rind, shell + -al, suff.]. See **memory**.

prelapsarian (pree-lap-sair'ri-ən) adj. (1. relating to any innocent or carefree period in the past—lit., before the fall {of Adam & Eve}.) 2. an extremely long time, ages ago, ancient, old. [pre-, pref., q.v., + L *lapsus* fall. The term refers to the period in the Garden of Eden before Adam and Eve lost their innocence]. See **past, time**. See **old**.

prepresbyophrenia (pree"prez"bee-ō-freen'ni-ə) n. before the onset of **presbyophrenia**, q.v. [pre-, pref., q.v., + presby-, presbyo- (prez'bi-ō-), comb., relating to old age < G *presbys* old man + *phren* mind]. adj. **prepresbyophrenic** (-phren'-ik). See **isolophobia** in relation to feelings of loneliness in the elderly as a precursor of **presbyophrenia**, q.v. See **intelligence**. See **past, time**. See **mentality, mentation, behavior**.

presbyacusis (prez"bi-ə-kyoos'siss) n. loss of ability to perceive or discriminate sounds, due to degenerative changes of the nerves and hair cells of the inner ear, as part of the aging process; the pattern and age of onset may vary. High frequency—3,000 to 4,000 Hz— consonant sounds such as "f", "p", "s", "sh", "t", are the most important sounds for speech recognition and are most affected in presbyacusis.
• Hearing loss, of varied etiology, but usually related to *presbyacusis*,

is the most common disability in the elderly. [presby-, presbyo-(prez-bi-ō-), pref., relating to old age < G *presbys* old man + *akousis* hearing < *akouein* to hear]. syn. = **presbyacousia** = **presbycusis**. See **ear, hearing**.

presbyatrics (prez-bi-at'trikss) n. geriatrics. [presby(o)-, pref., q.v. + < G *iatreia* medical treatment]. n. **presbyatrician** = geriatrician, gerontologist. syns. = **geriatrics, presbyatrics**, qv. See **old age**. See **role**.

presby(o)- (prez'bi-ō-), pref., relating to old age. [< G *presbys* old man].

presbyope (prez'bi-ōp) n. a person with presbyopia, i.e., the farsightedness of old age. [presby(o)-, pref., q.v., + *ops* eye]. n. **presbyopia**. syn. **hyperope**. See **eye**.

presbyophrenia (prez"bee-ō-freen'ni-ə)/**presbyphrenia**, n. one of the mental disorders of old age—senile dementia—marked by loss of memory, disorientation, and confabulation, but with relative integrity of judgment. [presby(o)-, pref., q.v., + G *phren* mind]. adj. **prsbyophrenic** (-fren'nik). syn. **Wernicke's dementia**. See **intelligence**.

presbyopia (prez"bi-ōp'pee-ə) n. the physiologic change in accommodation power in the eyes in advancing age. It's said to begin when the near point has receded beyond 22 cm. (9 inches). [presby(o)-, pref., q.v., + G *ops* eye]. adj. **presbyopic**. syns. (obs.) **presbytia** (prez-bish'i-ə) & (obs.) **presbytism** (pres'bee-tis-əm). See **eye**.

presenile (pree-seen'nīl) adj. pertaining to a condition resembling senility, but not certainly senile, and occurring in early or middle life. [pre-, pref., q.v., + *senilis* of old people, of an old man; aged; senile]. See **intelligence**.

presenile dementia (pree-seen'nīl dee-men'shee-ə, or -men'shə) n.phr. primary degenerative dementia of the **Alzheimer's** type, q.v., with presenile onset. [pre-, pref., q.v., + de-, pref, signifying down or away from < L away from, down from + *mens* mind + -ia, suff.]. n. **presenility**. See **intelligence**.

presenilin (pree-se-nil'lin) adj. pertaining to those human genes, shared by everyone, that are associated with senility, and certain mutations of which cause early **Alzheimer's disease**, q.v. [v.s.]. See **intelligence**.

presenium (pre-see'nee-əm) n. the period immediately preceding old age. [pre-, pref., q.v., + *senium* feebleness of age, decline, senility; decay; grief, trouble; gloom; crabbiness; old man]. Cf. **paracme**, q.v. (**proscenium** = the stage space in a theater between the curtain and the orchestra.). See **old age**.

preterist (pret'tur-ist) n. 1. one whose chief interest and pleasure is in the past; one who lives—may be lost—in the past. (2. in theology: one who believes that the prophecies of the Apocalypse have already been fulfilled.) [*preter-*, pref., before < L *praeter* < *prae* before + -ist, suff., practicing a specific skill or profession < L *-ista* < G *-istes*]. adj. **preterist** = pertaining to preterists, (or their interpretations of Biblical scriptures). See **old man**, **old woman**. See **past, time**. See **role**.

prevenient (pree-veen'yənt) adj. coming before; anticipatory; having in view the prevention of. • The purpose of so much of the medical care that seniors undergo is *prevenient*. [< L *praevenient-*, pres.p. of *praevenire* to precede < pre-, pref., q.v., + L *venire* to come]. See **therapy**.

pro-, pref., in favor of, for; before. [< L & G *pro* for; before].

probiotic (prō-bī-ot'tik) n. live microorganisms, which when administered (orally) in adequate amounts, confer a (supposed) health benefit. Probiotics are used for various gastrointestinal and immunologic conditions, maladies. Currently probiotics are unregulated; consumers don't know the dosage ingested, and manufacturers are not required to list the quantity added to a food product. • The **doyenne**, q.v., relied heavily on a yoghurt-laced *probiotic* for relief of bloating and constipation. [pro-, pref., q.v., + < G *biotikos* of life, lively < *bios* life]. See **therapy**.

procidentia (prōs"si-den'shee-ə, -den'shə) n. a prominent protrusion, displacement, or **prolapse**, q.v., of a part, viscus, or organ, e.g., the rectum, uterus, iris. [L, prolapse, a falling down]. See **gastrointestinal**. See **genitourinary**.

progenitor (prō-jen'ni-tōr) n. 1. a direct ancestor of somebody or some thing. 2. the originator of, or original model for, something. [L, *progenitor* begetter < *progenit*-, pp. of *progignere* < *pro*- before + *gignere* to beget]. See **old man**. See **role**.

progeria (prō-jeer'ri-ə) n. 1. premature senility. (2. Hutchinson-Gilford syndrome: a medical condition in which a relatively young person, usually a child, has some physical characteristics of senility, including severely arrested physical development, premature ageing, and premature arteriosclerotic heart disease. Death from coronary artery disease often occurs before 10 years of age.) [pro-, pref., q.v., + < G *geras* old age]. syn. **presenility**. See **intelligence**.

progerin (prō-jeer'in) n. a protein that accumulates slowly in people as they age. Its accumulation is very rapid in children with **progeria**, q.v., i.e., the Hutchinson-Gilford syndrome. Progerin may be a risk factor for heart disease according to a study by the National Institute of Health. [pro-, pref., q.v., + < G *geras* old age]. See **old age**.

prolapse (prō-laps', prō'laps) n. the falling down of or slipping of a body part or viscus from its usual position. [< L *prolapsus* < *pro*- before + *labi* to fall]. syn. **procidentia**, q.v. See **physique, appearance**.

prolix (prō-liks', prō'liks") adj. unnecessarily, tiresomely wordy; verbose. [< L *prolixus* that has flowed out < the pp. of *liquere* to flow]. n. **prolixity** (-liks'i-tee). n. **prolixness** (-liks'). adv. **prolixly** (-liks'). ● The **termagant's**, q.v. *prolixity* was unbearable. See **talk**.

prosopagnosis (prōs"sō-pan-ōs'siss) n. loss of memory for faces, inability to recognize familiar faces, face blindness. Can result from old age or brain injury. (A book on the topic and related ones is "The Man Who Mistook His Wife for a Hat" by Oliver Sacks.) [< G *prosopon* face, mask, person < *pros*- near + *opon* face + *ops* eye + *agnosia* ignorance < *a*-, privative pref., not, without + *gnosis* knowledge, investigation]. n., alt., **prosopagnosia**. n. **prosopagnosiac** = one who has lost memory for, can't recognize, faces. (A prosopagnosiac's motto might be "I don't take people at face value.") adj. **prosopagnostic** (-pan-ōs'tik). syn. = **prosopolethy**, q.v. See **memory**. See **role**.

prosophobia (prōs"sō-fōb'bi-ə) n. morbid fear of, or aversion to, progress. [< G *proso* forward + -phobia, suff., an exaggerated or irrational fear, < G *phobos* fear]. adj. **prosophobic**. n. **prosophobe**. See **phobias**. See innovation, misoneism.

prosopolethy (prŏs"sō-pō-lee'thee) n. inability to remember faces. [< G *prosopon* face, person + *lethe* forgetfulness]. adj. **prosopolethic**. syn. **prosopagnosis**. See memory.

prostatism (pros'tə-tis'əm) n. the symptoms and general condition induced by hypertrophy (hyperplasia, enlargement) or chronic disease of the prostate gland. Symptoms of benign prostatic hypertrophy (BPH) include a feeling of incomplete bladder emptying, urinary frequency, hesitancy, weakness of urinary stream, stream intermittency, urgency, and **nocturia**, q.v. [prostate(o)-, pref., relating to the prostate gland < L *prostata* < G *prostates* one standing before < *pro* before + *states* < *sta-* stand + -ism, suff.]. See genitourinary.

prostatomegaly (pros"ta-tō-meg'gə-lee) n. prostatic enlargement or hypertrophy, which could be benign, or due to cancer. [prostate(o)-, pref., relating to the prostate gland < L *prostata* < G *prostates* one standing before < *pro* before + *states* < *sta-* stand + *megas* large]. Cf. **benign prostatic hypertrophy**, **BPH**, q.v. See genitourinary.

prosthesis (pros-thees'siss), pl. **prostheses** (-sees) n. an artificial substitute for a missing body part, such as an extremity, eye, tooth, cardiac valve, etc., used for functional or cosmetic reasons or both. [G, a putting to]. adj. **prosthetic** (-the'tik). n. **prosthetics** (-the'tiks) = the field of knowledge relating to prostheses. n. **prosthetist** (-pros'thə-tist) = one skilled in prosthetics and practicing its application to individual cases. Cf. **orthosis**, q.v. See therapy. See role.

prosthodontics/prosthodontia (pros-thō-don'tikss)/(-don'shə) n. that branch of dentistry pertaining to the restoration and maintenance of oral function, comfort, appearance, and health of the patient by the replacement of missing teeth and contiguous tissues with artificial substitutes. Called also dental prosthetics, denture prosthetics, and prosthetic dentistry. [< G *prosthesis* a putting to + *odous* tooth + -ics/-ia, suff.]. adj. **prosthodontic**. n. **prosthodontist** = one practicing prosthodontics. See therapy. See mouth, gums, teeth. See role.

protervity (prō-tur'vi-tee) n. petulance; peevishness; perversity. [< L *protervitas* brashness, brazenness, impudence, boldness]. See mentality, mentation, behavior.

Proustian experience (prooss'ti-ən) n.phr. an involuntary extraordinarily clear and vivid memory that is triggered by something such as an odor. Marcel Proust, in his novel published in eight volumes between 1913 and 1927, *A la recherche du temps perdu* (variously translated as Remembrance of Things Past, In Search of Lost time, or Recovery of Lost Memory), describes such a flashback of extreme clarity in his boyhood. It was occasioned by the odor of a Madeleine cake dipped in green tea sweetened with lime blossoms. The recovered memory of a proustian experience evokes a deeper understanding and emotional reinterpretation of the situation that is apt to have current significance for one. See **memory**.

Prufrockian (proo-frok'ki-ən) adj. marked by timidity and indecisiveness, and beset by unfulfilled aspirations. [< the title character in T. S. Eliot's poem, "The Love Song of J. Alfred Prufrock". Prufrock is haunted by his cautious, hesitant approach to life, his conforming existence—"I have measured out my life with coffee spoons."—and the possible romances he didn't dare broach (a romance *manqué*, q.v.)—Anu Garg]. n. **Prufrock**. See **mentality, mentation, behavior**. See **role**.

prurient (proo'ree-ənt) adj. having, arising from, or intended to arouse, lewd thoughts, or an unwholesome interest in sexual matters. [< L *prurient-*, pp. of *prurire* itch, long for]. n. **prurience**. n. **pruriency**. adv. **pruriently**. Cf. **salacious, concupiscent**, q.v. See **sex, love**.

pruritus (proo-rīt'təs) n. itching: an unpleasant sensation that instinctively elicits attempts to scratch or rub. Pruritus is a common complaint among the elderly, and is due most frequently to **xerosis**, q.v., an extremely common condition in the elderly. (Systemic disorders such as liver disease, uremia, iron deficiency anemia, diabetes mellitus, hyperthyroidism, etc., and some drugs can cause pruritus.) [L, an itching < *prurio* to itch].

psellism (sel'liz-əm) n. defective or indistinct pronunciation: stammering, lisping, mispronunciation, substitution of letter sounds, mumbling, or garbling one's words. [< G *psellismos* a stammering]. adj. **psellistic** (sel-liz'tik). **psellistically** (-liz'tik-lee). See **talk**.

pseudomnesia (sood"dōm-neez'zi-ə, -zhə) n. memory for things that never happened. [pseud(o)-, pref., false, spurious; similar, < G *pseudes* false < *pseudein* lie + *mneme* memory + -ia, suff.]. n.

pseudomnesiac. adj. **pseudomnesic** (-ness'tik). syn. **paramnesia**, q.v. See **memory**. See **role**.

pseudophakic eye (soo-dō-fay'kik) n.phr. an eye with an intraocular lens implant. Cataract surgery usually involves replacement of the natural clouded lens with a plastic one: an intraocular lens implant. [pseud(o)-, pref., false, spurious; similar < G *pseudes* false < *pseudein* lie + *phakos* lentil or lentil-shaped object]. See **eye**.

pseudosmia (soo-doz'mi-ə) n. false smell-perception; an hallucination of smell. [pseud(o)-, pref., false, spurious; similar < G *pseudes* false < *pseudein* lie + *osme* odor + -ia, suff.]. **Cf. anosmia**, q.v. See **nose, smell**.

psilology (sī-lol'lə-jee) n. empty talk. [< G *psilos* bare, mere + -logy, suff., speech, expression; science, study < -*logia* < *logos* word, reason & < -*logos* speaking]. See **talk**.

psilosis (si-lōs'siss) n. 1. losing or falling out of the hair. (2. an old term for sprue: an intestinal malabsorption syndrome.) [< G *psilosis* a stripping < *psilos* bare]. adj. **psilotic** (sil-ot'-tik). See **hair**.

psittacistic (sit-ə-siss'tik) adj. speaking in a mechanical, repetitive, and meaningless way: like a parrot. ● "The old professor was a boring and *psittacistic* speaker." (Russell Rocke). [< G *psittakos* parrot + -ist, -istic, suff., practicing a special skill or profession < G –*istes* < -*izo* -ize + -*tes* an agent-suff.]. n. **psittacism**. See **talk**.

pterygium (tur-rij'ji-əm) n. 1. a triangular patch, growth of hypertrophied bulbar subconjunctival vascularized connective tissue extending from the inner canthus (corner of the eyeball) to the border of the cornea or beyond, with the pterygial apex pointing toward the pupil. (2. a forward growth of the eponychium (cuticle) with adherence to the proximal (upper) portion of the nail.) [< G *pterygion* little wing, wing-like, a disease of the eye—diminutive of *pteryx* wing]. adj. **pterygial**. See **eye**.

pultaceous (pul-tay'shəs) adj. of the nature of pap or a poultice, soft, pulpy. [< *pulse* (a collective singular sometimes with a plural verb) edible seeds of leguminous plants, e.g., peas, beans, lentils; (with plural) any kind of these < L *puls* -*ltis*, pottage of meal, etc.]. See **drink, food**.

pump head n.phr. a very informal and crude term for the short-term noticeable cognitive decline occurring in some patients after cardiac bypass surgery (in which a *pump* oxygenator is used). The term is used by medical personnel among themselves. Symptoms include memory loss, slowed responses, trouble concentrating, and emotional instability. [< the "pump" (the extracorporeal pump oxygenator) supplying blood to the body while the heart is isolated during bypass surgery]. syn. = **bypass brain**; **cognitive dysfunction**, q.v. See **intelligence**. See **mentality, mentation, behavior**.

purblind (pur'blīnd) adj. 1. an offensive term meaning partly or completely unable to see. 2. slow or unwilling to understand, unwitting. [< pure + blind]. Cf. **lusction**, q.v. See **eye**. See **intelligence**. See **mentality, mentation, behavior**.

purpura (pur'pyoo-rə) n. a condition characterized by hemorrhage into the skin, mucous membrane, or serosal surface (the outermost coat of a visceral structure that lies in a body cavity). [L, purple < G *porphyra* purple]. adj. **purpuric**. syn. **peliosis** [G, extravasation of blood]. See: **skin**. See **blood, circulation, glands**.

pursive (pur'siv) adj. (obs., arch.) breathing with labor and difficulty; short-winded; asthmatic. [< F *pousser* in the sense of to breath with labor or difficulty < L *pulsare* to agitate violently—frequentative of *pellere* to drive]. n. **pursiveness**. adv. **pursively**. syn. **dyspneic**, q.v. Cf. **pursy**, q.v. See **breathing**.

pursy (pur'see) adj. (obs., arch.) short of breath, especially because of being too fat. [See **pursive**]. Cf. **dyspneic**, **pursive**, q.v. See **breathing**.

Q

"Don't worry about avoiding temptation. As you grow older,
it will avoid you."—Winston Churchill.

QALYS (kwawl'ees) n., an acronym, or better, an initialism: quality-adjusted life-years, which is recently used by economists to decide medical treatment worthiness. QALYS is determined by a formula in which the cost of a treatment is divided by the number of years a patient is likely to benefit from it; the result = QALYS. A medical panel or official, usually governmental, determines whether the resultant quotient, the QALYS, is within or above the payer's (government's) ability to fund the treatment. Using QALYS is likely to deny treatment to older, in contrast to, younger patients, especially if a treatment is relatively expensive. See the term **Struldbrug** (stroold'broog) in this connection. See **therapy**. See **end-of-life, death**.

quaddle (kwad'dəl) vi. to grumble; mutter, complain. [E dialect]. n. **quaddle, quaddler.** See **talk**. See **role**.

quadragenarian (kwod"drə-jen-air'ri-ən) n. someone in his/her fourth decade, i.e., forties. [< L *quadragenarius* < *quadraginta* forty]. adj. **quadragenarian** = pertaining to someone in the fourth decade of life. See **role**.

quatrayle (kwot'trayl) n. a great-great-great grandfather. a male ancestor three generations earlier than one's grandfather. [< F *quatre* four < L *quattuor* four + < F *aïeul* grandfather]. Cf. **tresayle**, q.v. See **role**.

querent (kwer'ənt) adj. complaining. [< L *quaerere* ask]. (n. **querent** = 1. someone resorting to astrology. 2. a plaintiff.) See **talk**.

querier (kwee'ree-ər) n. 1. one who requests information, questions. 2. one who doubts or criticizes. [< L *quaere* ask < *quaerere* seek]. n. **query** (plural **-ries**) = 1. a question; a doubt or criticism. 2. a question mark. vt. **query**. Cf. **querist** (kwer'ist), q.v. See **talk**. See **role**.

querimony (kwer'ri-mōn"nee) n. a whiny or peevish complaint. [< L *querimonia* complaint]. adj. **querimonious** (kwer"ri-mōn'ni-əs). adv. **querimoniously** (kwer"ri-mōn'ni-əs-lee). See **talk**.

* **querist** (kwer'ist) n. one who asks questions. [< L *quaerere* ask]. Cf. **querier** (kwee'ree-ər), q.v. See **talk**. See **role**.

querulous (kwer'roŏ-ləs) adj. tending to complain, whine, peevishly find fault. "Be gentle in old age: peevishness is worse in second childhood than in first."—George D. Prentice. [< L *querulus* complaining, full of complaints, querulous; plaintive; warbling; cooing < *queri* to complain]. adv. **querulously**. n. **querulousness**. See **talk**. See **mentality, mentation, behavior**.

quetcher (kwech'er) n. A constant complainer; a bother. [1.? < quet, n., British dialect for guillemot (gil'mō) n. any one of various narrow-bellied arctic diving birds of the auk family + -er, suff., added to nouns meaning a person having to do with < ME -*er*, AS -*ere*—it's likely the **quetcher** makes constant noises, like the bird, that sounds complaining. 2. <?? quetch < OE *cweccan* to shake, stir, move + -er, suff.]. See **role**. See **talk**.

quidnunc (kwid'nunk) n. one who is curious to know everything that is going on; a busybody; a gossip. [< L *Quid nunc?* = What now?]. Cf. **spermologer**, q.v. See **role**.

quiescence (kwee-ess'ənz) n. a state of rest, inactivity, or quietude.
• It's not unusual to find the retirement-home's residents in a state of *quiescence*. [< L *quiescere* to become quiet, come to rest < *quies*, quiet]. adj. **quiescent**. See **mentality, mentation, behavior**.

quietist (kwī'ə-tist) n. 1. one who takes a passive attitude toward life, with devotional contemplation and abandonment of the will, as a form of religious mysticism. 2. one who believes in the principle of nonresistance. [< It *quietismo* < L *quietus* pp. of *quiescere* < *quies* quiet]. adj. **quietistic**. n. **quietism**. See **role**. See **religion, theology, morality**.

quietus (kwī-ee'təs) n., pl.n. **quietuses**, 1. final release from life; death, especially when viewed as a release from life. 2. something that brings an activity to an end. (3. a release given on payment of a debt or duty; a receipt for payment of a debt.) [< L *quietus est*. It is at rest. (This acknowledges receipt, or discharge of an obligation.)]. See **end-of-life, death**.

quinquagenarian (kwin"kwə-jen-nair'ri-ən) n. someone in his/her fifth decade, i.e., fifties. [< L *quinquagenarius* < *quinquaginta* fifty]. adj. **quinquagenarian** = pertaining to someone 50 to 60 years of age. See **role**.

quinquennium (kwin-kwen'ni-əm), pl. -ni-ums (əms), or -ni-a (-aa or ə) n. a period of fifty years. [< L *quinque* five + *annus* year]. adj. **quinquennial**. adv. **quinquennially**. See **ole age**.

quizzacious (kwiz-zay'shəss) adj. bantering. adv. **quizzaciously**. n. **quizzaciousness**. [< quiz, to question, interrogate < late 18th C. <?]. See **talk**.

quixotic (kwiks-ot'tik) adj. romantic by nature, idealistic, impulsive, and in pursuit of lofty, but impractical, goals. [Late 18th C. < Don Quixote, hero of a novel by Miguel de Cervantes, "*El ingenioso hidalgo don Quijote de la Mancha*" (The Ingenious Hidalgo Don Quixote of La Mancha), published in two volumes a decade apart: 1605 & 1615]. See **mentality, mentation, behavior**.

quodlibet (kwod'li-bet) n. 1. a subtle or scholastic argument. 2. a theological or philosophical issue for discussion. (3. A musical medley: a whimsical combination of popular tunes. 4. {formerly} a mock exercise in discussion.) • Seniors not infrequently engaged in *quodlibets* at their club's dining table. [L, *quod* what + *libet* it pleases]. See **talk**.

quodlibitarian (kwod"-li-bi-tar'ri-ən) n. one who raises or proposes a subtle, moot point, especially a scholastic or theological one, for argument. [< L *quodlibetum* < *quodlibet* whatever pleases]. n. **quodlibet**, q.v. See **role**. See **talk**.

quondam (kwon'dam) adj. that once had but no longer has the specified character, role, or relationship; having been earlier; onetime; sometime; former. • The *quondam* rake refused to believe his age now staring back at him in the mirror. [L, (adv.) once, at one time, formerly; at times, sometimes, once in a while; someday, one day (in the future)]. syn. **whilom**, **erstwhile**, q.v. See **past, time**.

quonking (kwon'king) n. side-line chatter that disturbs a speaker, performer. • *Quonking* from seniors, who are frequently hard of hearing and thus inattentive, disturbs speakers trying to entertain them. [slang, possibly onomatopoeic < duck-like chatter] See **talk**.

R

"Be gentle in old age: peevishness is worse
in second childhood than in first."
—George D. Prentice.

raconteur (rakɔ̄tœr), **-euse** (øz) n. someone (m. = -eur, f. = -use) who is noted for telling stories or anecdotes. [early 19ᵗʰ C. < F < OF *raconter* to recount, tell]. See **role**.

raddled (rad'dləd) adj. old and silly; aged, worn out appearance, and worsened by debauchery. [< E late 17ᵗʰ C. reddle, or raddle, or ruddle: red ocher, or coarse rouge—used to mark sheep—referring to the elderly roué's red cheeks.? < mid-16ᵗʰ C. E obs. *rud* redness]. See **old**. See **religion, theology, morality**.

raillery (rayl'lə-ree) n. (pl.n. **–ies**) 1. humorous, playful, or friendly ridiculing of somebody or something. 2. a remark that ridicules somebody or something jokingly and with good humor. [via F *railler* mock, tease < Old Provençal *ralhar* chat, joke < L *ragere* neigh, roar]. Cf. **persiflage, badinage**, q.v. See **talk**.

rake (rayk) n. one who indulges unrestrainedly in pleasantries and vices such as drinking, gambling, and womanizing; one who is debauched or immoral. • The old *rake* has difficulty admitting to old age. [< mid 17ᵗʰ C. shortening of E arch. *rakehell*, by folk etymology < *rakel* hasty, rash]. adj. **rakish** (ray'kish) = 1. stylish in a dashing or sporty way. 2. immoral or debauched. (3. having a streamlined look that suggests rapid movement through the water.) See **old man**. See **role**.

rale (raal) n. an adventitious and abnormal respiratory sound heard in auscultating the chest, a small rhonchus—usually used in the pl., rales are characterized as dry or wet, and by site of lung origin, i.e., right-basilar, left-apical, etc. They are found not infrequently in the elderly due to atelectasis (lack of expansion of alveoli {air sacks}) because of weak, superficial, feeble breathing, and disappear with forceful deep breathing. Rales can indicate lung pathology (disease). [F, rattle]. See **breathing**.

re-, pref., 1. again, anew. 2. back, backward. [< L *re-*, *red-* again, back, un-].

reable (ree-ay'bəl) vt. a British term meaning to restore to one's former condition or capacity. • Her fondest wish at eighty was to *reable* her twenty-year-old self. [< re-, pref., q.v., + < F (*h*)*able* < L *habilis* easy to hold or handle < *habere* to have, hold]. See **health, illness**.

recalcitrant (re-kal'si-trənt) adj. stubbornly resisting the authority or control of another; difficult to deal with. ●A few *recalcitrant* residents refused to vacate the nursing home in spite of the hurricane warning. [< L *recalcitrant*, pres.p. of *recalcitrare* kick back (used of horses) < *calcitrare* kick (with the heels) < *calc* heel]. n. **recalcitrant** = someone who stubbornly resists authority or control. n. **recalcitrance**. adv. **recalcitrantly**. See <u>mentality, mentation, behavior</u>.

recriminate (ri-krim'mə-nayt") vi. to accuse somebody who has already brought an accusation; indulge in countercharges. [< L *recriminat-* pp. of *recriminari* to accuse back, or again < *criminari*, *criminare* to accuse]. n. **recrimination** (-krim"mi-nay'shən). n. **recriminator**. adj. **recriminative**. adj. **recriminatory** (-krim'mən-ə-tawr"ree). See <u>talk</u>. See <u>role</u>.

recrudescence (ree-kroo-des'sənss) n. a breaking out or becoming active again of a disease, sore, or (fig.) of hostile feelings, discontent. [< L *recrudescere* become raw again < *crudus* raw, bloody]. vi. **recrudesce**. adj. **recrudescent**. n. **recrudescency**. See <u>health, illness</u>. See <u>mentation, mentality, behavior</u>.

rectopathic (rek-tō-path'ik) adj. easily hurt emotionally. ● The young fail to recognize the often *rectopathic* state of the elderly. [< L *rectus* direct, straight < *regere* to keep in a straight line or proper course + -*pathy*, suff., disease < G *pathos* suffering, disease]. n. **rectopathy** (-top'pə-thee). adv. **rectopathicly** (-path'ik-). See <u>emotion</u>.

recubation (rek-yoo-bay'shən) n. 1. lying down. (2. reclining while dining in ancient Greece, Rome—perhaps while talking to a **deipnosophist**, q.v.) [< L *recubare* to lie on one's back, lie down, rest]. See <u>tiredness, weakness</u>. See <u>work, activity</u>.

recusant (rek'kyoo-zant) adj. refusing to submit to authority, dissenting. [< L *recusant-*, stem of *recusans*, pres.p. of *recusare* to refuse or object]. n. **recusant** = 1. one who refuses to obey authority. (2. one of the Roman Catholics during the 16th C. who refused to attend services of the Church of England and was punished for it.) See <u>mentality, mentation, behavior</u>. See <u>role</u>.

reddition (red-dish'ən) n. 1. (arch.) a restoration to a previous condition. 2. ({obs.} a term for a comparative explanation.) ● **Juvenescent**, q.v., *reddition* is a forlorn hope of many elders. [<

L *redditionem*, n. of action < *reddere* to give back, to render]. See **health, illness**.

redintegrate (re-din'te-grayt, ree-din-) vt. (obs.) to restore to wholeness or unity; to fix or reassemble; renew or reestablish in united or perfect state. • If only his pre-Alzheimer's state could be *redintegrated*, we would be so pleased. [re-, red-, pref., q.v., + < L *integrare* make whole] n. **redintegration**. syn. **reintegrate**. See **health, illness**.

redivivous (red-i-vī'ves)—note: not re-div'i-ves—adj. (obs.) living again, revived, resuscitated, regenerated; reappearing. [< L *redivivus* (adj.) living again; {second-hand (building materials)} + -ous, suff.]. Cf. **redux**. See **health, illness**.

redux (reed'duks) adj. denoting renewed health after sickness. [< L *redux* guiding back, rescuing; brought back, restored]. Cf. **redivivous**, q.v. See **health, illness**.

refocillation (ree-foss"si-lay'shen) n. revival, revitalization; refreshment. [< L *refocillare* to rewarm, to revive < *focillare* to warm, to revive]. vt. **refocillate**. Cf. **redivivous**. See **health, illness**.

refractory (ree-frak'tawr-ee) adj. 1. stubborn, unmanageable, rebellious. 2. not yielding to treatment (of wound, disease). (3. hard to use, work.) 4. unresponsive to stimulus. (5. resistant to heat.) [< a variant of refractory < L *refractarius* stubborn < *refractus*, pp. of *refringere* break off, break back < *frangere* to break]. adv. **refractorily**. n. **refractoriness**. (pl.n. **refractories** = bricks used to line kilns.) See **mentality, mentation, behavior**. See **health, illness**.

regimen (rej'e-men, -i-mem) n. 1. a prescribed or recommended course or program of exercise, diet, etc., way of life intended to improve health, fitness, or stabilize a medical condition. (2. {archaic} a government; a regime.) (3. rule. 4.{gram.} relation of syntactic dependence between words, government.) • A dietary and exercise *regimen* becomes increasingly imperative in advanced years. [L, rule, government < *regere* to rule + -men, suff.]. See **health, illness**.

relic (rel'ik) n. 1. something surviving from a long time ago, often a part of something old that has remained when the rest of it has decayed or been destroyed (used fig., also, e.g., an old person). 2. a tradition, custom, rule that dates from some past time, especially one considered out of date, now inappropriate. 3. something that is kept for its interesting associations, e.g., with somebody famous, or with a historic event. (4. something that is kept and venerated because it once belonged to a saint, martyr, or religious leader, especially a part of his or her body. n.pl. **relics** {archaic} the corpse of a deceased person.) • Age rendered him a *relic* of his former self. [< L *reliquiae* remains (particularly of a dead saint), pl. of *reliquus* remaining]. See **end of life, death**. See **old age**. See **old man**. See **old woman**.

relics (rel'iks) n.pl. (archaic) the corpse of a deceased person. [< L *reliquiae* remains (particularly of a dead saint) pl. of *reliquus* remaining]. See **end-of-life, death**.

relict (rel'likt) n. (1. remnant of a preexisting land or rock formation left behind after a destructive event has taken place. 2. a mineral that did not change when the host rock metamorphosed. 3. a species of organism surviving long after the extinction of related species, or a once widespread natural population surviving in only isolated localities because of environmental changes.) 4. (archaic) a surviving person, especially a widow. [< ME *relike* < OF *relique* < *reliquiae* remains < L *relictus* remaining, left behind < *relinquere* to relinquish, not take along, to permit to remain, let remain, to leave alive, to abandon]. adj. 1. surviving in its original form when related organisms have become extinct, or its environment has changed completely. 2. (archaic) pertaining to a surviving person, especially a widow, i.e., widowed. syn. **relic** (1.), q.v. See **old man**, See **old woman**. See **old**. See **old age**. See **role**. See **end of life, death**.

religion, theology, morality: axiology, deisidaimonia, empyrean, enosimania, enosiphobia, entheal, entelechy, entheomania, epiolatry, eschatology, eschaton, eumoirous, exaugurate, fideism, hamartomania, hamartophobia, hemartia, heresiarch, heresyphobia, hieromania, hierophobia, irreverent, labefaction, labent, lector, metanoia, peccatiphobia, peccavi, perdition, quietism, raddled, reprobate, salvific, sanctiloquent, satanophobia, sententious, soterial, soteriology, sough, stygiophobia, supernal, theophobia, viaticum.

religion, theology, mortality: Subcategories

I. Divine inspiration:
    1. Belief one is divinely inspired: **entheomania**
    2. Divinely inspired (adj.): **entheal**
    3. Spiritual transformation: **metanoia**
    4. Vital force directing realization of full potential: **entelechy**

II. Faith:
    1. Belief in faith rather than reason: **fideism**
    2. Profound spiritual transformation, conversion: **metanoia**

III. God:
    1. Morbid fear of God, gods, wrath of God: **theophobia**
    2. Morbid fear of supernatural powers: **deisidaimonia**

IV. Heaven:
    1. Heavenly: **supernal**
    2. Sky, celestial sphere, heavens: **empyrean**

V. Hell, Satan:
    1 Morbid fear of hell: **stygiophobia**
    2. Morbid fear of the devil: **satanophobia**
    3. Punishment in hell for mortal sin; sin itself: **perdition**

VI. Heresy:
    1. Morbid fear of heresy: **heresyphobia**

VII. Last things, salvation:
    1. Communion given to someone dying: **viaticum**
    1. End of the world, time, last things: **eschaton**
    2. Pertaining to salvation: **soterial**
    3. Salvation through Jesus: **soteriology**
    4. Soul saving: **salvific**
    5. Study of last things: **eschatology**

VIII. Morality, moral, moralizing:
    1. Freely using aphorisms; moralizing; speaking tersely: **sententious**.
    2. Lucky or happy as a result of being good: **eumoirous**.
    3. Study of values & value judgment: **axiology**

IX. Religion, church:
    1. Biblical reader: **lector**
    2. Leader or founder of an heretical religious sect: **heresiarch**
    3. Morbid fear of religious or sacred objects: **hierophobia**

4. Religious belief in abandonment of will, devotional contemplation: **quietism**
5. Religious chant: **sough**
6. Religious insanity: **hieromania**
7. Speaking solemnly or of sacred things: **sanctiloquent**

X. Sin, sinning, immorality, irreverence, character defect:
1. Abnormal interest in sin: **hamartomania**.
2. admission of guilt or sin: **peccavi**
3. Aged, silly, and worsened by debauchery: **raddled**
4. Belief one has committed an unpardonable sin: **enosimania**
5. Disreputable, immoral (adj.): **reprobate**
6. Lacking reverence, respect: **irreverent**
7. Morbid fear of error, sin, sinning: **hamartophobia**, **peccatiphobia**
8. Morbid fear of having committed an unpardonable sin: **enosiphobia**
9. Punishment in hell for mortal sin; sin itself: **perdition**
10. Secularize, desecrate (vt.): **exaugurate**
12. Single character defect, classic tragic flaw; a mistake: **hemartia**
13. Slipping, falling (in sin) (adj.): **labent**
14. Weakening, undermining, especially of moral principles: **labefaction**

XI. 1. Worship of words: **epiolatry**

Rember® (rem'ber) n. The brand name of methyothioninium chloride, MTC, a drug of TauRx Therapeutics. It is said to be helpful in treating patients with mild and moderate **Alzheimer's disease**, q.v. Rember is aimed at counteracting an abnormal version of a protein, tau, that's linked to Alzheimer's. Normal tau supplies nutrients to brain nerve cells, while the abnormal tau of Alzheimer's creates tangles of aggregated protein that shut off nutrients. Cf. **Aricept/donepezil hydrochloride(HCI)**, **Exelon®Patch**. See <u>intelligence</u>. See <u>therapy</u>.

rememble (ri-mem'bel, ree-) n. a false memory, especially of some place. v.i.&vt. to remember incorrectly. [a portmanteau word: a blend of fumble & remember; coined by Elam Cole on the radio show "The Next Big Thing"]. See <u>memory</u>.

renidification (ree-nid"di-fi-kay'shən) n. the building of another nest. The word can be used fig. • Her daughter's offer to come live with her in California fulfilled the dowager's quest for *renidification*. [re-, pref., q.v., + < L *nidus* nest]. See **work, activity**.

renitent (ren'ni-tənt, ri-nī'tənt) adj. 1. resisting physical pressure rather than being flexible or pliant. 2. reluctant to have a change of mind or to concede to others; resisting or opposing stubbornly; recalcitrant. [< L *renitent-*, pres.p. of *reniti* to struggle against]. n. **renitence** = inflexibility. n. **renitency** = the ability to withstand constraint or pressure. See **mentality, mentation, behavior**.

rente (rãt) n. 1. annual income; annuity. (2. securities representing the French national debt; the interest paid on it.) [F. 1. nf. revenue, income; *vivre de ses rentes* (= to have a private income. 2. pension, annuity; *rente viagère* (rãt vjaʒɛr) = life annuity. 3. government bond]. n. **rentier** (rã tje) = one who receives or lives off of rents, an annuity, rather than working: a person of independent means. See **finance**. See **role**.

repine (ree-pīn') vi.&vt. to complain, fret, grumble, lament, express discontent (at, against, or abs.). [re-, pref., q.v., + < OE *pinean* to torment < L *poena* penalty, pain < G *poine* to long for, especially for the unobtainable; to become weak, lose vitality as a result of grieving, longing]. n. **repine** = complaint, lament, discontentment. adv. **repiningly**. See **mentality, mentation, behavior**. See **talk**.

reprobate (rep'prōb-bayt") n. 1. a disreputable or immoral person. 2. somebody whose soul is believed to be damned. [< L *reprobatus* < pp. of *reprobare* prove to be unworthy]. adj. **reprobate** = 1. disreputable or immoral. 2. with a soul that is damned. vt. **reprobate** 1. to censure or condemn somebody (formal). 2. to condemn somebody to supposed eternal damnation. n. **reprobater**. adj. **reprobative**. See **role**. See **religion, theology, morality**.

repullulate (ree-pul'-yoo-layt) vi. to sprout again; to recur, e.g., a disease. [< L *pullulare* to sprout]. See **health, illness**.

resipiscent (re-si-pis'sənt) adj. restored to sanity: learned from experience; to come to one's senses; having returned to a saner mind. [< L *resipiscere* to come to one's senses, < *re-* again + *sapere* to taste, to know]. n. **resipiscence** = a modification of belief or emotion that often results in readopting a previously abandoned correct view, position, or interpretation. Cf. **mumpsimus**, q.v. See **health, illness**. See **intelligence**.

resveratrol (res-ver'rə-trol) n. an antioxidant chemical contained in red wine and red grape extracts—it's located in the grape's skin. It activates a gene called SIRT-1, which is normally activated by near starvation. The gene extends life; it's a **gerontogene**, q.v. When resveratrol is fed to rats it counteracts their being overfed an American unhealthy diet and lets them live perhaps 12%-20% longer. Any certain resveratrol benefits to humans is conjectural, although it is being marketed not only for its longevity potential, but for warding off diabetes and heart disease. See **therapy**.

retardataire (rətardatɛr) adj. behind the times, or characteristic of an earlier period—used mainly about artistic styles. [F, nm.&f. meaning one who is late in arriving, a late-comer; loiterer, laggard]. n. *retardataire* = one who is behind the times. See **past, time**. See **role**.

retinitis (ret"tin-nī'tiss) n. inflammation of the retina. (In earlier ophthalmology the term was used much more generally.) [< L *rete* net (of retinal blood vessels) + < G –*itis*, a suff. denoting inflammation]. See **eye**.

retinol (ret'tin-ol) n. a vitamin A derivative that activates the gene that produces collagen, which forms the scaffolding that prevents wrinkles from forming. Sunlight breaks down retinol into an inactive molecule. Retinol cream, applied at night, when skin-cell processes are most active, and sun-screen lotion, applied during the day, are used to prevent wrinkles. [< G *rhetine* resin + -ol, suff., containing a hydroxyl, especially an alcohol or phenol]. See **skin**. See **therapy**.

retinopathy (ret"tin-op'pə-thee) n. 1. **retinitis**, q.v. 2. **retinosis**, q.v. [< L *rete* net (of blood vessels) + -pathy, suff., a morbid condition or disease, < G –*patheia*, a suff., < *pathos* disease]. See **eye**.

retinosis (ret"ti-nōs'siss) n. a general term for degenerative, non-inflammatory conditions of the retina. [< L *rete* net (of blood vessels) + -osis, suff., denoting a process, especially a disease or morbid process < G -*osis* < -*sis*, a suffix of action, process or condition]. See **eye**.

retirement: agathobiothik, aging in place, CCRC, ecesis, emeritus, *Opagefaengris*, pensioner, rusticate, rustication, snowbird, superannuated, ubiation, *villeggiatura*.

Retirement: Subcategories:

I. A northern retiree who migrates south for the winter: **snowbird**
II. A prison for retired male criminals in Singen, Germany: *Opagefaengris*
III. A retired, usually older, person receiving a stipend: **pensioner**
IV. A rural extended holiday, stay, or retirement: *villeggiatura*, **rustication**
V. Acclimatization to retirement: **ecesis**
VI. Remaining at home rather than living in a retirement home, etc. **aging in place**
VII. Retired and pensioned because of sickness or old age: **superannuated**
VIII. Retired from active service, usually due to age: **emeritus** (m.), **-ta** (f.)
IX. Retirement community with varied levels of care: **CCRC**
X. The act of occupying a new place: **ubiation**, **rusticate**
XI. The good life: **agathobiothik**

retrospective (ret"-trō-spek'tiv) n. a representative exhibition of the lifetime work of an artist or of a particular period of art. adj. 1. looking back over things in the past. 2. containing examples of work from many periods of an artist's life—a private showing or preview = a **vernissage**. 3. applying to things that have happened in the past as well as the present. [retro-, pref., back, backward; behind < L back, backwards, to the rear; past, + < *spectare* to watch < *specere* look at]. adv. **retrospectively**. See **past, time**.

revalescent (rev-əl-es'sənt) adj. recovering from illness or injury. [< L *revalescere* to regain one's strength, recover; to become valid again]. syn. **convalescent**. See **health, illness**.

revenant (rev'ven-ənt {F = rer-vər-nəN'}) n. 1. someone returning after a long absence. 2. a person whose character embodies qualities and traits appropriate to an earlier era. 3. somebody returning from the dead; a ghost. [F, < the pres.p. of *revenir* to return]. adj. **revenant** = remembering something long forgotten. See **memory**. See **role**.

rhagades (rag'gə-dees—not raa-gaads') n.pl. fissures, cracks, wrinkles, or fine linear scars in the skin, especially such lesions around the mouth or other regions subjected to frequent movement. [pl. of G *rhagas* rent {in the sense of a fissure, tear, hole}]. adj. **rhagadiform** (ra-gad'di-form) = resembling rhagades, wrinkles. See **skin**.

rhetor (reet'tor) n. 1. a mere talker. (2. a teacher of rhetoric. 3. an orator.) [< L *rhetor* rhetorician, teacher of rhetoric; orator]. See **role**. See **talk**.

rheum (room) n. a watery discharge coming from the eyes, nose, or mouth. [< G *rheuma* flow, bodily humor]. adj. **rheumy** (-mee). Cf. **gleet**. See **eyes**. See **nose, smell**. See **mouth, gums, teeth**.

rheumatic (roo-mat'tik) adj. affected with **rheumatism**, q.v. [< G *rheumatiko*s subject to flux < *rheuma* flux]. See **joint, extremities, back**.

rheumatism (room'mə-tiz-əm) n. any of a variety of disorders marked by inflammation, degeneration, or metabolic derangement of the connective-tissue structures of the body, especially of the joints and related structures, including muscles, bursae, tendons, and fibrous tissue. It is attended by pain, stiffness, or limitation of motion of the parts. Rheumatism confined to the joints is classified as arthritis. [< L *rheumatismus* < G *rheumatismos* < *rheuma* flux]. See **joint, extremities, back**.

rhinopathy (rī-nop'pa-thee) n. disease of the nose. (Nasal obstruction can be age-related: It's due to drooping of the nose tip with aging resulting in nasal elongation and narrowing.) [rhin(o)-, pref., relating to the nose < G *rhis*, gen. *rhinos* nose + *pathos* suffering]. See **nose, smell**.

rhinophyma (rhī-nō-fīm'mə) n. a severe form of **rosacea**, q.v., resulting in permanent thickening of the connective tissues and bulbous hypertrophy of the sebaceous glands of the nose, with resulting nasal enlargement and dilation; also called **hypertrophic rosacea**, copper nose, rum nose, brandy nose, hammer nose, toper's nose, rum-blossom (!). It can spread to the cheeks, and is usually seen in older men. [rhin(o)-, pref., relating to the nose, < G *rhis*, gen. *rhinos* nose + *phyma* tumor, growth]. See **nose, smell**.

rhinorrhea (rhī-nō-ree'ə) n. the free discharge of a thin nasal mucus. [rhino-, pref., denoting relationship to the nose or a nose-like structure < G *rhis*, gen. *rhinos* nose]. Cf. **rheum**, q.v. See **nose, smell**.

rhodomontade (rod"ə-mon-təyd') n., adj., & v., but almost always used as a n. extravagant boasting, vainglorious bragging, blustery self-glorification. [< *Rodomonte*, the vainglorious, bragging king of Algiers featured in the romantic epics *Orlando Innamorato* by Mattero Maria Boiardo (1431-1494) & its sequel *Orlando Furioso* by Ludovico Ariosto (1474-1553), both It, and based on Roland, the medieval legendary French hero celebrated in the 11th C. *Chanson de Roland*—Orlando is the It equivalent of Roland & rodomontade is the equivalent of Rhodomonte. Antonio Vivaldi created an opera, Orlando furioso—the f is not usually capitalized in It]. n. **rhodomontader**. syns. **braggadocio, fanfaronade, gasconade, & thrasonical**, q.v. See **talk**. See **role**.

rhonchisonant (rong'ki-sō"nənt) adj. snoring, snorting. [< L *rhonchus* snoring < G *rhegkhos* a snoring sound + E sonant, adj. & n. (sound, letter), accompanied by vocal vibration, voiced, not surd (e.g., b, d, g, j, v, z) < L *sonare* sound]. n. **rhonchisonance**. adv. **rhonchisonantly**. See **nose, smell**. See **breathing**.

rhonchus (rong'kuss, -kəss), pl **ronchi** (-kī) n. a rattling in the throat or a rattling sound like snoring, or a dry coarse **rale**, q.v., in the bronchial tubes heard on chest stethoscopy when the lung's air channels are partly obstructed. [L, *rhonchus* snoring < G *rhegkhos* a snoring sound < *rhegkein* snore]. See **breathing**.

rhytidectomy (rī-ti-dek'tə-mee) n. the surgical removal of wrinkles— **rhagades**, q.v.—especially from the face; face-lift. [G *rhytis* (*rhytid-*, pref.) a wrinkle + *ectome* excision]. syn. **rhytidoplasty**, q.v. See **skin**. See **therapy**.

rhytidoplasty (ri-tid"-dō-plas'tee) n. (plastic) surgery for elimination of wrinkles. [< G *rhytis* a wrinkle + *plasso* to fashion]. syn. **rhytidectomy**, q.v. See **skin**. See **therapy**.

rhytidosis (ri-ti-dōs'siss) n. 1. wrinkling of the face to a degree disproportionate to age. 2. laxity and wrinkling of the cornea, an indication of approaching death. [G *rhytis* (*rhytid-*) wrinkle + -*osis*, suff., a process, state or condition, usually diseased {alt., a parasitic invasion}]. syn. = **rutidosis**. See **skin**. See **end-of-life, death**.

rhytiphobia (rit"ti-fōb'bi-ə) n. a morbid fear of getting wrinkles. [< G *rhytis* a wrinkle + G *phobos* fear]. adj. **rhytiphobic**. n. **rhytiphobe**. See **skin**. See **phobias**.

rhytiscopia (rit"ti-skop'pi-ə) n. neurotic preoccupation with facial wrinkles. [< G *rhytis* a wrinkle + -scope, suff., observe; (an instrument for observing) < *skopion* < *scopein* to look, see + -ia, suff., connoting diseases or medical conditions < L < G]. See **mentality, mentation, behavior**. See **skin**.

rigescent (ri-jes'sənt) adj. growing rigid, rather stiff, or numb. • His osteoarthritis rendered him temporarily *rigescent* upon standing. [< L *rigescere* < *rigere* be stiff + -escent, suff., denoting the beginning of an actionv ccv < L pres. p. of inceptive verbs]. n. **rigescence**. See **physique, appearance**.

rimose (rīm'mōs, rīm-mōs')/**rimous** (rīm'məs) adj. full of fissures, chinks, or crevices. adv. **rimosely**. n. **rimosity** (rī-mōs'i-ti). • A complexion so *rimose* was not unexpected, especially in a formerly blonde **centenarian**, q.v. [< L *rimosus* < *rima* fissure, chink < I-E a scratch]. See **skin**.

rimple (rim'pəl) n. a wrinkle or crease. [< ME *rimpyl*]. vt.&i. **rimple**. syn. rumple. See **skin**.

rixatrix (riks-ay'triks) n. a scolding, nagging, shrill, shrewish, nasty old woman; a shrew or termagant. [< L *rixa* brawl, fight; quarrel, squabble < *rixor, rixari* to brawl, come to blows, fight; quarrel, squabble + -trix, suff., forming f.-agent nouns—corresponding to masculine nouns in -tor—< L *–trix –tricis* found chiefly in legal terms: *executrix, administratrix*]. syn. **termagant**, etc., q.v. See **old woman**.

roborant (rob'bō-rant) n. & adj. a refreshing, invigorating, stimulating medicine, drug, tonic, or physical agent; conferring strength, strengthening. [< L *roborans* strengthening, pres. p. of *roborare* to strengthen, invigorate]. See **therapy**.

robotic surgery (rō-bot'tik) n.phr. automated surgical therapy performed endoscopically with computer-programmed and controlled mechanical devices rather than by a relatively large incision and conventional direct inspection and manually held and directed instruments in the field. • The **graybeard**, q.v., was delighted with the only two-day hospital stay associated with his *robotically* done prostatectomy. [early 20ᵗʰ C. via Ger. < Czech *robota* forced labor; coined by Karel Čapek in his play R. U. R. (Rossum's Universal Robots) of 1820]. n. **robot** (rō'bot", rō'bət). adv. **robotically** (rō-bot'tik-). n. **robotism** (rō'bə-tiz'əm). adj. **robotistic** (rō-bə-tis'tik). adj. **robotlike** (rō'bət-līk) n. **robotry** (rō'bə-tree) n. **robotics** (rō-bot'tikss). vt. **robotize** (ro'bə-tīz). n. **robotization** (rōb"bə-ti-zay'shən). See **telepresence robots**. See <u>therapy</u>.

robots (rō'bots). See **telepresence robots**.

<u>role</u>: (Note: roles indicated by **old man**, **old woman**, **old person(s)**, q.v. supra, are usually listed under those terms rather than the following <u>role</u> category. Roles indicated by the suffix –**maniac** or –**phobe** are usually listed under the <u>manias</u> and <u>phobias</u> categories, q.v., respectively, rather than under the following <u>role</u> category.)

a dog in the manger, abderite, adjunct, agelast, agonist, alcoholomaniac, alector, *alieni juris*, **androgogue, antiquarian, antiquary, archaist, archaizer, artifact, atrabilarian, attercop, aurist, battologist,** *bien pensant*, **biogerontologist, blateroon, blatherer, blatherskite/blatherskate, bluenose, braggadocio, Briarius, burbler, burdalone, cachinnator, cacosomniac, Calypso, cataractist, cecutlent, centenarian, chiropodist, churl, claudicant, compotator, confabulator, conservative, coparcener, curmudgeon, cyclothyme,** *débrouillard*, **deipnosophist, desiccator, dewdropper, diabetic, dimbox, dipsomaniac, discalceate, dotard, dott(e)rel, dowager, doyen,** *doyen/doyenne*, **dragon, dromomaniac, dysphemist, dysuriac, emerita/ -ae, emeritus/-tii, epicene, epigone, ergophile, eristic, eschatologist, eulogizer, eupatrid, expatiator, fabulist, fainéant, famulus,** *fanfaron*, **fideist, franion, frugalista, gascon, gawkocracy, geriatric care manager, geriatric case manager, geriatrician, gerodontist, gerodontologist, gerontologist, gerontophile/gerontophilist, gerontotherapist, glusker, grouse/grouser, gudgeon, hakam, harpy, hemeralope, heresiarch, hesternopathic/-pothic, heteroclite, hunker, hyperope, idiopt, importuner, imprecator, inhumer, insomniac, intestate, intransigent, invaletudinarian, inveigher, irenicist,**

itinerant, Jeremiah, kvetch, languisher, *lécheur*, leptosome, lethologiac, lewdster, lipsanographer, logodaedalist, logorati, Luddite, macrobiote, magpie, mammothrept, mataeologian, mataeologue, matriarch, maunderer, mensch, methomaniac, micrographer, microlipet, misologist, misoneist, mnemonist, mnemotechnist, moirologist, monadnock, mulligrubs, musard, myope, nashgab, nazzard, necrologist, necromorph, nephalist, nihilarian, noctivagant, noctivagator, nonagenarian, noodge, nostologist, nostomaniac, nostalgic, obganiator, obituarist, objurgator, obtruder, octogenarian, oenomaniac, oikofuge, *old* birkie, oppugner, opsigamist, opsimath, orthotist, osophagist, otiant, otiatrus, otologist, otorhinolaryngologist, paleographer, palterer, paralogist, paramnesiac, pathocryptic, pathoneurotic, patriarch, Pecksniff, pedomorph (paedomorph), pensioner, peritoneoscopist, pettifogger, pharisee, philalethe, philobat, philodox, philopolemist, philosophaster, (all)-phobes, phrontistes, prosthetist, pickmote, platitudinarian, podiatrist, polyhistor, polyhistorian, polymath, poriomaniac, pornogenarian, posiomaniac, prater, prattler, precant, presbyatrician, presbyope, preterist, progenitor, prosopagnosiac, prosthetist, prosthodontist, Prufrock, pseudomnesiac, quaddler, quadragenarian, quatrayle, querier, querist, Quetcher, quidnunc, quietist, quinquagenarian, quodlibitarian, *raconteur/-tuse*, rake, recriminator, recusant, relic, relict, *rentier*, reprobate, *retardataire*, revenant, rhetor, rhodomontader, roué, rudas, rudesby, ruminator, rusticator, satyr, scatologist, seer, seneucia, septuagenarian, sermocinator, sexagenarian, siffilator, silentiary, Silenus, skinflint, slubber-degullion, smellfungus, somnipathist, splenetic, squintifego, stormy petrel, succorer, *sui juris*, sundowner, supercentenarian, surbater, *sussurator*, swelp, taphophile, tautologist, tergiversator, testator, testatrix, testudinarian, tetnit, thanatologist, toper, totterer, *traditionaliste*, traducer, tresayle, troglodyte, tropophobe, tutelary, twaddler, ubiquarian, umbratile, usufructuary, valetudinarian/valetudinary, vaticinator, verbigerator, *veuf*, *veuvage*, *veuve*, *vidua*, viduation, *viduité*, viduity, *viduus*, vituperator, voider, wallflower, wastrel, wellderly, wheezer, whinger, wowser, xanthodont, xeniatrophobe.

<u>role</u>: Subcategories

One (those) who (whose); or one who is, or who is a or an; one with:

I. Anger, complaint, criticism, fault-finding:
    1. Attacks in harshly abusive or critical language: **vituperator**
    2. Chides or scolds angrily: **objurgator**
    3. Constant complainer: **Jeremiah, kvetch, noodge, Quetcher**
    4. Counter accuses: **recriminator**
    5. Criticizes heavily, disparages someone: **traducer**
    6. Finds fault; is malcontent: **pickmote; smellfungus**
    7. Grumbles, complains, mutters; finds fault: **grouse/ grouser, quaddler whinger; smellfungus**
    8. Hates anything new: **misoneist**
    9. Invokes, calls down harm; curses: **imprecator**
    10. Mean-spirited, crotchety, cantankerous: **curmudgeon**
    11. Perennial complainer: **swelp**
    12. Protests or criticizes angrily; attacks violently or bitterly: **inveigher**
    13. Tries to prevent others from having or doing something that he or she can't have or do: **a dog in the manger**
    14. Uses unpleasant, offensive language, derogates: **dysphemist**
II. Age & antiquity:
    1. Concerned with very ancient things: **archaist, archaizer**
    2. Age by decade:
        a. In one's fourth decade: **quadragenarian**
        b. In one's fifth decade: **quinquagenarian**
        c. In one's sixth decade: **sexagenarian**
        d. In one's seventh decade: **septuagenarian**
        e. In one's eighth decade: **octogenarian**
        f. In one's ninth decade: **nonagenarian**
        g. In one's 100th year: **centenarian**
        h. Long-lived person: **macrobiote**
        i. Of a later generation: **epigone**
        j. Older than 100 years: **supercentenarian** (collectively = the **wellderly**)
III. Appearance:
    1. Barefooted: **discalceate**
    2. Dirty fellow who slobbers his clothing: **slubber-degullion**
    3. Fierce and formidable woman: **dragon**

4. Surviving trace of a person: **relic**
5. Thin, skinny person: **leptosome**
6. Yellow teeth: **xanthodont**

IV. Avocation, occupation, activity, engagement, inactivity, disengagement:
   1. Buries the dead: **inhumer**
   2. Composer of fables: **fabulist**
   3. Compulsive collector (fig., inf.): **magpie**
   4. Dealer in, or collector, scholar of antiques or antiquities: **antiquarian**, **antiquary**
   5. Diagnoses and treats the aged: **geriatrician**, **gerontologist**, **gerontotherapist**, **presbyatrician**
   6. Dormant, idle, unemployed: **otiant**
   7. Dries out, removes moisture from: **desiccator**
   8. Drunken, rollicking old man: **Silenus**
   9. Ear, nose, and throat specialist; ear specialist: **otorhinolaryngologist**; **aurist**, **otiatrus**, **otologist**
   10. Enforces peace and quiet: **silentiary**
   11. Engaged in a struggle: **agonist**
   12. Examines the abdominal contents with an inserted instrument: **peritoneoscopist**
   13. Fanatically opposed to technological innovation: **Luddite**
   14. Fellow drinker: **compotator**
   15. Female head of a family: **matriarch**
   16. Foot doctor: **chiropodist**, **podiatrist**
   17. Helps others: **succorer**
   18. Idler: **fainéant**
   19. Ill-tempered person: **mulligrubs**
   20. Imposes oneself or one's opinions: **obtruder**
   21. Insistent, demanding person: **importuner**
   22. Keeps state secrets: **silentiary**.
   23. Leader or founder of an heretical group: **heresiarch**
   24. Lives off of rents, an annuity, a financial portfolio: *rentier*
   25. Lives in the country: **rusticator**
   26. Looks after the care of the elderly: **geriatric care manager** or **geriatric case manager**
   27. Loves or longs to travel: **dromomaniac**
   28. Loves to work: **ergophile**
   29. Most senior, or respected, or experienced man, or man/woman in a group: **doyen**, *doyen/doyenne*

30. Person who goes everywhere: **ubiquarian**
31. Practitioner of gerodontics = geriatric dentistry: **gerodontist, gerodontologist**
32. Predicts the future, prophesizes, a soothsayer: **seer, vaticinator**
33. Private secretary, attendant, factotum: **famulus**
34. Promotes peace, compromise, a third way (*tertium quid*): **irenicist**
35. Protector, guardian: **tutelary**
36. Rake, debauchee, gambler, trickster: **roué**
37. Rich, or rich-looking, or respected woman of advanced years: **dowager**
38. Scientifically studies or cares for the aged: **nostologist**
39. Sits by a wall, or in solitude: **wallflower**
40. Skilled in memorization and memory retention: **mnemotechnist**
41. Skilled in orthopedic appliances, orthotics: **orthotist**
42. Skilled in restoring teeth: **prosthodontist**
43. Skilled in substituting artificial body parts for those missing: **prosthetist**
44. Sleeps by day and plays at night: **dewdropper**
45. Slow moving as a turtle: **testudinarian**
46. Smoothes things over amicably: **dimbox**
47. Solitary: **burdalone**
48. Spends his/her time indoors: **umbratile**
49. Spendthrift: **wastrel**
50. Studies death: **thanatologist**
51. Those who look at television frequently, or for long periods: **gawkocracy**
52. Tires, makes another footsore with walking: **surbater**
53. Treats cataracts: **cataractist**
54. Trouble maker: **stormy petrel**
55. Urinates: **voider**
56. Wandering from place to place: **itinerant**
57. Wanders by night: **noctivagant, noctivagator**
58. Writes about or studies ancient things: **paleographer**

V. Death:
1. Concerned with end of life, last judgment, heaven, hell: **eschatologist**
2. Feigns death: **necromorph**
3. Lover of funerals: **taphophile**

      4. Mourner: **moirologist**

      5. One who praises someone who has died: **eulogizer**

      6. One who studies death: **thanatologist**

      7. Returning after a long absence; returning from the dead: **revenant**

VI. <u>Family</u>:

      1. Child born of elderly parents: **tetnit**

      2. Child raised by its grandmother: **mammothrept**

      3. Female head of a family: **matriarch**

      4. Great-great grandfather: **tresayle**

      5. Great-great-great grandfather: **quatrayle**

      6. Hereditary (Greek) aristocrat: **eupatrid**

      7. Male family head: **patriarch**

      8. Marries late: **opsigamist**

      9. Spinster: *vidua*

      10. Unmarried man: *viduus*

      11. Widow: **relict**, *veuve*, *vidua*

         a. propertied or titled widow of advanced years: **dowager**

         b. widows: **viduage**

      12. Widower: *veuf*, *viduus*

      13. Widowerhood: *veuvage*

      14. Widowhood: **seneucia**, *veuvage*, **viduation**, *viduité*, **viduity**

VII. <u>Fear</u>: See –phobe under **phobias**.

VIII. <u>Law</u>:

      1. Entitled legally to use another's property: **usufructuary**

      2. Has died absent a legally valid will: **intestate**

      3. Joint heir to an undivided property: **coparcener**

      4. Makes a legally valid will: **testator** (man or woman); **testatrix** (a woman)

      5. One able to manage one's own legal, financial affairs: *sui juris*

      6. One under another's control due to mental incompetence: *alieni juris*

IX. <u>Mania</u>: See -maniac under **manias**.

X. <u>Memory</u>:

      1. Lost memory for, or can't recognize, faces: **prosopagnosiac**

      2. Remembers events that didn't happen: **pseudomnesiac**

3. Skilled in memorizing and not forgetting: **mnemonist**
4. Unable to recall the meaning of some familiar words, etc.: **paramnesiac**
5. Unable to recall words or a specific word: **lethologiac**

XI. Mental, psychological, or psychiatric problems:
1. Absent-minded dreamer or fool: **musard**
2. Dimwitted scoffer: **abderite**
3. Manifests confused, agitated, disruptive behavior in a nursig home at sundown: **sundowner**
4. Neurotically preoccupied with real illness: **pathoneurotic**
5. Silly in old age: **dotard**
6. Wanders aimlessly, acting incoherently: **maunderer**
7. Wanders away from home: **oikofuge**

XII. Morality:
1. Disreputable, immoral: **reprobate**
2. Excessively concerned with morals, morality; is puritanical: **bluenose**; **wowser**
3. Hypocritically self-righteous: **pharisee**

XIII. Old Man, Old People, Person(s), Old Woman: See under those categories.

XIV. Originator:
1. Direct ancestor or originator of something: **progenitor**

XV. Outdated:
1. Extremely out of date: **artifact**
2. Behind the times, old-fashioned; characteristic of another era: **retardataire**, **revenant**
3. Lives in the past: **preterist**
4. Opposes progress: **hunker**
5. Pathologically yearns for the good old days: **hesternopathic/-pothic**

XVI. Personality, trait, quirk, characteristic:
1. A devotee of oral intercourse: **lécheur**
2. A licker: **lécheur**
3. Aggressive, crusty, self-assertive, independent old person: **old birkie**
4. An adult who behaves like a child: **pedomorph**
5. Au fait and au courant: **Briarius**
6. Bad-tempered, malignant, venomous; spiteful person: **attercop**; **splenetic**

7. Bad-tempered old woman: **harpy**
8. Braggart: **braggadocio**, *fanfaron*, **gascon**, **rhodomontader**
9. Deals with things of no importance: **nihilarian**
10. Drinks a large quantity of alcohol: **toper**
11. Eccentric, maverick: **heteroclite**
12. Dupe, credulous person: **gudgeon**
13. Exhibits aggravated nostalgia, homesickness: **nostomaniac**
14. Fastidious eater: **osophagist**
15. Gloomy hypochondriac: **atrabilarian**
16. Good, kind, solid, honorable, decent, generous, human: **mensch**
17. Has bisexual or, a male having feminine, characteristics: **epicene**
18. Has prominent mood swings: **cyclothyme**
19. Hates reason, enlightenment: **misologist**
20. Indulges unrestrainedly in drinking, gambling, etc.: **rake**
21. Laughs loudly, noisily, unpleasantly: **cachinnator**
22. Learns late, is a late bloomer: **opsimath**
23. Loud-mouthed, ill-mannered boor: **rudesby**
24. Loves food critically, a gourmand: *lécheur*
25. Loves funerals: **taphophile**
26. Loves one's own opinions, a dogmatist: **philodox**
27. Loves to argue: **philopolemist**
28. Loves to forget: **philalethe**
29, Loves to travel widely: **philobat**
30. Loves to wander: **poriomaniac**
31. Makes up stories answers without regard to fact: **confabulator**
32. Miser; frugal person: **skinflint**; **frugalista**
33. Mood swings: **cyclothym**
34. Morbidly loves old people: **gerontophile/gerontophilist**
35. Never laughs: **agelast**
36. Never sleeps: **alector**
37. Of low birth, boorish, ill-bred: **churl**
38. Opposes, is contrary, antagonistic: **oppugner**
39. Over concerned with small details; trivia: **pettifogger**, **miccrolipet**

40. Perennial hedonist, reveler; a gay reckless fellow; a paramour: **franion**
41. Pines for something being denied: **languisher**
42. Predatory person: **harpy**
43. Reclusive, a hermit, living in seclusion: **troglodyte**
44. Recollects sentimentally; is homesick: **nostalgic**
45. Refuses to submit to authority, dissents: **recusant**
46. Resourceful, capable, clears things up, follows through: ***débrouillard***
47. Self-righteously hypocritical: **pharisee**
48. Silly, gullible, or senile person: **dott(e)rel**
49. Speaks at length, in detail; wanders, roams: **expatiator**
50. Stands out despite difficulties or amid surroundings: **monadnock**
51. Supports traditional ideas, values, and conservatism: **conservative**
52. Teetotaler: **nephalist**
53. Thoughtful and reflective: **ruminator**
54. Ugly, repugnant, foulmouthed old hag: **rudas**
55. Uncompromising, having a fixed attitude: **intransigent**
56. Unctuous hypocrite prating of benevolence: **Pecksniff**.
57. Unfulfilled, indecisive, timid, cautious, hesitant man: **Prufrock**
58. Whispers, wheezes, hisses in one's ear: **siffilator**

XVII. -Phobes: See under **phobias**
XVIII. Physical defect:
1. Declines steadily, loses vitality, strength: **languisher**
2. Far sighted: **presbyope**
3. Has diabetes mellitus: **diabetic**
4. Has difficult or painful urination: **dysuriac**
5. Insignificant or feeble person: **nazzard**
6. Leg pain (intermittent) on walking: **claudicant**
7. One with yellow teeth: **xanthodont**
8. Sees better in dim light, or has day blindness: **hemeralope**
9. Short-sighted: **myope**
10. Sickly, weak, unhealthy, feeble person: **invaletudinarian**

11. Squints: **glusker**, **squintifego**
12. Vision is less than perfect, has some vision peculiarity: **cecutient**, **idiopt**
13. Visually far-sighted: **hyperope**
14. Walks unsteadily, wobbling: **totterer**
15. Weak, sickly; convalescent; hypochondriacal: **valetudinarian/valetudinary**

XVIX. Religion:
1. Depending on faith for heavenly access: **fideist**
2. Prays: **precant**
3. Pious passivist: **quietist**

XX. Retired:
1. Receives a state stipend: **pensioner**
2. Reduced or secondary role: **adjunct**
3. With rank or title retained: **emeritus/-tii** (m.), **emerita/-tae** (f.)

XXI. Sex:
1. A devotee of oral intercourse: **lecheur**
2. Dirty old man: **pornogenarian**, **satyr**
3. One who is lewd: **lewdster**

XXII. Sleep:
1. One who has disturbed, disordered, bad sleep: **cacosomniac**, **insomniac**, **somnipathist**
2. One who sleeps by day and plays at night: **dewdropper**

XXIII. Substance abuser:
1. Abuses alcohol: **dipsomaniac**, **posiomaniac**, **alcoholomaniac**
2. Drinks a large quantity of alcohol: **toper**
3. Morbidly desires alcoholic beverages: **methomaniac**
4. Morbidly desires wine: **oenomaniac**

XXIV. Talking:
1. Answers one's own questions: **sermocinator**
2. Argues a minor, subtle or moot point: **quodlibitarian**
3. Argues illogically: **paralogist**
4. Argumentative, disputatious, contentious: **eristic**
5. Constant talker, chatterbox: **blateroon**
6. Criticizes or doubts: **querier**
7. Expresses disapproval; reasons or argues: **expostulator**
8. Full or platitudes: **platitudinarian**

9. Futilely repeats in speech or writing: **battologist**
10. Gossiper: **quidnunc**
11. Incurable chatterer (fig., inf.): **magpie**
12. Irritates with reiteration: **obganiator**
13. Loves to argue: **philopolemist**
14. Mere talker: **rhetor**
15. Mumbles, babbles: **palterer**
16. Noted for telling stories: *raconteur/-tuse*
17. One who babbles on: **burbler**
18. One who discourses unprofitably, unsuccessfully: **mataeologian, mataeologue**
19. One who is cunning with words: **logodaedalist**
20. One who pesters: **noodge**
21. One who whispers or mutters: *sussurator*
22. Pert chatterer: **nashgab**
23. Prophesizes, predicts: **seer**
24. Questioner: **querist, querier**
25. Reiterates persistently: **verbigerator**
26. Reverses constantly opinion, judgment, principles, etc.: **tergiversator**
27. Says the same thing in different words: **tautologist**
28. Skilled at dinner conversation: **deipnosophist**
29. Talks in a silly, purposeless way about nothing important: **prattler, twaddler**
30. Talks loquacious nonsense: **blatherer, blatherskite/ blatherskate**
31. Talks obscenely: **scatologist**
32. Talks volubly about nothing important: **prater**
33. Tells trite, hackneyed stories, jokes: **wheezer**
34. Those who are interested in or expert at words: **logorati**
35. Unctuous hypocrite prating of benevolence: **Pecksniff**
36. Unwilling to talk about or believe in one's illness: **pathocryptic**
37. Wheezes when talking: **wheezer**

XXV. Thinking, scholarship, philosophy, study, teaching:
1. Conformist: *bien pensant*
2. Conservative: *traditionaliste*
3. Deep thinker: **phrontistes**
4. Omniscient scholar: **polyhistor, polyhistorian, polymath**

5. One doing part time: **adjunct**
6. Pseudophilosopher: **philosophaster**
7. Questioner: **querist**
8. Sage: **hakam**
9. Studies why cells age. **biogerontologist**
10. Teacher of adults: **androgogue**

XXVI. Writing:
1. Futilely repeats in speech or writing: **battologist**
2. Obituary writer: **necrologist, obituarist**
3. Writes about relics, the elderly: **lipsanographer**
4. Writes small or increasingly smaller: **micrographer**

XXVII. Youth:
1. Promises perpetual youth: **Calypso**

rosacea (rō-zay'shee-ə) n. a disease found in the middle aged or elderly, particularly in men, marked by a large red nose; a "whiskey-nose", but not limited to topers—there is vascular and follicular dilation and proliferation of variable severity involving the nose and contiguous portions of the cheeks, with persistent erythema (redness), extensive hyperplasia (growth) of the sebaceous glands, and with deep-seated papules and pustules of the affected erythematous sites.) [< L *rosaceus* rosy]. syns. **acne rosacea**; most severe cases are called **hypertrophic rosacea, rosacea keratitis**, or **rhinophyma**, q.v. See **nose, smell**. See **skin**.

roué (roo-ay') (F = rue) a rake, profligate; trickster; one who regularly engages in drinking, gambling, womanizing; a romantic debauché. In use, the adj. "old" frequently precedes roué. (Originally *roué* was a nickname given to the dissolute companions of the *Duc d'Orléans*, c. 1720—New Orleans, Louisiana, was named for the Duc by John Law, the originator of the Mississippi-Bubble financial collapse occurring in the same period.) • The old *roué* continued to engage the ladies. [early 19th C. F-noun use of the pp. of *rouer* to break on the (torture) wheel—the word was applied, perhaps, to one thought deserving of this treatment—< L *rotare* to turn, whirl about]. See **old man**. See **role**.

rounceval (rəN-sər-vaal') n. 1. a bad-mouthed old woman. (2. anything huge. 3. the large marrowfat pea.) [< the huge prehistoric bones found in caves at *Roncesvalles*, France]. (adj. **rounceval** = large or strong.) syn. **termagant**, q.v. See **old woman**.

rudas (rood'dəs) n. a repugnant, ugly, foulmouthed old hag; a **beldam**, q.v. [< L *rudis–e*, adj., in the natural state, raw, undeveloped, unformed; inexperienced, unskilled, ignorant, awkward, uncultured, uncivilized < *rudere* to roar, bellow, bray; to creak]. adj. **rudas** = coarse, foulmouthed. See **old woman**. See **role**.

rudesby (roodz'bee) n. a loud-mouthed, ill-mannered boor; an uncivil, turbulent person. [< L *rudis –e*, adj., in the natural state, raw, undeveloped, rough, wild, unformed; inexperienced, unskilled, ignorant, awkward, uncultured, uncivilized < *rudere* to roar, bellow, bray; to creak]. See **mentality, mentation, behavior**. See **role**. See **old man**. See **old woman**. See **old person(s)**.

rugate (roo'gayt) adj. wrinkled. [< L *ruga* wrinkle < *rugare* to become wrinkled, become creased]. syn. **rugose**, q.v. Cf. **lirk**, **rhagades**, **rimose, rugulose**, q.v. See **skin**.

rugose (roo'gōs) adj. having wrinkles, marked by rugae, wrinkled. [< L *rugosus* wrinkled, shriveled; corrugated]. n. **rugae** = wrinkles. syn. **rimose, rugate**, q.v. Cf. **lirk, rugulose, rhagades**, q.v. See **skin**.

rugulose (roo'gyoo-lōs) adj. having many wrinkles. [< L *ruga* wrinkle < *rugare* to become wrinkled, become creased + -ose, suff., abounding in < -*osus* abounding in]. n. = **rugulosity**. Cf. **rhagades, rugate, rugose**, q.v. See **skin**.

ruminate (room'mi-nayt") vi.&vt. (followed by "over", "on", etc) 1. to meditate, ponder, reflect, chew over, muse, think carefully and at length about something. • The elderly woman's lawyer suggested that she *ruminate* over the codicil he advised. (vi. {of ruminants: cloven-hoofed, cud-chewing quadrupeds} to regurgitate partially digested food and chew it again: to chew the cud.) [< L *ruminatus* pp. of *ruminare* to chew over, chew the cud < *rumen* rumen, throat, gullet]. adj. **ruminant** (-nənt-) = (1. of animals that chew cud) 2. inclined to be thoughtful and reflective. (n. **ruminant** = a hoofed animal that chews cud.) n. **ruminator** (-nayt"-tor) = one who is thoughtful and reflective. n. **rumination** (room"mi-nay'shən). adj. **ruminative**. adv. **ruminatively** (-nayt'tiv-lee). See **mentality, mentation, behavior**. See **role**.

rusticate (rust'ti-kayt) v.i. to retire to or live in the country. [< L *rusticari* to live in the country]. n. **rustication** (-kay'shən). n. **rusticator**. vt. **rusticate**. See **retirement**. See **role**.

S

"Babies haven't any hair;/ Old men's heads are just as
bare;/ between the cradle and the grave/ Lies a haircut and
a shave."—Samuel Hoffenstein

sacchariferous (sak"kə-rif'fər-əss) adj. containing (or producing) sugar. [< sacchar(o)-, pref., sugar via L *saccharum* & G *sakkharon* < Sanskrit *sarkara* sugar + -ferous, suff., bearing, containing, producing < L *ferre* to bear, to carry]. • Such *sacchariferous* food shouldn't be on that **dotard's**, q.v., diet. See <u>drink, food</u>.

sacroiliitis (sayk"krō-il"li-īt'tiss) n. inflammation in the sacroiliac joint (joint between the sacrum, upper tail bone, and the ileum, a hip bone) and a common cause of lower backache. [sacro-, pref., denoting relationship to the sacrum < L *sacrum*, lit., sacred bone, neuter of *sacer* (*sacr*-) sacred + ili(o)-, comb., denoting relationship to the ilium (iliac bone, *os ilium*) L, groin, flank + -itis, adjectival suff., (usually) denoting inflammation < G, f. of *-ites* (agreeing with G *nosos* disease, understood)]. The adj. **sacroiliac** (say"krō-il'ee-ak) refers to the joint or articulation between the sacrum and the ilium and the ligaments associated therewith. See <u>joint, extremities, back</u>.

sagacious (sə-gay'shəss) adj. showing wisdom in one's understanding and judgment of things, wise. [< L *sagac*-, stem of *sagax* of quick perception]. n. **sagacity** (-gas'i-tee). adj. **sagaciousness**. adv. **sagaciously**. Cf. **sapient, percipient**, q.v. See <u>intelligence</u>.

salacious (sə-lay'shəss) adj. 1. erotic; intended to titillate or sexually arouse. 2. lewd, grossly indecent, obscene; showing crude sexual desire or interest. [< L *salac*- < *salire* to leap]. adv. **salaciously**. n. **salaciousness**. Cf. **prurient, concupiscent**, q.v. See <u>sex, love</u>.

sallow (sal'lō) adj. of an unhealthy or unnatural pale-yellow hue. • Increasing *sallowness* indicated a progression of old age and illness since they last met. [OE *salo* dark, dusky, < Gmc.]. vt. **sallow** = to make something unnaturally pale and yellowish. adv. **sallowly**. n. **sallowness**. See <u>color</u>.

salubrious (sə-loob'bree-əss) adj. wholesome, healthy, and beneficial. [< L *salubritas* healthiness, wholesomeness; health, soundness]. adv. **salubriously**. n. **salubriousness**. n. **salubrity**. See **health, illness**.

salvific (sal-vif'fik) adj. tending to help or promote safety or salvation, e.g., of one's soul. [< L *salvus* or *salvos* well, sound, safe, unharmed; living, alive < *salvere* to be well, in good health]. See **religion, theology, morality**.

sanctiloquent (sank-til'ō-kwent) adj. speaking solemnly or of sacred things. [< L *sanctus* holy, literally consecrated, pp. of *sancire* to confirm or consecrate + *loqui* to speak]. adj. **sanctiloquence** (-quenz). adv. **sanctiloquently**. See **talk**. See **religion, theology, morality**.

sapient (say'pee-ent) adj. having or pretending to have great wisdom, wise; learned. [< L *sapient-* < pres.p. of *sapere* to be wise]. adj. **sapiential** (-en'shel). n. **sapience**. n. **sapiency**. adv. **sapiently**. Cf. **sagacious, percipient**, q.v. See **intelligence**.

sarcopenia (sar-kō-peen'ni-e) n. loss of muscle mass—both the number and size of muscle fibers—associated with disuse, and with old age. About 10% of the elderly are affected by sarcopenia. Whether exercise is prophylactic is uncertain. The elderly are less able than the young to use insulin, which is stimulated by eating, to replenish muscle fibers. [sarco-, pref., muscular substance or resemblance to flesh < G *sarx* (*sark-*) flesh + *penia* poverty]. See **health, illness**. See **nerve, muscle, movement, touch**.

satanophobia (sayt"tan-ō-fōb'bi-e) n. morbid fear of the devil, Satan. [< Satan < pre-12th C. < L via Hebrew *satan* to accuse + < G *phobos* fear]. adj. **satanopnobic**. n. **satanophobe** (-tan'nō-). See **phobias**. See **religion**.

saturnine (sat'ter-nīn) adj. 1. gloomy and morose—said of a person and of his/her looks: saturnine facies. (2. {archaic} caused by the absorption of lead or suffering from lead poisoning). [< medieval L *saturninus* < L *Saturnus* Saturn < Roman mythology, the father of Jupiter and Juno, et al, and was the god of agriculture and ruler of the universe during the Golden Age]. adv. **saturninely** (-nīn"-). n. **saturninity** (sat'ter-nīn"ni-tee). n. **saturnineness** (sat'ter-nīn"ness). See **emotion**.

satyr (sat'tər, sat'tur, sat'yər) n. 1. a man who displays inappropriate or excessive sexual behavior. "Old satyr" is a frequent collocation: • He's such an old *satyr*. (2. in G mythology, a wood-dwelling creature with the head and body of a man and the ears, budding horns, and legs of a goat; the Roman version, was a man with ears and tail of a horse.) (3. a brown or gray butterfly with spotted wings.) [< G *saturos* or *satyros* a satyr]. See **old man**. See **sex, love**. See **role**.

satyriasis (sat"tə-rī'ə-siss, sat"yə-rī'ə-siss) n. excessive and uncontrollable sexual desire in a man. [< G *saturos* or *satyros* a satyr]. syns. **aidoi(o)mania, cretomania, edeomania, erotomania, hyperprosexia, lagnesis, paraprosexia, satyrism, satyromania,** q.v. Cf. **concupiscence, prurience,** q.v. See **sex, love**.

satyromania (sat"tir-ō-may'ni-ə) n. satyriasis; excessive sexual desire in a man. [< G *saturos/satyros*, satyr + *mania* frenzy]. adj. **satyromaniacal** (-mə-nī'ə-kəl). n. **satyromaniac**. syn. **aidoi(o)mania, cretomania, edeomania, erotomania, lagnesis, satyrism,** q.v. Cf. **concupiscence, prurience,** q.v. See **manias**. See **sex, love**.

scabrous (skab'brəs) adj. 1. indecent, salacious, obscene. 2. behaving indecently or immorally. 3. having a rough surface due to scales or short stiff hairs; **scurfy**, q.v. 4. of a subject or situation, hard to handle with decency; requiring tactful treatment. • He's a *scabrous* old goat. [< L *scabrosus* < L *scaber* scurfy, scaly]. adv. **scabrously**. n. **scabrousness**. See **sex, love**.

Scamander (skə-man'dur) n., v.i. to wander about. [< G *Skamandros*, a river in Homer's Iliad < the river Menderes, formerly Maiandros, located now in north-west Turkey]. syn. **meander**. (The origin of the famous Greek-key design was supposedly suggested by the sharp turns of the Maiandros River.) See **standing, walking, wandering**.

scatology (skə-tol'lə-jee) n. 1. vulgar language related to excretory functions. 2. preoccupation with excrement or obscenity. (3. the scientific study of excrement especially for diagnostic purposes. 4 Language or literature dealing with excretory matters in a prurient or humorous manner.) • The more annuated the old **roué**, q.v., became the more *scatological* were his intended jests. [< G *scato-*, pref., excrement < *scat-*, stem of *skor, scatos* dung, excrement + *-ology* < *-o-*, comb., + *-logos*, suff., who speaks in a certain way]. n. **scatologist**. adj. **scatological** (ska-tō-loj'jə-kəl). See **role**. See **talk**.

Schadenfreude (shaa'den-froy"də) n. taking pleasure in others' misfortune. [< Ger. *Schaden* harm, damage + *Freude* joy, pleasure]. Cf. **epicaricacy**, q.v. See **mentality, mentation, behavior**. See **emotion**.

schizophasia (skiz"ō-fay'zi-ə/ -fay'jə) n. a meaningless mixture of words and phrases characteristic of advanced schizophrenia; also known informally as the slang, **word salad**. [schiz(o)-, pref., divided, or denoting relationship to division < G *schizein* to divide + *phasis* speech]. See **talk**.

schizothemia (skiz"zō-thee'mi-ə) n. digression by a long reminiscence. [< G *skhizo* split + *thema* proposition]. See **talk**.

Schlimmbesserung (shlim-bes'ser-ung) n. an attempted improvement that makes things worse. • He was convinced that **arthroscopy**, q.v., with lavage could best be deemed a *Schlimmbesserung*, but total **arthroplasty**, q.v., was a success. [Ger. < *schlimm*, bad, awful + *Besserung* improvement]. See **therapy**.

sciatica (sī-at'ti-kə) n. neuralgia of the sciatic nerve, felt at the back of the thigh and running down the side of the leg. It's can be due to a herniated lumbar disc, but sometimes is due to sciatic neuritis, or **spinal stenosis**, q.v., which is common in the elderly; pain anywhere along the course of the sciatic nerve. [L, < *sciaticus*, a corruption of G *ischiadikos* < *ischion* the hip joint]. adj. **sciatic** = 1. relating to or situated in the neighborhood of the ischium or hip, ischiatic. 2. relating to sciatica. See **joint, extremities, back**. See **pain**.

sclerotherapy (skler'rŏ-ther"rə-pee) n. injecting a chemical solution into a small vein in order to destroy it—usually as a treatment for varicose veins. An endovascular procedure may be needed for larger veins, i.e., threading a catheter into the varicose vein and directing a heat source, e.g., a laser or radio-frequency device, into the vein to destroy it. See **therapy**.

screed (skreed) n. a tirade or diatribe; long tiresome harangue or letter (among other definitions). [ME variation of shred, to tear or cut into]. See **talk**.

-scopy (skō-pee) a word termination denoting the act of examining. In more recent years the suffix is used to indicate examining a part, such as the peritoneum (peritoneo*scopy*) or a knee joint (osteo*scopy*), with an instrument (osteoscope) inserted surgically, via a very small incision, in lieu of widely opening the part, thus affording direct inspection; corrective surgery is often possible using specialized instruments inserted through the osteoscope. Robotic instrumentation is frequently combined with various -scopic procedures. ● Osteos*copy* of the knee is a relatively frequent procedure in the elderly. [< G *skopein* to view, examine]. n. **-scope**. adj. **-scopic**. adv. **-scopically**. See **therapy**.

scurfy (skurf'fee) adj. pertaining to or covered with dandruff (scurf). [OE *scurf* < Scand. *sceorf* < root of *sceorfan* gnaw, or *scurfa* crust]. n. **scurf** = scales or flakes such as dandruff. See **skin**.

scurrilous (scur'ril-ləss) adj. 1. containing abusive language or defamatory allegations. 2. using or containing coarse, vulgar, or obscene language. 3. behaving in ways thought to be wicked, evil, or immoral. *La nouvelle vague* (new wave) in the lexicon of **scurrility** is related to the computer and the internet. Cyber swearing as in: "Up your USB!" (USB = a plug-in computer port.), or "What a load of appping (app = application), synching, twittering balls!", or "Blog off!"— *The Decline of Cursing* by Jan Morris, Wall Street Journal, 10/13/10. [< F *scurrile* < L *scurrilis* < *scurra* buffoon]. adv. **scurrilously**. n. **scurrilousness**. n. **scurrility** (-ril'li-tee) = coarseness, vulgarity, or language that is so. Cf. **billingsgate**, **scatology**, q.v. See **talk**.

sear (seer) adj. withered, dried up—lit., of flowers, leaves, etc.; fig., of the aged (". . . the sear, the yellow leaf;"—Macbeth V, iii, 22), etc. [OE *saerian*]. vt. **sear** = to wither up; scorch; cauterize; make callous (a seared conscience). syns. **old**, **aged**, q.v. See **old**.

seborrhea (seb-ōr-ree'ə) n. 1. excessive secretion of sebum— the secretion of the sebaceous glands of the skin. 2. seborrheic dermatitis. The scalp may be affected (with dandruff) in any age group, but seborrheic dermatitis of the face and chest is rare prior to middle age and is most common in the elderly. Besides its relation to excessive sebum secretion, seborrheic dermatitis may be due to a hypersensitivity response to the usually nonpathogenic yeast, *Pityrosporum ovale*. [< L *sebum* suet, tallow + < G *rhoia* flow]. adj. **seborrheic**. syn. **hypersteatosis**, q.v. See **skin**.

seborrheic keratoses (se-bor-ree'ik ker-ə-tōs'seess) n.pl. (n.s. **keratosis**) benign flesh-colored or pigmented, waxy, raised, verrucous (warty) lesions of quite variable size, seen in the elderly; they look as if pasted on the skin, and consist of proliferating epidermal cells enclosing horned cysts. [seb(o)-/seb(i)-, pref., meaning sebo, sebaceous < L *sebum* suet, tallow + < G *rhoia* a flow + -ic, suff., and kerat(o)-, pref., meaning horny tissue or cells < G *keras* horn + -oses, pl. suff.]. See **skin**.

sedens (sed'dens) n, a person, often an old-timer, who remains in the vicinity where he was born. [< L *sedere* to sit]. npl. = **sedentes** (-dent'tees). n. **sedentation** (sed'den-tay'shen) = staying, living in one place, or adoption of a sedentary habits. Cf. **sessile**, q.v. See **old man**, See **old woman**. See **old person(s), people**.

sedentary (sed'den-tar'ee) adj. inclined by nature, driven by occupation, or characterized by, much sitting. [< L *sedentarius* sedentary < *sedere* to sit]. n. **sedentary** = a person who sits a great deal (also refers to spiders lying in wait for prey). n. **sedentariness** (sed'den-tar"ri-ness). adv. **sedentarily** (sed'den-tar"ri-lee). See **old man**, See **old woman**. See **old person(s), people**.

sedentarize (sed-den'tər-īz) vi. to take up, or cause to take up, a permanent residence after a life of nomadic wandering. • The salubrious climate there tempted the previously nomadic old couple finally to *sedentarize*. [< L *sedentarius* sedentary < *sedere* to sit; to settle, to be fixed; to be established + -ize, suff.]. See **standing, walking, wandering**.

seer (seer, see'ər) n. a prophet, predictor of future events; a person with supernatural powers. The term is frequently associated with someone elderly, perhaps venerated. (A famous seer was Tiresias in Sophocles's plays "Oedipus The King" and "Antigone".) [ME *seon* < OS, OHG *sehan* <ON *sja* < *sea* < Goth. *saihwan* < Gmc. *sehw-*]. See **role**.

semisomnous (sem-ee-som'nəs) adj. half asleep. • Not infrequently one finds the very elderly having left the conversation, drifted off, *semisomnous*. [semi-, pref., denoting half < L, cognate with G *hemi-* + L *somnus* sleep]. Cf. **hypnopompic**, q.v. See **sleep, wakefulness**.

senectitude (se-nek'ti-tood) n. old age; the final phase of the average life span. • A relevant apothegm is: "*Senectitude* is not for the faint of heart." [< L *senex* advanced age + suff. –tude: state, condition, or quality, via F < L -*tudo*]. See **old age**.

senescence (se-ness'enss) n. a term applied to cells that have died. Such cells accumulate in the aged in tissues such as arthritic cartilage, cataracts, and arterial plaques, and cause low-level inflammation that is thought to promote the aging process; relatively few of these cells are found in both mice and humans. Researchers have recently generated a strain of mice that can be purged of their senescent cells by administration of a drug that causes such cells to self-destruct—the drug activates a gene, which is more highly expressed in aged cells, such that a "suicide gene" causing senescent cell death is triggered. The tissues in such mice subsequently showed major improvement in their burden of old-age-related disorders such as cataracts, spinal arthritis, and loss of muscle mass and strength. Experiments have yet to be done in humans, but there is the possibility of delaying cancer, dementias, atherosclerosis, diabetes, obesity, etc., in man by ridding him of senescence. (< AMA Morning report, 11/5/11.) See adj. **sencescent**.

senescent (sen-ess'sent) adj. approaching an advanced age, growing old, aging. [L *senescent*-, pres.part., < *senescere* to grow old; to decline, to become feeble, lose strength; to wane, draw to a close < *senex* advanced in age, aged, old]. n. **senescence**, q.v. n. **senescent** = an old man or old woman. vi **senesce**. ant. **juvenescent**, q.v. See **old age**. See **old man**. See **old woman**. See **old person(s)**. See **physique, appearance**.

seneucia (sen-yoo'zee-e, -zhe) widowhood. [< L *senere* to be old— widow in L = *vidua* & widowhood = *viduitas*; widower = *viduus*]. syns. = **viduage**, **viduation**, *viduité*, q.v. See **old woman**. See **marriage**.

senex (sen'eks) n. L m. old man, f. old woman. [L]. (*Senex psittacus negligit ferulam* = an old parrot does not mind the stick. *Senex bis puer* = An old man (or woman) is twice a child.) adj. *senex* = aged. See **old man**.

senicide (sen'ni-sīd) n. killing old men, especially as a tribal custom. [< L *senex* old man + -cide, suff., meaning slayer of, or slaughter of < L *caedere* to kill]. See **end-of-life, death**.

senile (seen'nīl"/se'nil") adj. 1. pertaining to or characteristic of old age. 2. forgetful, confused, or otherwise mentally less acute in old age. [< L *senilis* of old people, old man; aged; senile]. n. **senility** (sə-nil'lə-tee). adv. **senilely** (seen'nīl"lee). See **old**.

senile delirium (seen'nīl" di-leer'ree-əm) n.phr. a syndrome occurring in old age, usually of acute onset, and characterized by disorientation, restlessness, insomnia, hallucinations, and aimless wandering, sometimes associated with senile psychosis. [< L *senilis* of old people, old man; aged; senile]. See **delirium**. See **nerve, muscle, motion, touch**.

senile elastosis (seen'nīl" ee-las-tō'siss) n.phr. senile atrophy or actinic (solar) atrophy, ageing, wrinkling of the skin's elastic and/or connective tissue. [< L *senilis* of old people + < G *elastiko-* < *elastikos* driving, *propelling* < *elaunein* to drive + < G *-osis*, a suff. denoting especially a diseased or morbid process]. syn. **senile keratosis**, q.v.

senile keratosis (seen'nīl" ker-ə-tō'sis) n.phr. photoaging of the skin due to chronic UV (ultra violet) radiation. The lesion is a **dyskeratotic**, q.v., (premalignant) scaly, warty lesion occurring on the sun-exposed skin of aged, light-skinned persons. Senile keratosis is extremely common in the elderly. [< L *senilis* of old people, old man; aged; senile + kerat(o)-, suff., denoting horny tissue or cells < G *keras* horn + -osis, suff.]. syns. **keratosis senilis, acanthosis verrucosa, actinic keratosis**, q.v.—the more current and preferred terms—and **senile keratoma, senile wart, solar keratosis, verruca plana senilis**, and **verruca senilis**. syn. **senile elastosis**, q.v. See **skin**.

senilism (seen'nil"-iz-əm) n. premature old age. [< L *senilis* of old people, old man; aged; senile]. See **old age**.

senility (se-nil'li-tee) n. old age; the physical and mental deterioration associated with old age. [< L *senilitas* old age]. See **old age**.

senior (seen'yər) n. 1. person of advanced age or comparatively long service, etc.; one's elder or superior in length of service, membership, etc.; a senior citizen. (2. a final-year student.) [< L, older, old(ish), the comparative < the stem of *senex, senis* old (man)]. adj. **senior** = 1. more advanced in age or older, superior in age or standing to, or of higher or highest degree (opposed to junior). 2. used to distinguish in a family the elder of two members with the same name from the younger person of that name. n. **seniority** = status accorded to greater age, higher rank, or longer service or employment; the state of being of greater age or higher rank than another. See **old man**, See **old woman**. See **old**. See **old age**.

senior moment n.phr. an instant, a moment, or small interval of time during which an elder is absent minded, has a period of memory lapse or befuddlement—forgetting a name, losing a thought, misplacing keys or glasses. Such lapses are not medically very well understood. In the aged, only the very slightest thought interruption, intrusion, can annihilate concentration. In contrast, such thought interruptions and intrusions in the young are quite easily ignored and the main train of thought is held. Good internal brain communications are essential for proper attention span, focus, and memory. Memory gradually breaks down beginning in middle age, and genes controlling brain function in the prefrontal cortex become less active, thus reducing the deftness with which thoughts are orchestrated. Further, frontal-cortex myelin, the insulation of the brain's nerve fibers, is progressively lost with age. Other moment collations include "teachable moment", "defining moment", and the triumphal "aha! moment", as perchance when a senior unexpectedly remembers. See **intelligence**. See **mentality, mentation, behavior**. See **memory**.

senium (seen'nee-əm) n. old age; the period of life marked by the weaknesses and deterioration that may accompany advanced years. [L, the weakness, feebleness of old age, decline, senility; decay; grief, trouble; gloom; crabbiness]. See **old age**. See **tiredness, weakness**.

senopia (sen-ōp'pi-ə) n. second sight: an apparent decrease in presbyopia in the elderly, which is related to the development of nuclear (lens) sclerosis (hardening and thickening) and resultant myopia (inability to see distant objects) that compensates for presbyopia (inability to see near objects). [< L *senilis* aged, of old people; senile + < G *ops* eye]. syn. **gerontopia**, q.v. See **eye**.

sententious (sen-ten'shəss) adj. 1. tending to use or be full of aphorisms, maxims. 2. inclined to moralize more than is merited or appreciated. 3. expressing much in few words; pithy. [< L *sententiosus* meaningful < *sententia* feeling, opinion < *sentient-* pres.p. of *sentire* to feel]. adv. **sententiously**. n. **sententiousness**. See **talk**. See **religion, theology, morality**.

September (sep-tem'bər) n. the ninth month (of the Gregorian calendar—Pope Gregory XIII introduced the calendar by a 1582 papal bull), i.e., occurring late in the year, thus used as a metaphor for the arrival or imminent approach of old age, the end of life. September marks Shakespeare's seventh age of man ending in "second childishness and mere oblivion; sans teeth, sans eyes, sans taste, sans everything." [< L September < *septem* seven, because September was the seventh month of the early pre-Julian, i.e., pre-46 B.C., Roman year that had 10 months]. syn. **evening of life**, q.v. See **old age**. See **end-of-life, death**.

septuagenarian (sep-too"ə-jen-air'ri-ən, -ree-ən) n. someone in his/ her seventh decade, seventies. [< L *septuaginarius* (*septuageni* seventy each < *septuaginta* seventy + -an, suff.)] See **old man**. See **old woman**. See **old person(s), people**. See **role**.

sepulcher/–ker (sep'pul/pəl-kur) n. tomb—especially one cut in rock or built of stone or brick—burial vault, or cave. [< L *sepulc(h) rum*, grave, tomb < *sepelire* to bury]. adj. **sepulchral** (se-pul'krəl) = of sepulcher(s) or sepulture; suggestive of a tomb, funereal, gloomy, dismal. [< L *sepulcralis* of a tomb, sepulchral, funeral]. adj. **sepulchral** (se-pul'krəl) = of sepulcher(s). adv. **sepulchrally** (-pul'). n., vt. (U.K) **sepulchre = sepulcher**. See **end-of-life, death**.

sepulture (sep'pul-tur) n. 1. burying, putting in a grave; the act of interring a body. 2. a **sepulchre**, q.v., or grave. [< L *sepultura* burial < *sepelire* to bury, (fig.) to suppress]. vt. **sepulture** = to inter, bury, put in the grave. See **end-of-life, death**.

sermocination (ser-mōs"si-nay'shən) n. speaking, questioning, and quickly answering one's own questions. [< L *sermocinari* to talk, converse]. n. **sermocinator**. See **talk**. See **role**.

sermunculus -ī (ser-moŏn'koŏ-loŏs -ī) n. small talk, chit-chat. [L, nm., pl.nm. = *sermunculi* (-*lī*)]. See **talk**. syns. **blether/blather, faff, glossolalia, piffle**, etc. Cf. **badinage, persiflage**, q.v.

serotine (ser'ə-tin, -tīn) adj. late in occurring, forming, or flowering. [< L *serotinus* belated < *serus* late]. (**serotine** n. a small brown bat {Eptesicus serotinus} native to Europe and Asia—named after its habit of appearing late in the evening.) Cf. **opsimathic**, q.v. See **mentality, mentation, behavior**.

serotonin (ser-ə-tōn'nin) n. a neurotransmitter, i.e., any of a group of substances released from neurons of the central and peripheral nervous systems and which excite or inhibit target cells linked to mood regulation. Exercise stimulates serotonin and thereby lessens inertness and depression—especially useful in the elderly. [sero-, pref., meaning serum or serous < L *serum* whey + < G *tonikos*, tonic]. See **health, illness**. See **emotion**.

sessile (ses'sīl) adj. (1. attached directly to a base, without a stalk (as a leaf or flower). 2. permanently attached, immobile, as an animal, e.g., a barnacle, or, fig., a person who is habituated to a certain place. • The *sessile* Mrs. Ubiety—See **ubiation**.—was invariably at her habitual place by the front door as one entered the geriatric center. [< L *sessilis* relating to sitting < *sedere* to sit]. Cf. **sedens**, q.v. See **standing, walking, wandering**.

sex, love: acarpous, acedolagnia, acolasia, acokoinonia, acyesis, ADAM syndrome, agapism, agennesic, aidoi(o)-mania, anagapesis, anandrious, anaphroditous, andropause, anililagnia, aphanisis, apogenous, atocia, azygophrenia, azygous, cacemphaton, capripede, coimetrophilia, concupiscence, cretomania, deosculate, detumescence, dysgenesia, dysgonesis, dyspareunia, edeomania, effete, elumbated, epicene, erotomania, Ewig-Weibliche, evancalous, exosculate, gerontolagnia, gerontophilia, gynecomania, hyperprosexia, hypogonadism, *impotentia*, improcreant, lagnesis, lalochezia, *lécheur*, lenocinant, lewdster, libido, libidopause, lovertine, lupanarian, matronolagnia, medomalacophobia, neanilagnia, obsolagnium, opsimatria, opsipatria, opsiproligery, paraprosexia, piss-proud, pornogenarian, prurience, salacious, satyr, satyriasis/satyrism/ satyromania, scabrous, shunam(m)itism, sphallolalia, viripause, xeronisus.

sex, love: Subcategories

I.   Abnormal genital function, procreation ability:
     1. Functional disorder of the genital organs: **dysgonesis**
     2. Impaired powers of procreation; inadequate gonadal function: **andropause, dysgenesia, hypogonadism**
II. Children:
     1. Ability to have children late in life: **opsiproligery**

2. Bearing a child late in a woman's life: **opsimatria**
3. Becoming a father late in life: **opsipatria.**
III. Decadence, indecency, lewdness:
    1. Decadent, over refined: **effete**
    2. Indecent, salacious, obscene: **scabrous**
    3. Lewd allusion: **cacemphaton**
    4. Lewd; lascivious, lubricious: **lenocinant**; **lupanarian**, **salacious**
    5. Talking dirty to relieve tension, anxiety: **lalochezia**
    6. That which arouses, or is intended to arouse, lewd thoughts: **prurience**, **salacious**
IV. Gender differentiation:
    1. Eternal-feminine characteristics: **Ewig-Weibliche**
    2. Having sexual characteristics of both sexes or sexless: **epicene**
V. Hormones:
    1. Androgen deficiency in the aging male: **ADAM syndrome, andropause, viripause**
    2. Time of life when a man loses interest in sex and/or is unable to perform sexually: **andropause, viripause**
VI. Impotence:
    1. Erectile dysfunction: **detumescence**, *impotentia*, **improcreant**
    2. Morbid fear of losing an erection during lovemaking: **medomalacophobia**
    3. Sterile, impotent: **agennesic, anandrious, apogenous, effete**
    4. Time of life when a man loses interest in sex and/or is unable to perform sexually: **viripause, andropause, detumescence**, *impotentia*, **improcreant**
VII. Intercourse:
    1. One who likes oral intercourse: *lécheur*
    2. Painful (for women) intercourse: **dyspareunia**
VIII. Kissing, loving, embracing:
    1. Kiss affectionately: **deosculate**
    2 Kiss heartily: **exosculate**
    3. Pleasant to embrace: **evancalous**
IX. Non-sexual love:
    1. Doctrine exalting non-sexual love: **agapism**

      2. Flirtatious talk that does not lead to amorous action: **sphallolalia**

      3. Fondness for & interest in cemeteries, tombstones, and collecting tombstone epitaphs: **coimetrophilia**

X. Orgasm:

      1. Inability to reach orgasm: **xeronisus**

XI. Sexual drive:

      1. Sexual drive: **libido**.

      2. Time of life when libido wanes: **libidopause**.

      3. Waning sexual desire due to age: **obsolagnium**.

      4. Weak in the loins, weak genital response: **elumbated**.

      5. Without sexual desire: **anaphroditous**.

XII. Sexual indifference:

      1. Complete sexual indifference: **acedolagnia**

      2. Loveless, passionless sex: **acokoinonia**

      3. Time of life when a man loses interest in sex and/or is unable to perform sexually: **viripause**

      4. Time of life when libido wanes: **libidopause**

      5. Waning sexual desire due to age: **obsolagnium**

XIV. Sexual attraction re: those older:

      1. Attraction to older, especially married or widowed women: **matronolagnia**

      2. Love of a much older woman: **anililagnia**

      3. Morbid love of old persons: **gerontophilia**

XIII. Sexual attraction re: those younger:

      1. Attraction to nymphets: **neanilagnia**

      2. Nymphomania (or satyriasis): **lagnesis**

      3. Possible rejuvenation of old men's sexuality by contact—sexual or otherwise—with young girls: **shunam(m)itism**

XV. Sterility:

      1. Female sterility: **acyesis**, **atocia**

      2. Fruitless, sterile: **acarpous**

XVI. Strong sexual desire, addiction, intemperance:

      1. Addicted to lovemaking: **lovertine**

      2. Lecherous elder man: **pornogenarian**

      3. Morbid or excessive sexual desire in a male: **gynecomania**, **cretomania**, **lagnesis** (or nymphomania), **satyriasis/satyrism/satyromania**

      4. One who is lewd: **capripede**, **lewdster**, **satyr**, **pornogenarian**

5. Powerful or excessive feelings of physical desire, sexual intemperance, lust, being oversexed: **acolasia, aidoi(o)mania, concupiscence, edeomania, erotomania, hyperprosexia, paraprosexia**

6. Strong sexual desire in an older man: **gerontolagnia**

XVII. Unmarried:

1. Neurosis due to living singly: **azygophrenia**
2. Unpaired, unmarried, widowed: **azygous**

XVIII. Waning sexual desire, love, prowess:

1. False, faltering erection: **piss-proud**
2. Fear of losing sexual power: **aphanisis**
3. Flirtatious talk that does not lead to amorous action: **sphallolalia**
4. Lack of interest in former loved ones: **anagapesis**
5. Lacking in vitality, worn out, spent: **effete, epicene**
6. Time of life, due to age, when libido wanes: **andropause, libidopause obsolagnium**

sexagenarian (seks"sə-jən-nair'ri-ən) n. someone in his/her sixth decade, i.e., sixties. [< L *sexagenarius* sixty-year-old (*sexageni* 60 each < *sexaginta* sixty < *sex* six + *generare* to beget, procreate, produce, engender) + -an, suff.]. n. (syn.) **sexagenary** (-jen'nə-ree) = someone in his/her sixth decade. adj. **sexagenarian**. See **old man, old woman**. See: **role**.

shamble (sham'bəl) vi. to walk or run in an awkward, shuffling, or decrepit way. [origin uncertain]. n. **shambling**. See **standing, walking, wandering**.

shibui (shi-boo'i) n. refers to beauty that only time can reveal: the impression—a distinct but ineffable sensation—that one gets, e.g., from looking at the face of a certain kind of older person. Such a visage conveys *shibui* to the degree that it reflects the person's personality and his or her experiences in life. • "*Shibui* successfully contradicts the ravages of time." [Japanese]. See **old age**. See **physique, appearance**.

shingles (shing'gəlz) n. See **zoster**.

shpilkes (shpil'keeys) pl.n. inability to sit still, ants in one's pants, feeling antsy, fidgeting, on pins and needles, unpleasant nervousness, impatience; upset stomach. Inability to sit quietly still, unmoving, for long periods has been shown in a study by the American Cancer Society and in a large Australian study (2010) to increase longevity. The ACS study showed women who sat for greater than six hours per day increased their risk of premature death by 37%, and men did so by 18%. The Australian study found a similar correlation between immobile time watching TV and premature death. Too much idle time decreases production of lipoprotein lipase necessary for healthy processing of fat. Physical movement boosts thinking and problem solving, while sitting for long periods can even negate the benefits of vigorous exercise. [Yiddish, pins < Polish *szpilka* pin & < Russian *shpelka* hairpin, tack, or little pivot]. See **end-of-life, death**. See **nerve, muscle, movement, touch**. See **work, activity**.

shrew (shroo) n. (1. a small nocturnal animal that resembles a mouse but is an insectivore with velvety fur, a long pointed snout, and small eyes and ears. Family: Soricidae.) 2. an offensive term for a woman who is regarded as quarrelsome, nagging, or ill-tempered; it is frequently preceded by *old*. (There was a folktale that a shrew's bite is venomous. Originally the term applied metaphorically to both men and women having a spiteful nature, but over time the word referred exclusively to women). [O.E. *screawa*]. See **old woman**.

shunam(m)itism (shyoo-nam'mi-tis"səm) n. contact—visual, tactile, or carnal—with younger girls by old men to encourage or restore their (old men's) sexual vigor; the act of old men sleeping with young girls in the belief that the closeness of youthful bodies can have a rejuvenating effect. The practice was common in biblical times. (The Old Testament, I Kings, 1., relates that King David, when quite old, could not keep warm. His attendants sought all over Israel for a beautiful maiden to look after him and to keep him warm. Abishag of Shunam was their choice. She attended the king, but did not have sexual relations with him. Supposedly it was her *pneuma*—G, air, breath, spirit {Holy Spirit of the Christian Trinity}—that kept King David warm. In ancient medical practice, the elderly were believed to become naturally cold due to gradual loss of innate heat; it was this that resulted in senescence and death. In the 17th C., a Latin forgery that attracted considerable attention indicated one L. Clodius Hermippus lived to be 115 years of age thanks to the vital **pneuma** of young maidens. [< Shunam, the home of Abishag the Shunamite, I Kings 1.]. See **sex, love**.

sialoquent (sī-al'lō-kwənt) adj. spraying saliva when speaking. [sial(o)-, pref., indicating saliva or salivary gland < G *sialon* saliva + < L *loqui* to speak]. n. **sialoquence.** adv. **sialoquently.** Cf. **slubber-degullion, slaver,** q.v. See **talk.** See **mouth, gums, teeth**

sideromonomania (sid"dər-ō-mōn"nō-may'ni-ə) n. abnormal interest in traveling by railroad. [sidero-, pref., denoting iron < G *sideros* iron + *monos* single + *mania* frenzy]. adj. **sideromonomaniacal** (-ma-nī'ə-kəl). n. **sideromaniac.** See **manias.**

siffilate (sif'fi-layt) vi. to whisper; wheeze; whizz; hiss; talk in soft sibilant tones. [< F *siffler* to whistle; wheeze; whizz; hiss; boo; catcall]. n. **siffilator** = one who whispers, etc. syn. **susurrate,** q.v. See **talk.** See **role.**

silential (sī-len'shəl) adj. pertaining to or performed in silence. [< L *silent-*, pres.p., of *silere* to be silent + -al, suff., relating to or characterized by < L -*alis*]. n. **silentium** (sī-len'shee-əm) = a place where silence is imposed. n. **silentiary** (sī-len'shee-air"ree) = 1. someone who enforces peace and quiet. 2. someone who keeps state secrets. • a *silential* atmosphere usually prevails in the seniors' residence. See **role.** See **loneliness, solitude, silence.**

Silenus (sī-leen'nus), pl. **Sileni** (-nee) n. drunken old man, rollicking old drunkard. [G, a god representing the spirit of untamed nature. (Silenus was the tutor, perhaps foster father, of Dionysus. Sileni were represented artistically as half-man and half-horse, with horse's ears, tail, and sometimes legs. Sileni were sometimes confused with the god Pan, but more often with satyrs, which, in contrast, were young, half-goat, half-man, and were lecherous rather than inebriated)]. See **old man.** See **role.**

Silurian (sil-yoor'ri-ən) adj. (1. of the Silures, a people of ancient Britain.) 2. terribly old: Mark Twain used the word to indicate doddering old age. (3. of a series of rocks forming a subdivision of the Paleozoic immediately underlying the Devonian, named as first investigated in the district of the Silures.) [< L *Silures* an ancient people in what is now Wales where rocks from the period were discovered]. n. **Silurian** = that period of geologic time, a subdivision of the Paleozoic age, when fishes first appeared > 400 million years ago; it immediately underlies the Devonian. n. **Silurian** = old age; old person. See **old.** See **old man.** See **old woman.** See **old person(s).**

silver alert n.phr. (informal) a recent collocation: an announcement that can be placed in various media, directing the attention of the elderly to something occurring of interest to or affecting them particularly. See **ole age**.

silver surge n.phr. (informal) a recent collocation indicating the large number of elderly in proportion to other age groups in the population and the increasing influence of the elderly due to their number. See **old age**.

sinistrophobia (sin"nis-trō-fōb'bi-ə) n. morbid fear of the left or things on the left. [sinistr(o)-, pref., indicating left, or toward the left < L *sinister* left + < G *phobos* fear]. adj. **sinistrophobic**. n. **sinistrophobe**. syn. **levophobia**, q.v. ant. **dextrophobia**, q.v. See **phobias**.

Sirtum 1 (sir'tum)/**SirT1**/**SIRT1** n.phr./acronym/acronm a member of the sirtuin family of genes. Sirtum 1 is a protein that in humans is encoded by the SIRT1 gene. It's a homologue of Sir 2, the first of the sirtuin genes to be discovered. Inducing Sirtum 1's expression increases insulin sensitivity and decreases the need for insulin, thus expediting carbohydrate metabolism. Sirtum 1 can break up the protein of amyloidal plaques that form in **Alzheimer's-disease**, q.v., patients. Sirtum 1, along with caloric restriction, is important for promoting longevity; it's sometimes called the "longevity gene". **Resveratrol**, q.v., found in red wine, may switch the gene on. Old-age genes are found in a certain region of chromosome 4. [< Sir, acronym, < silent-information-regulator (gene)]. See **old age**.

Sisyphean (sis-sə-fee'ən) adj. endlessly laborious and fruitless, unproductive activity, effort. • Ultimately, preventing the adversities of old age is a *Sisyphean* task. [< G *Sisyphus*, a mythological cruel king of Corinth who was cursed for eternity by having repetitiously to push a huge boulder to the top of a hill only to have it roll down again]. See **work, activity**.

skeuomorph (skyoo'ə-mawrf) n. "a design feature copied from a similar artifact in another material, even when not functionally necessary" (< A.Word.A.Day), e.g., the click sound of an analog camera's shutter in currently produced digital cameras by playing a sound clip. • (fig.) That **mossback's**, q.v., radical socialism is a *skeuomorph* in today's pseudo-liberal Democratic politics. [< G *skeuos* vessel, implement + -*morph* form]. adj. **skeuomorphic** (skyoo'ə-mawrf"ik). adv. **skeuomorphically** (skyoo"ə-mawrf"ik-lee/ kə-lee). See **past, time**.

skin: acanthosis verrucosa, achrochordons, actinic elastosis, actinic keratosis, basal cell carcinoma, Bowen's disease, callositas, callosity, cereous, cernuous, chaetophorous, cherry angioma, cinerescent, clavus, compursion, dealbate, decubital, decubitus (ulcer), desquamate, dropsy, dyschroia, dyschromia, dyskeratoma, ecchymosis, ecdysiast, effleurage, elastosis, embrocation, emollient, erubescence, erugate, etiolate, excoriate, flavescent, furfuraceous, geroderma, heloma, heloma molle, heloma durum, hematoma, herpes zoster, hyperkeratosis, hypersteatosis, icterical, illinition, irrugate, Kaposi's sarcoma, keratocanthomas, keratoma, keratosis, lentigo maligna, lepidic, lepidote, lichen simplex chronicus, lirk/lerk/ lurk, luteolus, malactic, marcescent, marcescible, melanocyte, melanoma, passulation, pediculosis, petechia, poroma, pruritus, purpura, retinol, rhagades, rhytidectomy, rhytidosis, rhytidoplasty, rhytiphobia, rhytiscopia, rimose, rimple, rosacea, rugate, rugose, rugulose, scurfy, seborrhea, seborrheic keratoses, senile elastosis, senile keratosis, stasis dermatitis, snurp/snerp/ snirp, squamous, squamous cell carcinoma, stasis dermatitis, tyloma, UVA & UVB rays, venous ulcer, xanthelasma, xanthoma, xeroderma, xerosis, zoster.

skin : Subcategories

I. **Aged**:
   1. Aged, atrophied, withered: **geroderma, marcescent, marcescible, senile elastosis**
   2. Photo (sun)-aged skin, horniness: **acanthosis verrucosa, actinic elastosis, actinic keratosis, hyperkeratosis, keratosis, lentigo maligna, senile elastosis, senile keratosis, UVA & UVB rays**

II. **Color, covering**:
   1. A reddening; a blush: **erubescence**
   2. Color: **cinerescent, dyschroia, dyschromia**
   3. Covered with white powder: **dealbate**
   4. Degenerative changes: **elastosis**
   5. To make sickly, white: **etiolate**

     6. Yellowish cast to the skin: **flavescent, icterical, luteolus**

III. <u>Corns</u>: **callositas, callosity, clavus, heloma, heloma durum, heloma molle, keratoma, melanocyte, poroma, tyloma**

IV. <u>Drooping, pendulous</u>: **cernuous**

V. <u>Dryness, scaliness</u>:
    1. Dryness: **xeroderma, xerosis**
    2. Peel, shed: **desquamate, ecdysiast, furfuraceous, scurfy**
    3. Scaliness: **lepidic, lepidote, scurfy, squamous**

VI. <u>Edema</u>: **dropsy, stasis dermatitis**

VII. <u>Eruption</u>:
    1. Acute eruption, eczema, dermatitis, vascular dilatation: **herpes zoster** (shingles), **lichen simplex chronicus, rosacea, seborrhea, stasis dermatitis**
    2. Vesicular eruption along one side of the chest (usually): **zoster, herpes zoster** (shingles)

VIII. <u>Hemorrhage</u>:
    1. <u>Hemorrhage into the skin</u>: **purpura**
    2. <u>Localized mass of extravasated blood</u>: **hematoma**
    3. <u>Patch of extravasated blood in the skin</u>: **ecchymosis**.
    4. <u>Pinpoint skin hemorrhage</u>: **petechia** (pl. = **petechiae**)

IX. <u>Infected</u>:
    1. infested with lice: **pediculosis**

X. <u>Itching</u>: **pruritus**

XI. <u>Rubbing</u>: **effleurage**
    1. Agent that softens, soothes the skin: **emollient, malactic**
    2. Using liniment, oil, etc., to rub on the body, lubricate: **embrocation, illinition**

XII. <u>Shaving, abrading</u>:
    1. Needing a shave (bristle bearing): **chaetophorous**
    2. Removing, peeling off, stripping skin: **excoriate**

XIII. <u>Tumors</u>:
    1. Benign tumors: **dyskeratoma, achrochordons, cherry angioma, keratocanthomas, seborrheic keratosis, xanthelasma, xanthoma**
    2. Premalignant lesions: **acanthosis verrucosa, actinic keratosis, Bowen's disease, dyskeratoma, lentigo maligna, senile keratosis**.

3. Malignant lesions: **basal cell carcinoma, dyskeratoma, Kaposi's sarcoma, lentigo maligna, melanoma, squamous cell carcinoma**

XIV. Ulcer, soreness:
1. Caused by pressure from lying down: **decubital, decubitus** (ulcer)
2. Caused by venous blockage: **venous ulcer**

XIV. Waxy lesions: **hypersteatosis, seborrhea, seborrheic keratosis, -ses**
1. Waxen: **cereous**

XVI. Wrinkle(s): **rimple(s), lirk/lerk/lurk**
1. Dried up & wrinkled: **passulation**
2. Early facial wrinkling: **rhytidosis**
3. Fine cracks around the corners of the mouth: **rhagades**
4. Freed from wrinkles, smoothed, smooth: **erugate**
5. Full of wrinkles: **rimose, rugulose**
6. Morbid fear of getting wrinkles: **rhytiphobia**
7. Neurotic preoccupation with wrinkling: **rhytiscopia**
8. Preventive: **retinol**
9. Surgical removal of wrinkles: **rhytidectomy, rhytidoplasty**
10. To become wrinkled, shriveled (vi): **snurp/snerp/ snirp**
11. To wrinkle: **irrugate**
12. Wrinkled: **rimpled, rugate, rugose**
13. Wrinkled by: **UVA & UVB rays**
14. Wrinkling one's face: **compursion**

skinflint (skin'flint) n. a miser, niggard. It is often preceded by *old*. [17th C. < someone miserly enough to try taking the skin off a flint, or to use a flint until it was as thin as a skin. < ON *skinn*]. See **old man**. See **old woman**. See **old person(s)**. See **role**.

slaver (slav'ver, slay'ver) vi. 1. to dribble saliva from the mouth. 2. to behave obsequiously to somebody, to fawn. [? < Ger. *slabbern or* Scand. *slafra*]. n. **slaver** = dripping saliva. adj. **slavery**. syns. **salivate, slobber, dribble, drool**. Cf. **sialoquent, slubber-degullion**, q.v. See **mouth, gums, teeth**. See **physique, appearance**.

sleep, wakefulness: **accumbent, agrypnia, agrypnocoma, agrypnotic, ahypnia, akathisia, alector, anypnia, aypnia,**

bruxism, cacosomnia, circadian sleep, dysrhythmia, decubital, decubitus, dewdropper, diurnation, dormition, dysania, dyskoimesis, dysnystaxis, dysphylaxia, dyssomnia, egersis, euania, euneirophrenia, hypersomnia, hypnodia, hypnolepsy, hypnomogia, hypnopathy, hypnophobia, hypnophrenosis, hypnopompic, hypnosia, hypnosophy, hyposomnia, ignavy, insomnia, insomnolence, jacent, languescent, languid, latibulize, levisomnous, narcolepsy, nid-nod, nutation, oneiric, oscitancy, pandiculation, parahypnosis, parasomnia, pernoctation, PLMD, polysomnography, semisomnous, sleep apnea, somnifacient, somniferous, somnific, somnifugous, somnipathy, somnolence, somnolency, somnolentia, sopient, sopor, soporific, soporose/ soporous, soporiferous, *veilleuse*, zoara.

sleep: Subcategories

I. Any generalized sleep disorder, problem: **dyssomnia, hypnopathy, parahypnosis, parasomnia, somnipathy**
II. Awakening:
    1. Difficulty waking up: **dysania**
    2. Easy awakening: **euania, levisomnous**
    3. Waking too soon: **dysphylaxia**
    4. Wakefulness: **egersis**
III. Between sleep and wakefulness: **hypnopompic, levisomnous, semisomnous, somnolence, somnolency**
    1. Uncontrolled drowsiness: **hypnosia**
IV. Beginning sleep:
    1. Becoming tired, faint: **ignavy, languescent**
    2. Nodding: **nid-nod, nutation**
IV. Dreams:
    1. Pleasant dreams: **euneirophrenia**
    2. Relating to or like a dream: **oneiric**
VI. Hibernate: **latibulize**
VII. Lethargy:
    1. Apathy, apathetic: **agrypnocoma, ignavy, sopor**
    2. Slow moving, sluggish: **languid**
VIII. Light sleep: **dysnystaxis, levisomnous**
IX. Role:
    1. One who is sleepless: **alector**
    2. Day sleeper: **dewdropper**

X. Sleep inducing: **somnifacient, somniferous, somnific, sopient, soporific, soporose/soporous**

XI. Sleep position; recumbent: **accumbent, decubital, decubitus; jacent**

XII. Sleep vigil: **pernoctation,** *veilleuse*

XIII. Sleeping: **dormition**

XIV. Specific sleep problems:
1. Constantly sleepy: **hypnodia**
2. Difficulty getting to sleep: **dyskoimesis**
3. Dispelling sleep: **akathisia, somnifugous**
4. Disturbed sleep: **cacosomnia, hypnophrenosis, parahypnosis, parasomnia**
5. Excessive sleep: **hypersomnia, sopor**
6. Fear of sleep: **hypnophobia**
7. Habit of sleeping, being dormant during the daytime: **diurnation**
8. Insomnia, unable to sleep: **agrypnia, agrypnotic, ahypnia, anypnia, aypnia, hypnomogia, insomnia, insomnolence, zoara**
9. Periodic leg movement disorder: **PLMD**
10. Repeated temporary cessation of breathing during sleep: **sleep apnea**
11. Rhythmic: **circadian sleep dysrhythmia**
12. Sleep epilepsy: **hypnolepsy, narcolepsy**
13. Teeth grinding: **bruxism**
14. Too little sleep: **hyposomnia, somnolentia**

XV. Study of sleep: **hypnosophy, polysomnography**

XVI. Yawning: **oscitancy, pandiculation**

sleep apnea (ap'nee-ə) n.phr. temporary cessation of breathing that happens in some people during sleep. The longer the apneic periods, the more severe the disorder. There are three types: central (brain), obstructive (palate, respiratory tract), and mixed. Obstructive sleep apnea is common in the elderly, especially in those who are obese, who sleep supine, and are men. Temporary collapse of the oropharyngeal airway during inspiration is the cause. Cacophonous snoring suggests the condition. **Bruxism**, q.v., may coexist. Side effects of prominent apneic episodes include sleeplessness, decreased oxygenation, pulmonary and systemic hypertension, cardiac arrhythmias, etc. Sleep study, **polysomnography**, q.v., is confirmatory of apneic episodes, i.e., > 10 sec. of sleep apnea. [See **apnea** for etymology]. See **sleep, wakefulness**. See **breathing**.

slubber-degullion (slub'ər-dee-gul'yən) n. One who slobbers his clothing, **slavers**, q.v., is **sialoquent**, q.v., a dirty fellow. [< slubber, vt. & vi., do carelessly or bunglingly; slaver, slobber, prob. < LG *slubbern* + de-, pref., completely, in a bad sense, < L adv. & prep. *de* + gull, a dupe, fool <? gull, a young bird < ON *gulr* yellow + -ion, suff., forming nouns of condition or action < F *–ion* < L *–ionem* (nom. *-io*)]. Cf. **sialoquent**, **slaver**, q.v. See **mouth, gums, teeth**. See **role**.

SM a chat and text-message initialism or acronym = **s**enior **m**oment, q.v. (An initialism should properly, strictly be composed of the initial letter only of each word represented, while an acronym does not have this restriction, but there are some who would restrict acronyms only to initials that in themselves compose a recognized relevant word, e.g. RADAR = radar {**r**adio **d**etection **a**nd **r**anging}, now a word.) [See www.NetLingo.com for a list of such acronyms]. Cf. **CRAFT**, **CRAT**, **CRS**, **CRTLA**, & **OSIF**, q.v. See **memory**.

smellfungus (smel'fung"gəss) n. a malcontent; a grumbler or fault-finder. [<? slang]. See **role**. See **mentality, mentation, behavior**.

snowbird (snō'burd") n. 1. a person, usually a retired senior, who lives, usually in a northern area with snowy winters, but moves south in winter to a warmer place without snow. (2. a bird that is seen chiefly in winter, e.g., a snow bunting). See **old man**. See **old woman**. See **old person(s)**. See **retirement**.

snurp/snerp/snirp (snurp) vi to become shriveled or wrinkled. [of Scandinavian origin, Cf. Norwegian dial. *snurpa*, *snyrpa* to draw together in wrinkles]. See **physique, appearance**. Cf. **irrugate**, q.v. See **skin**.

solivagant (səl-liv'ə-gənt) n. one who wanders alone. [< L *solus* alone + *vagus* wandering]. adj. **solivagant** = wandering alone. See **loneliness, solitude, silence**. See **standing, walking, wandering**. See **role**.

solophobia (sōl"lō-fōb'bi-ə) n. morbid fear of being alone, of loneliness. [< L *solus* alone + < G *phobos* fear]. adj. **solophobic**. n. **solophobe**. syns. **autophobia**, **eremophobia**, **isolophobia**, **monophobia**, q.v. See **phobias**. See **loneliness, solitude, silence**.

somnifacient (som"ni-fay'shent, som"ne-) adj. describes a sleep-inducing, **soporific**, q.v., drug. [< L *somnus* sleep + *facere* to make]. n. **somnifaeient** = a drug that induces sleep; a hypnotic. syn. **soporific**, q.v. See **sleep, wakefulness**.

somniferous (som-nif'er-es) adj. sleep inducing. [< L *somnus* sleep + *ferre* to bear; bring forth]. syns. **somnifacient, somnific, soporific**, q.v. See **sleep, wakefulness**.

somnific (som-nif'ik) adj. inducing sleep. [< L *somnus* sleep + *ferre* to bear; bring forth]. syns. **somnifacient, somniferous, soporific**, q.v. See **sleep, wakefulness**.

somnifugous (som-nif'fyoo-gess) adj. dispelling sleep. [< L *somnus* sleep + *fugare* to put to flight; drive away, chase away]. See **sleep, wakefulness**.

somnipathy (som'nip'a-thee) n. 1. any disorder of sleep. Insomnia affects almost 50% of those 60 years of age or more. In one recent study of those living in assisted-living facilities, 65% had significant sleep problems. Sleep problems are associated with an increased incidence of depression and a lower quality of life. Elders get sleepy earlier and awaken earlier than younger adults, and may require somewhat less sleep to remain awake during the day. Elders who sleep as well as they did in middle age remain physically and mentally healthier longer than those who don't. (2. hypnotism.) [< L *somnus* sleep + -pathy, suff., < G *pathos* suffering, disease]. n. **somnipathist** = one affected by or under the influence of somnipathy. adj. **somnipathic** (-path'ik). syn. **parahypnosis**, q.v. See **sleep, wakefulness**. See **role**.

somnolence/somnolency (som'nō-lenss/som'nō-len-see) n.1. drowsiness; sleepiness. 2. a condition of semiconsciousness approaching coma; asleep. [< L *somnolentia* somnolence]. adj. **somnolent**. adv. **somnolently**. See: **sleep, wakefulness**.

somnolentia (som-nō-len'ti-e, -shi-e). n. sleep drunkenness caused by severely insufficient sleep—not too much sleep or alcoholic stupor. [L < *somnolentus* sleepy < *somnus* sleep + -ia, suff, diseases or medical conditions < L, G]. See **sleep, wakefulness**.

sonorous (son'nər-əs, sə-nawr'əs) adj. 1. producing or possessing sound. 2. sounding with loud, deep, clear tones; resonant. 3. speaking, spoken or expressed in a full, rich, and impressive manner. • The old woman's *sonorous* breathing periodically interrupted her **somnolence**, q.v. [< L *sonorus* noisy, loud < *sonar* sound < *sonare* to make a sound]. adv. **sonorlusly**. n. **sonority** (son-nawr'ri-tee). n. **sonorousness**. Cf. **stertorous**, q.v. See **talk**. See **breathing**.

sopient (sōp'pee-ənt) adj. **soporific**, q.v. [L, pres. p. (active) of *sopire* to lull to sleep]. See **sleep, wakefulness**.

sopor (sōp'pawr) n. stupor; an unnaturally deep sleep; lethargy. [L, deep sleep]. See **sleep, wakefulness**.

soporiferous (sō"pawr-if'ər-əs) adj. **soporific**, q.v. [< L *soporifer* < *sopor* deep sleep + *ferre* to bring forth; bear]. See **sleep, wakefulness**.

soporific (sō-pōr-if'ik) adj. 1. causing sleep or drowsiness. 2. experiencing sleep or drowsiness. 3. dull and boring; tedious. [< L *sopor* deep sleep + *facere* to make]. n. **soporific** = an agent that produces sleep. adv. **soporifically**. syns. **somnifacient, somniferous, somnific, sopient, soporiferous, soporose/ soperous**, q.v. See **sleep, wakefulness**.

soporose/soperous (sō'pawr-ōz, sō'pawr-əs) adj. relating to or causing **sopor**, q.v., comatose; stuporous. [< L *soper* deep sleep]. See **sleep, wakefulness**.

sororate (sawr'or-ayt) n. marrying one's wife's sister after one's wife dies. [< L *soror* sister + -ate, suff.]. See **marriage**. Cf. **anilojuvenogamy, anisonogamia, dysonogamia, isonogamia, nomogamosis**, q.v.

soterial (sō-ter'ri-əl) adj. pertaining to salvation. [< L *soteria* salvation]. See **religion, theology, morality**.

soteriology (sō-ter"ri-ol'lə-jee) n. the Christian doctrine that salvation has been brought about by Jesus Christ. [< L *soter*, savior, deliverer, protector < *soteria* salvation; (a party for a person recovering from an illness) < G *soter* deliverer, savior—applied to Zeus, Poseidon, etc. + -logy, suff., study, science < G *logos* word, reason]. adj. **soteriologic**

(-ō-loj'jik), **soteriological** (-ō-loj'ji-kal). **See religion, theology, morality**.

sough (suf, sow) n. 1. a sighing, moaning, whistling, or rushing sound, as of the wind. 2. a vague rumor. 3. a religious chant. (4. a swamp). [< OE *swogan* < Old Saxon *swogan*, move with a rushing sound]. vi. **sough** 1. to sigh, as the wind sounds. 2. to breathe heavily. 3. used with *away*: to breathe one's last. 4. to preach in a whining tone. **sough** vi. 1. to hum, to chant. (2. to dig a drainage ditch). See **breathing**. See **emotion**. See **end-of-life**. See **religion, theology, morality**. See **talk**.

spavined (spayv'vind) adj. (1. suffering from spavin, a disease involving swelling of the hock joints in a horse.) 2. (fig.) old, over-the-hill; decrepit; broken-down, unfit—perhaps even having joint problems, e.g., **osteoarthritis**, q.v. [< ME < OF *espavain* swelling]. See: **old**. See: **health, illness**.

spermologer (spur-mol'lo-gər) n. one who gathers seeds. By extension (fig.), one who is a trivia-monger, a gatherer of gossip. [sperm(o)-, irregular pref. for sperm(o)-, male generative fluid < G *sperma* –*matos* seed, semen + -loger, suff., used to form personal nouns corresponding to words in –logy (but now is superseded by –logist) < -*logos* < *logos* word, reason < *lego* to speak]. Cf. **quidnunc**, q.v. See **talk**. See **role**.

sphallolalia (sfal"lō-layl'li-ə) n. flirtatious talk that does not lead to amorous action—perhaps due to **andropause**, q.v., or **medomalacophobia**, q.v., or **agapism**, q.v., etc. [< G *sphaleros* slippery, uncertain + -lalia, suff., speech, speech disorder < G *lalia* < *lalein* to talk]. See **talk**. See **mentality, mentation, behavior**. See **sex, love**.

spinal stenosis (spī'nəl sten-ōs'siss) n.phr. a narrowing of the spinal canal resulting in pressure on the sciatic nerve from bony encroachment with resultant claudication, aching pain, **sciatica**, q.v., i.e., pain running down the lateral thigh, lower leg; there may be associated low-back pain, also. Diagnosis can be confirmed by CT (computerized tomography) scan, or MRI (magnetic resonance imaging), but many asymptomatic elderly people have the pathologic changes of spinal stenosis on such imaging studies. (Another cause of spinal stenosis is a herniated vertebral disc.) [< L *spina* a thorn; the backbone, spine. < G, *stenosis* a narrowing]. See **joint, extremities, back**. See **pain**.

splenetic (sple-net'tik) adj. 1. of a person who is ill-tempered, peevish, irascible, spiteful. (2. of the spleen.) • That old gal is a *splenetic* if there ever was one. [< L *spleneticus* < *spleen* spleen]. n. **splenetic** = a bad-tempered or spiteful person. adv. **splenetically**. See **mentality, mentation, behavior**. See **role**.

spoffish (spof'fish) adj. (slang) upset at trifles; fussy; bustling [origin unk.]. See **mentation, mentality, behavior**.

spondyloarthropathy (spoon"di-lō-awr-thop'pe-thee) n. a general term for inflammatory disease of the joints of the spine. Ankylosing spondylitis, < G *ankylos* bent or crooked, is a form of spondyloarthropathy in which joint fusion occurs. [spondyl(o)-, a pref. denoting relationship to a vertebra or to the spinal column + < arthr(o)-, a comb. denoting a relationship to a joint(s) < G *arthron* joint + -pathy, suff., denoting a morbid condition or disease < G *-patheia* < *pathos* disease]. See **joint, extremities, back**.

spondylosis (spon"di-lōs'siss) n. a general term for degenerative changes due to osteoarthritis of the spine; stiffening or fixation (ankylosis) of a vertebral joint. Sometimes there is pain or paresthesia (morbid or perverted sensation) the location of which depends on the area of the spine that is affected. [< G *spondylos* vertebra + -osis, suff.]. See **joint, extremity, back**.

spry (sprī) (sprier or spryer, spryest or spriest) adj. 1. markedly brisk and active, especially at an advanced age. 2. said in reference to "any senior citizen who is not in a wheelchair or coma", as defined by John Leo's *Time* essay on "Journalese for the Lay Reader" < *Dickinson's Word Treasury*, Ch. 24, *Journalese*. [mid 18th C. <?]. adv. **spryly**. n. **spryness**. See **mentality, mentation, behavior**. See **work, activity**.

squamous (skwaym'mess) adj. covered with scales. • **Actinic keratosis**, q.v., results in *squamous* skin in sun-exposed areas. [< L *squamosu* covered with scales, scaly < *sqama* scale]. See **skin**.

squamous-cell carcinoma (skwaym'mess-sel kaar"sin-ōm'me) n.phr. Cancer that arises from malpighian cells (< Marcello Malpigi, It. anatomist {1628-1694}) known as keratinocytes, i.e., keratin-producing (horny) cells of the epidermis. There is a modest propensity to metastasize (spread to distant sites). Such cells may arise from **actinic keratoses**, q.v., or Bowen's disease (pre-cancerous dermatitis or dermatosis), and occur in sun-exposed areas, especially in fair-complected individuals. The lesions are erythematous (reddened), scaly; they become ulcerated and crusted. [< L *squamosu* covered with scales, scaly < *sqama* scale + < L *cella* cell. < G *karkinoma* < *karkinos* crab]. See **skin**.

squamulose (skwaym'yoo-lōss) adj. covered with minute scales. [< L *squamosus* covered with scales, scaly < *sqama* scale]. See **skin**.

squintifego   (skwin-ti-feeg'gō)/**squintefuego**   (skwin-tee-fway'gō) n. (obs. or rare) a person who squints a great deal. [< mid 16ᵗʰ C., shortening of *schuinte* <? Du *asuqinte* slope, slant +? -ifego, suff.]. See **eye**. See: **role**.

standing, walking, wandering: abasia, afforient, ambulophobia, **astasia, astasia-abasia, ataxia, basiphobia, basistasiphobia, basophobia, circumforaneous, claudicant, claudication, climacophobia, dinic, disequilibrium, divagate, dotty, double stance/double support, dwaible/dwaibly, dysbasia, dysdiadochokinesia, dysergia, dysmetria, dysstasia, dyssynergia, dystaxia, dystonia, ecdemomania, errabund, expatiate, maunder, noctivagant, noctivagation, obambulate, oberrate, oikofugic, oxter, planeticose, podalgia, pododynia, poriomania, Scamander, sedentarize, sessile, shamble, solivagant, stassibasiphobia, stasiphobia, surbate, surbater, tardigrade, tarsalgia, testudineous, titubation, totter, vertiginous, wamble**

standing, walking, wandering: Subcategories

I.   Balance, falling, climbing:
   1.   Altered   balance: derangement   of   balance:
        disequilibrium
   2.   Fear: morbid fear of climbing or falling down stairs:
        climacophobia
   3.   Unsteadiness: move unsteadily, stagger about:
        wamble
   4.   Walk unsteadily, wobble, be about to fall: **totter**
II.   Dizziness: **vertiginous, dinic**

III. Movement, moving:
    1. Slow: as slow-moving as a turtle: **testudineous**
    2. Difficulty in quickly moving a limb, hand in opposite directions:**dysdiadochokinesia**
    3. Slow-moving, sluggish: **tardigrade**
    4. Unable to arrest a muscular movement at a desired point: **dysmetria**
    5. Unstable, weak, shaky movement: **dwaible/dwaibly**
    4. Voluntary: lack of harmonious voluntary muscle movement: **dysergia**

IV. Muscles:
    1. Inability to stand or walk due to muscular incoordination: **astasia**
    2. Involuntary muscle contraction as in Parkinson's disease: **dystonia**
    3. Lack of harmonious voluntary muscle movement: **dysergia**
    4. Loss of muscular coordination: **ataxia, dyssynergia**
    5. Loss of tonicity in any of the tissues: **dystonia**
    6. Mild loss of muscular coordination: **dystaxia**
    7. Voluntary: lack of harmonious voluntary muscle movement: **dysergia**

V. Pain:
    1. Footsoreness: **podalgia, pododynia, tarsalgia**
    2. Intermittent leg pain: **claudication**
    3. Make or become footsore: **surbate**
    4. Re: limping, lameness, intermittent leg pain on walking: **claudicant**

VI. Role:
    1. Someone with intermittent leg pain on walking: **claudicant**

VII. Standing:
    1. Difficulty in standing: **dysstasia**
    2. Morbid fear of standing: **stasiphobia**
    3. Morbid fear of standing and walking: **stassibasiphobia**
    4. Time spent in walking when both feet are on the ground: **double stance/double support**
    5. Unable to stand or walk due to muscular incoordination: **astasia**
    6. Unable to stand or walk normally: **astasia-abasia**

VIII. Walking, gait:

1. Difficulty:
   a. difficulty walking: **dysbasia**
   b. inability to stand or walk normally: **astasia-abasia**
   c. limping or impaired gait due to pain: **claudication**
   d. shaky gait: **dotty**
   e. to walk or run awkwardly, decrepitly: **shamble**
   f. to walk unsteadily, wobble, be about to fall: **totter**
   g. unsteady, wobbling gait: **titubation**
2. Fear:
   a. morbid fear of standing and walking: **basistasiphobia**, **basiphobia/basophobia**, **stassibasiphobia**
   b. morbid fear of walking: **ambulophobia**
3. Inability:
   a. inability to stand or walk due to muscular incoordination: **astasia**
   b. inability to walk: **abasia**
   c. one who tires another with walking: **surbater**
4. Support:
   a. support with an arm another's walking: **oxter**.

IX. <u>Wandering</u>:
1. Compulsive wandering: **ecdemomania**.
2. Liking to wander—on foot or (fig.) in talking: **planeticose**
3. Losing one's way: **oberrate**
4. Not wandering, habituated to one a certain place: **sessile** 4. 5. Obsessive wandering: **oikofugic**
6. State of confusion, wandering: **afforient**
7. To stay put, take up residence after wandering: **sedentarize**
8. To wander or roam at will: **expatiate**
9. Wandering alone: **solivagant**
10. Wandering by night: **noctivagant**, **noctivagation**
11. Wandering from place to place; to and fro or about: **circumforaneous**, **divagate**, **errabund**, **maunder**, **Scamander**; **obambulate**
12. Wanderlust: **poriomania**

stasiphobia (stas"si-fōb'bi-ə) n. morbid fear of standing (for fear of falling). [< G *stasis* a standing still + phobos fear]. alt. **stasophobia** (stas"sō-). adj. **stasiphobic**. n. **stasiphobe**. syn. **basistasiphobia**, q.v. Cf. **stasibasiphobia**, q.v. See **phobias**. See **standing, walking, wandering**.

stasis dermatitis (stay'siss dur"mə-tī'tiss) n.phr. inflammation associated with venous hypertension in the lower legs. The skin there is eczematous (characterized by papules {small circumscribed, superficial, solid elevations of the skin} and vesicles {small sacs containing liquid}) and usually edematous (swollen), with hemosiderin (extravasated blood) pigmentation, and dilatation of superficial venules (little veins) around the ankles. It can be exacerbated by edema (swelling), scratching, and topical medication. [G, a standing still + derma-, pref., denoting relationship to the skin < *derma*, gen. *dermatos* skin + *-itis* inflammation]. syns. **gravitational eczema**, **varicose eczema**. See **skin**.

stassibasiphobia (stas"si-bay"si-fōb'bi-ə) n. morbid fear of standing and walking. [< G *stasis* a standing still + *basis* step + *phobos* fear]. alt. **stasobasiphobia** (stas"sō-). adj. **stassibasiphobic**. n. **stassibasiphobe** (-bay'si-). See **phobias**. See **standing, walking, wandering**.

staunch (stawnch) adj. firm in attitude, opinion, loyalty, dependability.
• His *staunch* behavior coincides with old age. [< OF *estanchier* to stop, dam up, make water tight]. adv. **staunchly**. n. **staunchness**. vt. **staunch/stanch** = check the flow of or from. See **mentality, mentation, behavior**.

steatopygous (stee"a-tō-pi'jəs) (stee'aa-top'pi-guss) adj. pertaining to or characterized by protuberant buttocks; fat-rumped. [steato-, pref., relating to fat < G *stear* (*steat-*) tallow, fat, grease + *pyge* buttocks]. n. **steatopygia** (stee'a-tō-pij'jee-ə) (stee-at"tə-pij'jee-ə) alt. **steatopyga** (-pī'jə). adj. **statopygic** (-pi'jik). adj. **steatopygous** (stee"ətə-pī'-gəss). See **physique, appearance**. See **joint, extremities, back**.

stereotypy (ster'ee-ə-tīp"pee, -ee-ō-tip"pee) n. a pattern of persistent, fixed, and repeated speech or movement that is apparently meaningless and characteristic of some mental conditions; monotonous repetition. [< stere-, stereo- (before vowels), pref., solid;

(three-dimensional) < G *stereos* solid + *tupos* blow, impression]. See **nerve, muscle, movement, touch**. See **talk**.

stertorous (stur'tawr-əss) adj. characterized by loud, rasping, inspiratory breathing or snoring. [< L *stertere* to snore + -or-, comb., + -ous, suff.]. adv. **stertorously**. n. **stertor** = loud snoring. n. **stertorousness**. Cf. **sonorous**, q.v. See **breathing**.

sthenobulia (sthen-ō-bool'li-ə) n. strong will power. [< G *sthenos* strength + *boule* will]. adj. **sthenobulic**. See **mentality, mentation, behavior**.

stomachous (stum'ə-kəs) adj. obstinate, angry. [< G *stomakhos* gullet < *stoma* mouth]. See **mentality, mentation, behavior**.

stormy petrel (stor'mee pet'trəl) n.phr. (1. any of various small sea birds of the family Hydrobatidae having dark feathers and lighter underparts, also known as Mother Carey's Chicken.) 2. One who brings trouble, or whose appearance is a sign of coming trouble. [The birds got the name *storm petrel* or *stormy petrel* because old-time sailors believed their appearance foreshadowed a storm. It's not certain why the bird is named petrel. (One unsubstantiated theory is that it is named after St. Peter who walked on water in the Gospel of Matthew. The petrel's habit of flying low over water with legs extended gives the appearance that it's walking on the water—Anu Garg.)]. See **role**.

stridulous (strid'yoo-ləss) adj. 1. making a creaking, shrill, or squeaky sound. 2. pertaining to stridor, a whistling during respiratory blockage. [< L *stridulus* < *strideo* to creak, to hiss < *stridor* shrill sound, hiss, shriek, scream, whine; harsh noise, grating, rattle, buzz]. n. **stridor** (strī'dər) = a high-pitched, noisy, sound due to airway obstruction, especially in the trachea or larynx. See **breathing**. See **talk**.

Struldbrug (stroold'broog) adj. 1. as applied recently, the term indicates the difficulties governmental social and medical programs encounter with the expense of providing continuing care to the decrepit elderly. 2. the equivocal benefit of social planners' frantic efforts to prolong life in the very old by increasingly restricting many of life's enjoyments such as eating "unhealthy" foods, smoking, imbibing alcohol, etc. (Meltzer, P.E.). 3. relating to the so-called "death panels" mandated in recently passed federal health-care legislation, i.e., measuring the cost of medical procedures, drugs vs. the life expectancy of prospective recipient patients. [The term is based on characters Gulliver met in Swift's "Gulliver's Travels" who, as they age, become increasingly sick, decrepit, "are opinionated, peevish, covetous, morose, vain, talkative", and are "incapable of friendship and dead to all natural affection, which never descended below their grandchildren." Struldbrugs live on wretchedly at the state's expense—they are immortal, but their minds are free of the apprehension of death]. n. **Struldbrug**, pl. **Struldbrugs**, an old, decrepit, shuffling person. See **QALYS**. See **old** man. See **old** woman. See **old person(s)**. See **end-of-life, death**.

stultiloquence (stul-til'lō-kwəns) n. foolish or senseless talk; idiotic babble; twaddle. [< L *stultiloquentia* silly talk < *stultus* foolish (literally immovable) + *loqui* to talk]. adv. **stultiloquently**. adj. **stultiloquent**. syns. **piffle**, **prattle**, q.v., **twaddle**. Cf. **delirament**, q.v. See **talk**.

Stygian (sti'jee-ən) adj. 1. of or relating to the River Styx. 2. gloomy and dark. 3. infernal, hellish. (4. totally binding or inviolable, as was an oath sworn beside the River Styx in Greek mythology.) (Styx {G, hate} was the daughter of Okeanos and Tethys who, having had innumerable children, presumably ran out of names and called their last daughter Styx. She, and her four sons, won Zeus's favor by supporting him in the war of the Titans {Titanomachia}. As a reward, Zeus granted Styx the largest river in Hades, and Zeus instituted the Stygian Oath there. It conferred immortality on those taking it—not taking the oath required drinking the River Styx's freezing-cold water, resulting in loss of one's spirit and voice, having to lie breathless for one year, and being denied the gods' ambrosia and nectar. Souls of the dead were required to cross the River Styx into Hades, or Tartarus, by being ferried across by the ferryman, Charon. A glittering gold coin, meant as payment to Charon, was inserted by relatives in a corpse's mouth. Those unfortunates without a coin would have to wander in Stygian darkness for eternity. Water from the Styx river conferred invaluable strength on those whom Styx permitted to be immersed in it. Achilles was one; his only bodily areas of vulnerability were his ankles held by his mother during his immersion. [via L *Stygius* < G *stugios* < *Stux-ugos* the Styx River (< G mythology: the river encompassing Hades)]. n. **Styx**, q.v. See **end-of-life, death**. See **color**.

stygiophobia (stīg"ee-ō-fō'bi-ə) n. morbid fear of hell. [< G *stugios* < *Stux-ugos* the Styx River (< G mythology: the river encompassing Hades or Tartarus) + -phobia, suff., fearing < G -*phobia* < *phobos* fear]. adj. **stygiophobic.** n. **stygiophobe.** Cf. **Hadephobia,** q.v. See **Stygian.** See **phobias.** See **religion, theology, morality.**

Styx (stikss) n. in Greek mythology, the river—one of five in Hades— the entrance to which was guarded by the three-headed dog, Cerberus, and across which the souls of the dead were ferried into the underworld, Hades. Lethe (lee'thee) was a river in Hades, the waters of which caused forgetfulness, oblivion. [< G *Stux-ugos*]. adj. **Stygian,** q.v. See **end-of-life, death.**

subintelligitur (sub"in-tel-ij'ji-tur) n. a subtle wording with meaning implied but not stated. [sub-, pref., under, below, beneath < L, under + *intellegere* to perceive, understand < *inter-* between + *legere* to choose, read]. See **talk.**

subvention (səb-vensh'ən) n. (formal) (1. a grant of money given by an official body, e.g., a government, especially to an institution of learning, study, or research.) 2. the giving of help, aid, or support, especially financial. [< LL *subventionem* < *sub-*, pref., under + *vent-*, pref., < *venire* to come + -ion, suff.] adj. **subventionary.** syns. allocation, allotment, annuity, appropriation, grant, subsidy. See **finance.** See **therapy.**

succorance {Br. = **succourance**} (suk'kər-ans) n. the state of needing assistance from another. • Such *succorance* resulted from his progressive **parkinsonism**, q.v. [< L *succurrere* run under < *currere* to run]. n. **succor** {Br. **succour**} = help given or somebody giving help. vt. **succor** = to give help, assistance. n. **succorer.** adj. **succorable.** adj. **succursal** (-kurs'səl) = providing subsidiary, additional, or limited support, or help as an offshoot or branch (usually used in relation to a chapel). (The adj. **succorless** = the state of being without help.) syn. **tendsome,** q.v. See **health, illness.** See **role.** See **finance.** See **therapy.**

sui juris (soŏ'ī' joŏ'riss) adj.phr. legally competent to manage one's own affairs or assume responsibility. [L, *sui* of one's own + *juris* right]. ant. *alieni juris*, q.v. See: **end-of-life, death.** See: **finance.** See **role.**

sulforaphane (sul-for'rə-fayne) n. a phytonutrient (plant nutrient) found in cruciferous vegetables such as broccoli, particularly, and cauliflower, Brussels sprouts, cabbage, and wallflower. Sulforaphane activates antioxidant pathways at the cellular level by activating antioxidant genes and enzymes to counteract free radicals of oxygen and thus raises the immune response. Free radicals are important in aging; the immune function tends to diminish in the elderly. In sulforaphane-treated elderly mice, the immune response equals that of young mice. [L, *sulfur, sulphur* sulfur + -phane, suff., a substance having the appearance or qualities of < G –*phanes*, suff., < *phainesthai* appear < *phainein* bring to light. (Cruciferous {< L –*cruc* cross + -*fer* bearer} vegetables—their four-petal flowers are cross shaped—have a sulfurous smell, unattractive to many.)]. See **therapy**.

sundowning (sun'down'ing) n. the exacerbation of confusion and disruptive behaviors at sundown, or early evening, in which agitation is prominent, e.g., as seen in aged patients with delirium. n. **sundowner** = 1. a patient with sundowning symptoms. (2. an alcoholic drink in the UK and S. Africa drunk at sundown.) See **mentality, mentation, behavior**. See **role**.

sunset clause n.phr. the collation indicates a date certain when a will's stipulations of a donor's intent will no longer prevail, e.g., when a funded foundation will go out of business, having accomplished its mission, rather than continuing indefinitely after a founder's death and being at risk of having its mission changed or distorted. See **end-of-life, death**. See **finance**.

superannuated (soop"pur-an'nyoo-ayt"təd). adj. 1. made obsolete; disqualified due to old age, past work or use. 2. retired and pensioned because of sickness or old age. [< super-, pref., of higher kind, or degree, expressing addition, in higher than the ordinary sense < L, over, beyond + *annus* year + -ed, suff., having, characterized by, like < OE -*ede* < -*od*, Gmc.]. vi. **superannuate** = become too old for a former activity. vt. **superannuate** = declare too old for work or use or continuance; dismiss or discard as too old; send into retirement with pension. n. **superannuation**. See **old age**. See **work, activity**. See **retirement**.

supercentenarian (soop"pur-sent"ten-ayr'ri-ən) n. one who is 110 or more years of age. The world's oldest supercentenarian—not surprisingly a woman—is Jeanne Calment of France, who died at age

122 in 1997; she is recognized by Guiness-World-Records standards. None has surpassed her as of Nov.24, 2012. The title has turned over 17 more times from 1997 to 24 July, 2010, according to a Wall Street Journal column of that date, but by then no one reached even 120 years. Currently, Nov. 24, 2112, the oldest-living person is Bessie Cooper of the U.S: 116 years; Jiroeman Kimura of Japan, 115 years of age, is the oldest living man. Nine documented women have lived to be older than the oldest documented man ever, Christian Mortensen of the U.S., who died at age 115 years, 252 days, in 1998. By 2010, the number of **centenarians**, q.v., in the U.S had increased 32% in just the preceding five years. The New England Supercentenarian Society, as of 2010, had enrolled 108 supercentenarians since 1997. [< super-, pref., of higher kind, or degree, expressing addition, in higher than the ordinary sense < L, over, beyond + *centum* "hundred" + -ian, suff., belonging to, coming from, being involved in, or being like something < *-ianus*, suff.]. Cf. (plural) **wellderly**, q.v. See **old man**. See **old woman**. See **role**.

supernal (soo-pur'nəl) adj. 1. celestial, heavenly, lofty. 2. of or coming from on high, the sky, heaven. [<L *supenus* heavenly < *super* over, above]. syn. **empyrean**, q.v. See **end-of-live, death**. See **religion, theology, morality**.

superseptuagenarian (soop"pə-sep-too"ə-jə-ner'ree-ən) n. someone over seventy. [< super-, pref., of higher kind or degree, expressing addition, in higher than the ordinary sense < L, over, beyond + *septuagenarius* (*septuageni* seventy each < *septuaginta* seventy + -ian, suff.)]. See **old man, old woman**.

sura (soor'raa) n. a leg's calf or *regio suralis* (sural region), i.e., the muscular swelling, made up chiefly by the bellies of the gastroconemius and soleus muscles, of the posterior portion of the leg below the knee. [L, calf of the leg]. adj. **sural**. n.phr. **nocturnal sural pain** = pain in the calf that awakens one from sleep and occurs particularly in older adults: a **charley** (or **charlie**) **horse**. adj. **sural**. See **pain**. See **joint, extremities, back**.

suralgia (soor-al'ji-ə) n. sural, i.e., calf, pain. [a neologism: < L **sura**, calf + -algia, suff., denoting a painful condition < G *algos* pain + -ia, suff.]. adj. **suralgic**. See **sura**. See **pain**. See **joint, extremities, back**.

surbate (sur'bayt) vt. (obs.) to make or become footsore. [< OF *surbatre* to beat excessively]. n. **surbate** = footsoreness. adj. **surbated**: said of feet that have become sore due to extensive walking. Cf. **podalgia, pododynia, tarsalgia**, q.v. See **standing, walking, wandering**. See **pain**. See **joint, extremities, back**.

surbater (sur-bay'tər) n. (obs.) someone who tires another person with walking. [See **surbate** + -er, suff.]. See **standing, walking, wandering**. See **role**. See **joint, extremities, back**.

surdity (sur'di-tee) n. deafness. [< L *surditas* < *surdus* deaf, unheard, silent, mute]. (n. **surd** = a voiceless consonant, as is the k̲ in k̲nife, the first m̲ in m̲nemonic, the t̲ in whis̲tle, the c̲ in c̲nemial (pertaining to the shin), etc.). See **ear, hearing**.

suspirious (sus-pir'ree-əss) adj. producing a long, audible breath; breathing heavily; sighing. [< L *suspirium* a deep breath, sigh < *suspirare* to sigh, heave a sigh]. See **breathing**.

susurration (soo-sur-ray'shən) n. an onomatopoeic word mimicking a whisper, a murmuring, a soft rustling or muttering sound. • Age had rendered her voice a mere *susurration*. [< L *susurrare* to whisper < *susurrus* whisper]. n. **susurrus** (soo-sur-əss) = **susurration**. n. *sussurator* [L], q.v. = a whisperer, a mutterer. adj. **susurrous** (soo'sur-roŏr-əss). adj. **susurrant** (soo'sur-ənt). vi. **susurrate** (soo'sur-ayt). n.phr. *susurrus aurium*, q.v. = a whisper in the ear. syn. v.i. **siffilate**, q.v. See **talk**. See **breathing**. See **role**.

swelp (swelp) n. a perennial complainer. [< liaising "So help (me God)."]. Cf. **grouse/grouser, quaddler**; **smellfungus, whinger**, q.v. See **role**. See **talk**.

swivet (swiv'vət) n. a state of anxiety, discomposure, or agitation. [unk.]. • It's not unusual for that **old duffer**, q.v., to be in a *swivet* about one thing or another. See **mentality, mentation, behavior**.

synoikismos (sin-oy-kiz'moss)/**synoikism** (-ki'zəm)/**synœcism** (sin'noy-si-z əm) n. to come together as one (usually applied to nations, states, or political subdivisions, but used fig. re: groups, persons.) • The two factions that had developed at the **gerontocomium**, q.v., finally achieved a *synoikismos* that seemed lasting. [G, *synoikismos* noun of action meaning to cause to dwell

with, to unite under one capital city in re: city states]. See **mentality,**
mentation, behavior.

T

"Senex bis puer." [L] (The old man is twice a child.)

tabes (tay'beez) n. wasting away. [L *tabes, -is* wasting, melting, decay,
dwindling, shrinking; decaying matter, rot; disease, pestilence]. vi. & vt.
tabefy (ta'bee-fī). n. **tabescence** (ta-bes'sens), q.v. adjs. **tabescent**
(tə-bes'ənt), **tabetic** (tə-bet'ik), **tabic** (ta'bik) **tabid** (ta'bid). See
physique, appearance.

tabescence (tə bes'ənz) n. the state of progressive wasting, withering
away, decay; becoming emaciated. • The tabescence he suffered
from terminal cancer was startling. [< L pres. p. of *tabescere* to begin
to decay, begin to melt away < *tabes* wasting, decay]. adj. **tabescent.**
See **physique, appearance.** See **health, illness.**

tabefaction (ta-bee-fak'shən) n. emaciation due to disease. [< L
tabefacere < *tabere* to waste away < *tabes* wasting, shrinking, decay,
melting + -faction, suff., forming nouns of action: making, producing <
L. *–faction-* < *fact-* pp. of *facere* to do, make]. See **health, illness.** See
physique, appearance.

tabefy (tab'ə-fī) vt. & vi. to waste away gradually. [< L *tabes* wasting,
shrinking, decay, melting < *tabere* to waste away, to melt away]. See
physique, appearance. See **health, illness.**

tachophobia (tak"ō-fō'bi-ə) n. morbid fear of speed. [tachy-, pref.,
rapid < G *tachys* quick, rapid + *phobos* fear]. adj. **tachyphobic.** n.
tachyphobe. See **phobias.**

tachyarrhythmia (tak"ki-ə-rith'mi-ə) n. any disturbance of the heart's
rhythm, regular or irregular, resulting in a heart rate over 100 beats
per minute at rest, in adults. [tachy-, pref., meaning rapid < G *tachys*
quick, rapid + *a-*, priv., + *rhythmos* rhythm]. See **heart, rhythm.**

tachycardia (tak"ki-kaar'di-ə) n. rapid beating of the heart, usually
at a rate greater than 100 beats/min. in adults; "heart hurry". [tachy-,

pref., meaning rapid < G *tachys* quick, rapid + *kardia* heart]. syns. **polycardia, tachysystole**. See **heart, rhythm**.

tachylogia (tak"ki-lōj'ji-ə) n. 1. rapid or voluble speech. 2. speech that tends to become more rapid until words run together into a grumble or mumble, as seen in parkinsonism. [tachy-, pref., meaning rapid < G *tachys* quick, rapid + *logos* word]. syn. **tachyphemia**, q.v., **tachylalia, tachyphasia, tachyphrasia**. See **talk**.

tachyphemia (ta"chi-fee'mi-ə) n. **tachylogia**, q.v. [tachy-, pref., meaning rapid < G *tachys* quick, rapid + *pheme* speech]. See **talk**.

taciturn (tas'si-turn) adj. 1. habitually saying very little. 2. reserved in speech. [< L *taciturnus* < *tacitus*, pp. of *tacere* to be silent]. n. **taciturnity** (-turn'ni-). adv. **taciturnly** (tas'si-). See **talk**. See **loneliness, solitude, silence**.

tai chi (tī chee')/*Tai Chi, T'ai Chi* /*tai chi chuan* (tī"chee-chwaan')/*Tai Chi Chuan*/ *T'ai Chi Ch'uan* n. a Chinese form of physical exercise characterized by a series of very slow and deliberate balletic body movements. • It's said that *tai chi* reduces the likelihood of falls, a serious problem in the elderly, by 55%. [mid 18th C. < Chinese, lit., extreme limit]. See **work, activity**.

taisch (tīsh) n. the phantom or apparition experienced by a living person who is about to die. [Gaelic folklore < Gaelic *taibsh* phantom]. See **end-of-life, death**.

talk: adianoeta, alieniloquence, alogism, amadelphous, ambagious, amphibology/amphiboly, anfractuous/anfractuosity, animadversion, aristarchian, asseverate, atrophic laryngitis, auricular, badinage, balbutient, balderdash, baragouin, battology, befuddle, bemuse, billingsgate, blateroon, blatherskite/ blatherskate, blether/blather, blithering, bradylogia, bradyphemia, braggadocio, breviloquent, bruit, burble, cacemphaton, cachinnation, *cacoethes loquendi*, cacology, calando, cantankerous, captious, catachresis, cataphasia, catarolysis, chivvy/chivy/chevy, commatic, commentitious, comploration, confabulation, conspue, contumelius, coprolalia, costive, crassilingual, crusty, cuggermugger, darraign, deblaterate, deipnosophist, delirament, Delphic, dicacity, dilogical, dittology, diversivolent, dixit, doctiloquent, *double entendre*/*double* *entente*, drimble/drumble, dulciloquy, dysarthria, dyseneia, dysfluency, dysgrammatism, dyslalia, dyslogia, dyslogistic, dysphasia/dysphrasia, dysphemia, dysphemism, dysphonia, dysprosody, dyssyllabia, dystimbria, echolalia, edipol, elder rap, embolalia, encephalophonic, *enfin*, epilegomenon, epiolatry, epizeuxis, equivoque, eristic, errabund, ethnophaulism, eulogy, eulogize, exaugurate, excoriate, execrate, execration, expatiate, explaterate, expostulate, fabulist, factious, faffle, fanfaronade, flannel, fremescent, fuddle, fustigate, gadzookary, galimatias, garrulous, gasconade, gerontiloquence, glossolalia, gnome, gnomic aorist, grouse, idiolalia, idioticon, importunate/ importune/importunity, imprecate, inaniloquence, ingeminate, insusurration, inveigh, ipsedixitism, jabberwocky, jactancy, jactitation, jeremiad, jobation, kompology, kvetch, laconicism/ laconism, lalochezia, lalorrhea, lamprophony, *lapsus linguae*, latrinalia, lector, lexaphasia, linguacious, lingual titubation (See titubation.), linsey-woolsey, logagnosia, logamnesia, loganamnosis, logaphasia, logasthenia, logoclonia, logodaedaly/ logodaelus, logokophosis, logomania, logomonomania, logoneurosis, logoneurotic. logopathy, logoplegia, logorati, logorrhea, logospasm, longiloquence, *lubricum linguae*, maffle, magniloquent, magpie, mataeology /mateology, maunderer, *megillah/ganz megillah*, moider, monepic, multiloquent, Munchausenism, Munchausen syndrome, mussitation, mythopoeic, natter, nominal aphasia, noodge/ nudzh/nudge, nuncupate, obganiation, objurgate, objurgator, obloquy, obmutescence, obnubilate, obtrude, omniloquence, onology, onomatomania, opprobrious, oppugn, pallid, palter, paralogize, paralogizer, paraphasia/paraphrasia, pathocryptia, pauciloquence, peccavi, Pecksniffian, periphrase/ periphrasis, perissology, persiflage, perspicacity, phatic, philopolemist, philosophastering, phonasthenia, Pickwickian, piffle, planeticose, platitudinarian, pleniloquence, pleonastic, polylogy, polyloquence, prate, prattle, prolix, psellism, psilology, psittacistic, quaddle, quaddler, querent, querier, querimony, querist, querulous, Quetcher, quizzacious, quodlibet, quodlibitarian, quonking, raillery, recriminate, recrimination, repine, rhetor, rhodomontade, sanctiloquent, scatology, schizophasia, schizothemia, screed, scurrility, scurrilous, sententious, sermocination, *sermunculus*, sialoquence, siffilate, sonorous, sough, spermologer, sphallolalia, stereotypy, stridulous, stultiloquence, subintelligitur, susurration, swelp, tachylogia, tachyphemia, taciturn, tautology, telepresence robots, tendentiousness, tergiversate, thersitical, thetic, thrasonical, tootlish, traduce, trumpery, twaddleize, vaticinate, verbal apraxia, verbiage, verbigeration, verbomania, verbose, vitilitigate, vituperate, voluble, waffle, waspish, wheeze, whinge, whinger, wolly, yammer, yatter, zoilism.

talk: Subcategories

I. Amount of talk (See also Duration of Speech, Talk below.):
    1. Increased:
        a. compulsion to talk: *cacoethes loquendi*
        b. talkative, loquacious, wordy; excessive talk; verbose, unnecessarily wordy; excessive & incoherent; talking about everything: **garrulous, lalorrhea, linguacious, logomania, logomonomania, multiloquent; perissology, pleniloquence, polylogy; prolix, verbiage, voluble; logorrhea, verbose, yammer; omniloquence**
    2. Decreased: **taciturn, obmutescence**
II. Content:
    1. Angered scolding: **objurgate**
    2. Coarse, abusive, foul, vituperative language: **billingsgate**
    3. Complaint, complain:
        a. whiney or peevish complaint; to whine: **querimony; noodge/nudzh/nudge**
        b. complain, complaining, grumble, grumble, fret, whine; complaining, peevishly finding fault: **kvetch, natter, quaddle, repine; querent, querulous, whinge, yammer**
        c. to complain self-servingly: **grouse**
        d. to pester, nag: **noodge/nudzh/nudge**
    4. Conversation characterized by playful, joking remarks: **badinage, persiflage**
    5. Criticism:
        a. censorious comment, adverse criticism: **animadversion**
        b. criticize angrily, attack violently or bitterly in words: **inveigh**

    c. criticize severely, censure, berate severely, rebuke: **fustigate**,   **excoriate**

    d. having or creating factions: **factious**

    e. long, tedious criticism,: **jobation**

    f. nagging, carping, destructive criticism: **zoilism**

    g. one who questions, or criticizes, doubts: **querier**

    h. trivial criticism, fault-finding, sophistical, carping, caviling: **captious**

6. Defamation: **obloquy**
7. Derogatory; unfavorable: **dysphemism**; **dyslogistic**
8. Detest, loathe, denounce: **execrate**
9. Dogmatic statement: **dixit**.
10. Emotional, non-informative language conveying feelings, sociability, good will: **phatic**
11. Flirtatious talk not leading to amorous action: **sphallolalia**
12. Foolish story; a raving: **delirament**
13. Full of aphorisms, maxims; pithy: **sententious**
14. Full of platitudes: **platitudinarian**
15. Good-humored ridicule: **raillery**
16. Guilt: **peccavi**
17. Hypocritically benevolent and of high moral principle: **Pecksniffian**
18. Imaginary or fabricated: **commentitious**
19. Invoke harm, evil, a curse upon someone: **imprecate**
20. Lamentation: **jeremiad**
21. Lacking in color, intensity, spirit: **pallid**
22 Light or teasing, good-natured talk, banter: **persiflage**, **badinage**.
23. Making up stories, sometimes fabulous, fantastic, and answers without regard to fact: **confabulation**, **Munchausenism, Munchausen syndrome**
24. Mental state characterized by invented language: **idiolalia**
25. Myth making: myth-making or things related to it: **mythopoeic**
26. Non-literal, meaningless, contrary: **Pickwickian**
27. Obscene talk: **scatology, scurrility**, **scurrilous**
28. Predict: **vaticinate**
29. Repetition, reiteration; repetitiousness:.

a. emphatic verbal repetition: **epizeuxis**
b. futile repetition in speech or writing: **battology**
c. general: **ingeminate**; **pleonastic**
d. involuntary, meaningless repetition of the same word: **cataphasia**
e. irritation by reiteration: **obganiation**
f. monotonously repeated speech (or movement): **stereotypy**
g. repeatedly reversing one's opinions: **tergiversate**
h. repeating another's words: **echolalia**
i. saying the same thing in different words: **tautology**
j. senseless reiteration of clichés, the same words: **verbigeration**

30. Scholarly or subtle argument: **quodlibet**
31. Scurrilous jest: **cacemphaton**
32. Secularize; desecrate: **exaugurate**
33. Settle an argument (at law): **darraign**
34. Speaking about the aged: **gerontiloquence**
35. Talk about many things: **polyloquence**
36. Talk foolishly, incoherently; senseless, empty, or pointless talk (or writing); talking nonsense; chatter; senseless, idle, and childish; to dither: **balderdash, flannel, moider**; **psilology**; **blether/blather, blithering, glossolalia, inaniloquence, jabberwocky, stultiloquence, trumpery**; **linsey-woolsey, onology, piffle, prate, *sermunculus*, waffle**; **prattle, tootlish, twaddleize**
37. Talk illogically: **paralogize**
38. Uncontrollable use of obscene language; talking dirty: **coprolalia, latrinalia**
39. Unwillingness to talk about (or believe in) one's illness: **pathocryptia**
40. Urge to do something: **chivvy/chivy/chevy**
41. Verbal legerdemain: **logodaedaly/ logodaelus**
42. Wailing, weeping together: **comploration**
43. Without a past tense to express a general truth: **gnomic aorist**
44. Whispered gossip: **cuggermugger**
45. Word misunderstanding or forgetfulness: **lexaphasia**

46. Word worship: **epiolatry**

III. Diction, elocution (not due to a speech defect):

1. Disturbed stress, pitch, rhythm of speech: **dysprosody**
2. Garbled diction, or incorrect, defective, or indistinct pronunciation; bad choice of words; improper use of words: **psellism; cacology; catachresis**
3. Slip of the tongue: *lapsus linguae, lubricum linguae*
4. Spoken clearly, loudly, deeply, sonorously: **lamprophony, sonorous**
5. Stammering: **balbutient, lingual titubation** (See **titubation**.)

IV. Duration of speech, talk:

1. Long: speak (or write) about a subject at great length; speak lengthily, babble or bubble; long winded, loquacious: **expatiate, explaterate**; **burble, deblaterate**; **longiloquence,** *megillah/ganz megillah*
2. Short: **laconicism/laconism, pauciloquence, breviloquent**
   a. having short phrases or sentences, brief: **commatic**
   b. reserved: **taciturn**

V. Form, using a form:

1. Added on to a speech: **epilegomenon** \
2. Admission of guilt: **peccavi**
3. Any racial pejorative: **ethnophaulism**
4. Consisting of one word or one-word sentences: **monepic**
5. Countercharge; controvert: **recriminate, recrimination; oppugn**
6. Declare orally, make an oral will: **nuncupate**
7. Detestation, loathing, denunciation: **execration, execrate**
8. Dialectical dictionary, i. e., used only in one region: **idioticon**
9. Diatribe, harangue, tirade: **screed**
10. Digression by a long reminiscence: **schizothemia**
11. Discourse done in vain, useless: **mataeology/ mateology**
12. High praise: **eulogy,** *eulogize*

13. Indicating the end, finish of a speech, talk, comment: *enfin*
14. Lamentation: **jeremiad**
15. Made up, confected stories—sometimes fabulous, fantastic—and answers without regard to fact: **confabulation, Munchausenism, Munchausen syndrome**
16. Maxim, aphorism, proverb: **gnome**
17. Mild oath or asseveration: **edipol**
18. Story, true or not, passed around: **bruit**
19. Trite, hackneyed saying, story, joke: **wheeze**

VI. Manner of speaking (See below: Pronunciation; Speech Disorder, also):

1. Bantering: **quizzacious**
2. Boasting, bragging, vainglorious talk, bluster, arrogant bravado, ostentatious talk: **braggadocio, fanfaronade, gasconade, jactancy, jactitation, kompology, rhodomontade, thrasonical**
3. Calculated to entrap or entangle: **captious**
4. Chat, chatter idly, rapidly: **natter, yatter**
5. Circumlocutory, circuitous, tortuous, twisting, winding: **ambagious, anfractuous/anfractuosity, periphrase/periphrasis**
6. Complain: **quaddle**
7. Confuse, perplex someone: **befuddle, fuddle, maffle**
8. Declared dogmatically, imposed arbitrarily; authoritative assertion as if factual: **thetic; ipsedixitism**
9. Disparage, abuse severely; attack critically, harshly, abusively: **traduce; vituperate**
10. Emotional release via cursing, talking dirty; cursing to relieve anxiety: **catarolysis; lalochezia**
11. Exaggeratedly solemn, pompous, dignified, using impressive words, boastful: **magniloquent**
12. Express disagreement, disapproval; reason or argue: **expostulate**
13. Extremely critical: **aristarchian**
14. Frequent hesitations, meaningless insertions in speech: **embolalia**
15. Gruff, curt, candid in speech: **crusty**
16. Impose one's opinions or oneself on others: **obtrude**

17. Improper use of words; bad choice of words: **catachresis; cacology**
18. Indistinct speech, speak indistinctly:
    a. growling, muttering speech: **fremescent**
    b. drone or mumble, babble, mutter: **drimble/ drumble, palter; maffle**
    c. grumble to oneself: **mussitation**
    d. garbled diction, or incorrect, defective speech, substitution of letter sounds, or indistinct pronunciation; **psellism**
19. Insolent: **contumelius**
20. Irritate by reiteration: **obganiation**
21. Looking for trouble, or an argument: **diversivolent**
22. Loud immoderate or convulsive laughter: **cachinnation**
23. Loudly verbally abusive, foul-mouthed, cursing: **thersitical**
24. Making insistent requests, often requiring immediate attention: **importunate/importune/importunity**
25. Morbid talkativeness: **verbomania**
26. Oracular: **Delphic**
27. Oral, word playfulness: **dicacity**
28. Questioning, and answering one's own questions: **sermocination**
29. Reads aloud to congregation usually from a Bible: **lector**
30. Scold angrily: **objurgate**
31. Scornful or reproachful words, talk: **opprobrious**
32. Sharp in retort: **waspish**
33. Sigh, sighing; whistling: **sough**
34. Silently imitating the lip movements of those speaking: **mussitation**
35. Slow or stiff to express opinion or to act: **costive**
36. Speaking solemnly or of sacred things: **sanctiloquent**
37. Speaking to, about, or among the elderly: **gerontiloquence**
38. Spraying saliva while speaking: **sialoquence**
39. Straying from the point, wandering:
    a. speaking discursively: **alieniloquence**

        b. erratic, random, wandering: **errabund**, liking to wander—on foot or (fig.) in talking: **planeticose**

40. Use of archaic words, expressions: **gadzookary**
41. Whispering or talking into the ear, insinuation; whisper, wheeze, hiss: **auricular**, **insusurration**; **siffilate**, **susurration**

VII. Meaning:

1. Ambiguity: **amphibology/amphiboly**, **Delphic**, **dilogical**
2. Double meaning: **cacemphaton**, **Delphic**, **dilogical**, **dittology**, *double entendre/double entente*, **equivoque**
3. Hidden meaning: **subintelligitur**
4. Illogical statement or thought: **alogism**
5. Implied meaning, meaning not stated: **adianoeta**
6. Insight, astuteness: **perspicacity**
7. Meaningless, unintelligible, garbled, gibberish: **baragouin**, **galimatias**; **glossolalia**; **psittacistic**, **schizophasia**, **wooly**
8. Pun: **equivoque**
9. Stupefy, bewilder, befuddle: **bemuse**.

VIII. Memory:

1. Obsession with trying to recall a forgotten words; names: **loganamnosis**, **onomatomania**
2. See the categorical headword <u>memory</u>.

IX. Pronunciation, quality of voice:

1. Breathe heavily: **sough**
2. Garbled diction, or incorrect, defective, or indistinct pronunciation; bad choice of words; improper use of words: **cacology**; **psellism**; **catachresis**
3. Hoarseness: **dysphonia**
4. Lack of speech ease, fluency: **dysfluency**
5. Last breath, breathe one's last: **sough**
6. Making a creaking, shrill, or squeaky sound: **stridulous**
7. Making a whistling expiratory sound while speaking: **wheeze**
8. Thick-tongued, indistinct: **crassilingual**
9. Weak or hoarse voice; abnormal voice production with enunciation too high, low, or loud; functional voice fatigue: **phonasthenia**

X. Role:
1. One who asks questions: **querier, querist**
2. One who complains: **quaddler, whinger**
3. One who complains constantly: **Quetcher**
4. One who complains perennially: **swelp**
5. One who composes fables, apologues: **fabulist**
6. One who draws illogical conclusions from a series of facts: **paralogizer**
7. One who grumbles, speaks incoherently, confusingly: **maunderer**
8. One who is a gossip-gatherer: **spermologer**
9. One who is a skilled dinner conversationalist: **deipnosophist**
10. One who is a trivia-monger: **spermologer**
11. One who is an incurable chatterer (fig., inf.): **magpie**
12. One who loves argument, controversy: **philopolemist, quodlibitarian**
13. One who merely talks: **rhetor**
14. One who scolds angrily: **objurgator**
15. One who talks constantly, a babbler, prater, motormouth: **blateroon**
16. One who talks loquacious nonsense: **blatherskite/ blatherskate**
17. One who wanders aimlessly in talking: **maunderer**
18. One who whispers gossip: **cuggermugger**
19. Those interested in or expert at words: **logorati**

XI. Sound volume:
1. Gradually decreasing sound volume and tempo: **calando**
2. Loud: **thersitical**.
3. Soft: speaking softly: **dulciloquy**
4. Variable: with abnormal voice production, i.e., enunciation too high, low, or functional voice fatigue: **phonasthenia**
5. Weak or hoarse voice: **phonasthenia** See herein: XIV Speed, 3.

XII. Speaking conditions:
1. Side-line chatter disturbing to a speaker: **quonking**

XIII. Speech disorder, abnormality, defect, aphasia:
1. Any neurosis associated with a speech defect: **logoneurosis, logoneurotic**

2. Auditory inability to comprehend speech: **logokophosis**
3. Central* difficulty in speech articulation due to lack of muscle control: **dysarthria**
4. Central* impaired speech due to incoordination and failure of word-arrangement: **dysphasia/dysphrasia**
5. Central* impairment of grammatical speech: **dysgrammatism**
6. Central* impairment of speech power: **dyslogia**
7. Central* inability to comprehend speech: **logasthenia**
8. Central*inability to speak: **logagnosia**
9. Central* inability to speak or write: **logaphasia**
10. Central* inability to understand speech or its written or tactile symbols: **logamnesia**
11. Central* speech disorder, in general: **logopathy**
12. Defective use of the names of objects: **nominal aphasia**
13. Difficulty in initiating speech and articulation errors: **verbal apraxia**
14. Difficulty in speech articulation due to a hearing abnormality: **dyseneia**
15. Disturbance of speech's stress, pitch, and rhythm: **dysprosody**
16. Emotionally caused disorder of phonation, articulation, or hearing: **dysphemia**
17. Impaired reasoning ability: **dyslogia**
18. Impairment of speech due to structural abnormality of the auditory organ: **dyslalia**
19. Impairment of or defect in vocal quality or resonance: **dystimbria**
20. Laryngitis due to old age: **atrophic laryngitis**
21. Paralysis of the speech organs: **logoplegia**
22. Partial aphasia (speech defect) in which wrong words are used in wrong and/or senseless combinations: **paraphasia/paraphrasia**
23. Refers to hearing talking, noise, voices in one's head: **encephalophonic**
24. Spasmodic repetition of the final syllables of words: **logoclonia**
25. Spasmodic talking, speech: **logospasm**

26. Stuttering, stammering: **faffle**, **lingual titubation** (See **titubation**.), **balbutient**
27. Syllable stumbling: **dyssyllabia**
* originating in the central nervous system, the brain, i.e., aphasia

XIV. Speed:

1. Gradually decreasing sound volume and tempo: **calando**
2. Rapid, or increasingly rapid, speech: **tachylogia**, **tachyphemia**
3. Slow: **bradylogia**, **bradyphemia**
   See herein: XI Sound Volume, 5.

XV. Style:

1. Argumentative, controversial, quarrelsome, disputatious: **eristic**
2. Attack, abuse: **vituperate**
3. Authoritative assertion, factual or not: **ipsedixitism**
4. Bantering: **quizzacious**
5. Befog, confuse: **obnubilate**
6. Engrossing talk: **elder rap**
7. Gregarious, sociable, talkative: **amadelphous**
8. Having and promoting a particular viewpoint or ideology: **tendentiousness**
9. Lacking in color, intensity, spirit: **pallid**
10. Preach in a whining tone: **sough**
11. Prejudiced speech: **ethnophaulism**
12. Pseudo-philosophizing: **philosophastering**
13. Quarrelsome, bad tempered, perverse: **cantankerous**, **vitilitigate**
15. Robotic: **telepresence robots**
16. Speaking learnedly: **doctiloquent**
17. Spurn contemptuously: **conspue**
18. State earnestly or solemnly: **asseverate**

Re: auditory difficulty related to talk, speech, see Category: <u>ear, hearing</u>.

taphephobia (taf''fee-fōb'bi-ə) n. morbid fear of being buried alive; fear of cemeteries. [< G *taphos* grave + *phobos* fear]. adj.

taphephobic. n. **taphephobe**. alt. **taphophobia**. See <u>phobias</u>. See <u>end-of-life, death</u>.

taphophilia (taf"fō-fil'li-ə) n. love of funerals. [<G *taphos* grave + *philos* love < *phileo* to love]. n. **taphophile**. adj. **taphophilic**. See <u>end-of-life, death</u>. See <u>role</u>.

tardigrade (taar'di-grayd) adj. slow-moving, sluggish. [< L *tardare* to slow down, delay, hinder; to go slow, take it easy + *gradus* step, pace, walk, gait]. See <u>standing, walking, wandering</u>. See <u>mentality, mentation, behavior</u>.

tarsalgia (taar-sal'jee-ə) n. pain in the foot. [tars(o)-, pref., denoting relationship to the instep, the tarsus, (or edge of the eyelid) < G *tarsos* a flat surface, sole of the foot (or edge of the eyelid) + *algos* pain]. Syns. **podalgia**, **pododynia**, q.v. See <u>standing, walking, wandering</u>. See <u>pain</u>. See <u>joint, extremities, back</u>.

Tartarus (taar'-tər-əss) n. in G mythology, either Hades (underworld, hell, HELL < Hades, god of the underworld) in general, or the place there where the worst evildoers were imprisoned. [< G *Tartaros* hell]. See <u>end-of-life, death</u>.

tautegorical (taw-tə-gor'ri'kəl) adj. saying the same thing, but in different words—the opposite of allegorical. [< tauto-, pref., the same, identical < G *t'auto* the same thing < *to* the + *autos* same + *agoreuein* to speak in public]. See <u>talk</u>.

tautology (taw-tol'lə-jee), pl. **–gies** n. 1. saying the same thing in different words, especially as a stylistic fault; redundancy. ● Lapsing easily into *tautology* seems to be a further impairment of ageing (= aging). 2. an instance of redundant repetition. 3. a proposition that, in itself, is logically true. [tauto-, pref., the same, identical < G *t'auto* the same thing < *to* the + *autos* same + -logy, suff., speech < G *–logia* < *-logos* speaking]. adj. **tautological** (-loj'ji-). adj. **tautologic** (-loj'ik). adj. **tautologous** (-tol'lə-gəss). adv. **tautologically** (-loj'ji-). adv. **tautologously** (-tol'lə-). n. **tautologist**. syn. **pleonasm**, q.v. See <u>talk</u>. See <u>role</u>.

taxophobia (taks"sō-fōb'bi-ə) n. morbid fear of taxes. ● *Taxophobia* is characteristic of elders living on a fixed income. [13th C via F *taxer* <

L *taxare* to censure; assess < *tangere* to touch]. adj. **taxophobic**. n. **taxophobe** (taks'sŏ-). See **phobias**.

technophobia (tek"nō-fōb'bi-ə) n. morbid fear of computers or high technology. [< G *techne* an art + *phobos* fear]. adj. **technophobic**. n. **technophobe**. See **phobias**. See **innovation, misoneism**.

Teiresias/*Teiresias*/Tiresias (tī-rees'si-əss) a mythological Theban seer who, having seen Athena bathing, was blinded by her, but Athena, in compensation, gave him the gift of prophecy. In Sophocles's "Oedipus the King", Teiresias is portrayed as an old prophet who tries to shield Oedipus from his parentage and past history, hence fig., Teiresias = an old wise prophet. See **old man**.

telamnesia (tel"lam-neez'zi-ə, -zhə) n. poor memory for events long past. [< tele-, pref., distant, operating at a distance < G *tele* far away + a-, priv., not, without < G *a-*, *an-* not, without + *mneme* memory]. Cf. **mneme**. ant. **paleomnesia**, q.v. See **memory**.

telepresence robots (tel'lee-prez"zənss rōb'botss) n.phr. robots that augment human users, mainly the old and infirm, by enhancing their senses, such as vision, hearing, and face recognition. The robots are on wheels and contain a computer, keyboard, and joy stick that control their movement, stereophonic "hearing", and a camera on the monitor, so Skype-like monitoring between users is possible. Doctors can communicate with patients using the robot, and medical devices such as electronic stethoscopes, otoscopes, and ultrasound can be employed for patient examination. Thus, from anywhere with a computer and a Wi-Fi connection the operator can use the robot to hear, talk, see, be seen, and move around a distant location. Telerobotics enables seniors to remain independent longer, stay in contact with family and friends, and to visit museums and theaters. One such anthropomorphic robot, from Vgo Communications, is nicknamed "Celia". (Telerobots currently cost $5,000-$15,000.) [< G *tele-*, pref., distant, operating at a distance, + < L *praesentia* < -*praesent*-, comb. pres.p. of *praeesse* be in front of < *esse* be + early 20th C. via Ger. < Czech < *robota* forced labor (coined by Karel Čapek in his play *R.U.R.* (Rossum's Universal Robots) in 1920]. n. **telerobotics** (tel'ee-rō-bot'tikss). See **ear, hearing**. See **eye**. See **talk**. See **therapy**.

telomere (tel'lō-meer) n. DNA sequences at either free end of eukaryotic (nuclear in contrast to cytoplasmic) chromosomes, which sequences shorten as humans age. One key to longevity is having telomeres that shorten more slowly, on average, than those of other people. Multivitamins taken daily are said to result in telomeres 5.1% longer, on average, than those of non-vitamin users. Vitamins C and E seem to be involved, but the role of other vitamins is currently uncertain. There is an association between multivitamin dosing and telomeric behavior, but not proof so far of a cause-and-effect relationship. The telomere is just one of apparently many factors contributing to ageing. Low levels of telomerase, an enzyme, leads to erosion of telomeres. In recent experiments with prematurely-aged mice, an estrogen-based drug introduced into them was used to switch on the mice's dormant telomerase gene called TERT. This procedure led to their rejuvenation—the first instance of this ever happening—in terms of their telomeres lengthening, smell sense returning, new neuron formation resulting in better brain function, and their return of fertility. Trying the technique on normal-age mice to see if they live longer is the next experimental step. A telomere-length test is being developed to allow individuals to estimate their longevity and perhaps make lifestyle changes that would increase live expectancy. [< tele-, pref., connoting distant, operating at a distance < G *tele* far away + -mere, suff., denoting a segment or a part < G *meros* part]. adj. **telomeric**. See **old age**.

tendsome (tend'sum) adj. (obs.) requiring much attendance, being attended to [? < L *attendere* reach toward < *tendere* to stretch + -some, suff., characterized by a particular quality, condition, or thing, < OE *sum*; cited in *Webster*, 1847 & 1864, & *Century Dictionary*, 1891]. Cf. **succorance**, q.v. See **health, illness**. See **therapy**.

tendentious (ten-den'shəs) /**tendencious/tendential** (-shəl) adj. having a particular tendency or viewpoint; promoting a particular viewpoint, cause, or ideology to which one is partial. • His *tendentiousness* was off putting to many of the other residents of the retirement home. [early 20th C. < tendency < L *tendentia* < *tendere* to tend, be inclined to]. adv. **tendentiously**. adv. **tendentially** (-den'shal-lee). n. **tendentiousness**. See **talk**.

tenebrous (ten'nə-brəss) adj. dark, gloomy. • Entering the old **fuddy-duddy's**, q.v., dark and gloomy quarters awakened **revenant**, q.v., thoughts of his grandmother's *tenebrous* surroundings. [<

L *tenebrosus* < *tenebrae* darkness]. See **color**. See **mentality, mentation, behavior**.

tergiversate (ter-giv'vur-sayt) vi. to keep reversing one's opinions, attitudes, principles, causes, theories, religious preference, etc.

• When the elderly woman vacillated, she was criticized for her *tergiversation*, but she quoted Ralph Waldo Emerson saying: "A foolish consistency is the hobgoblin of little minds . . ." [< L *tergiversare* to turn one's back < *tergum* back + *versatus*, pp. of *versare* to turn about often < *vertere* to turn]. n. **tergiversation** (-giv"ver-say'shen) = double-talk. adj. **tergiversatory** (-se-taw"ee). n. **tergiversator** (-say"tawr) or **tergiversant** (-sant/sent). See **talk**. See **role**.

termagant (tur'me-gent) (hist. **Termagant**) n. 1. a brawling, bullying, or overbearing woman, a schrew, a scold, a virago. 2. an offensive term that deliberately insults a woman's temperament suggesting a propensity for arguing, criticizing, and quarreling. (3. an imaginary deity of violent and turbulent character, often appearing in mortality plays.) [13th C. ME *Tervagant* < OF *Tervagan* (in *Chanson de Roland*), an overbearing non-Christian deity supposedly worshipped by the Saracens and figuring in medieval mystery plays of the 15th & 16th Cs. His dress in flowing robes led the public to mistake him for a turbulent female. < It *Trivigante*]. n. **termagancy**. adj. **termagant** = boisterous, turbulent, schrewish. adv. **termagantly**. syns. & Cf. **catamaran, rixatrix, rounceval, virago, Xanthippe**, q.v. See **old woman**.

tessera hospitalis (tes-ser'ra hos-pi-taal'liss) n.phr. a square tablet, which was divided as a tally or token between two friends in order that they, or their descendants, might thereby ever afterwards recognize each other. [L, *tessera* a chequer, tally, token; cube; die; watchword, countersign; ticket + *hospitalis* host's, guest's; hospitable]. See **togetherness**.

testate (tess'tayt) adj. having made a legally valid will. [< L *testatus*, pp. of *testari* bear witness, make one's will < L *testis* witness—testis, pl. testes, = male paired reproductive organs, so named because of "bearing witness" to a man's virility]. n. **testacy** = being testate. ant. **intestate**, q.v. See **testator** (-tay'tawr). See **testatrix** (-tay'trikss). See **finance**. See **end-of-life, death**. See **role**.

testator (tes'stay"tər/tawr, tes-tay'tər/tawr) n. someone, especially a man, who has made a legally valid will. [< L *testatus*, pp. of *testari* bear witness, make one's will < *testis* witness + -or, suff., somebody who performs < L -(*at*)or]. See **finance**. See **role**.

testatrix (tes'tay"triks, tes-tay'triks) a woman who has made a legally valid will. [< L *testatus*, pp. of *testari* bear witness, make a will < *testis* witness + -trix, suff., a woman who performs a particular function < L fem. form of -(*at*)or]. See **role**. See **finance**.

testudineous (tes"stoo-din'nee-əss) adj. 1. as slow-moving as a turtle, tortoise. (2. curved like a tortoise shell; vaulted.) [< L *testudo* tortoise]. adj. **testudinate** (-stoo'-din-). n. **testudinarian** (-din-air'ee-ən) = one who is as slow moving as a turtle. See **standing, walking, wandering**. See **role**.

tetchy (tech'ee) **-i-er**, **-i-est** adj. easily upset or annoyed, oversensitive. [probably < F *tache* blemish, defect]. adv. **tetchily**. n. **tetchiness**. See **mentality, mentation, behavior**.

tetnit (tet'nit) n. a child born of elderly parents. [Slang. Possibly tetnit is derivative of **teknonymic**, the name of the offspring used in identifying the parent, e.g., *Odysseus*, who is well known, can be a teknonymic used to identify the less known *Laërtes*, his father. (**teknonymy** = naming, or the practice of naming, the parent after the child.)]. See **youth, younger generation**. See **role**.

thanatoid (than'nə-toyd) adj. death-like, deadly. [< G *thanatos* death + -oid, suff., like, resembling, related to < G *oeides* < *eidos* form, shape]. See **end-of-life, death**.

thanatology (than"nə-tol'lə-jee) n. the study of the medical, psychological, and sociological aspects of death and the ways in which people deal with it. ("Death is not an event in life."—Ludwig Wittgenstein.) [< G *thanatos* death + *logos* word, reason, study]. n. **thanatologist**. adj. **thanatological** (-tō-loj'ji-kəl). See **end-of-life, death**. See **role**.

thanatomania (than"nə-tō-may'ni-ə) n. abnormal interest in, preoccupation with, death. [< G *thanatos* death + *mania* frenzy]. adj. **thanatomaniacal** (-mə-nī'ə-kəl), q.v. n. **thanatomaniac**. Cf. **thanatophobia**, q.v. See **manias**. See **end-of-life, death**.

thanatophobia (than"nə-tō-fōb'bi-ə) n. a morbid fear of death. [< G *thanatos* death + *phobos* fear]. adj. **thanatophobic**. n. **thanatophobe** (-nat'tŏ-). See **phobias**. See **end-of-life, death**.

thanatopsis (than-ə-tŏp'siss) n. a musing on or contemplation of death. (Joseph Stalin (1879-1953), the Russian communist dictator who caused countless deaths infamously said, "One death is a tragedy, a million is a statistic." [< G *thanatos* death + *-opsis* appearance, view]. See **end-of-live, death**.

thegosis (theeg'gō-siss) n. Grinding of teeth as a means of sharpening them. Cf. **bruxism**, q.v. [< G *thegos* to sharpen]. See **mouth, gums, teeth**.

theophobia (thee"ŏ-fōb'bi-ə) n. morbid fear of God, the gods, or the wrath of God. [theo-, pref., relating to God < G *theos* god + *phobos* fear]. adj. **theophobic**. n. **theophobe**. syn. **thanatophobia**, q.v. Cf. **deisidaimonia**, q.v. See **phobias**. See **religion, theology, morality**.

therapy: acopic, aesthetics/esthetics, anatripsis, apocatastasis/apokatastasis, Aricept®, balneal, balneology, bots, cannabanoids, capromorelin, carminative, catholicon, CCRC, chiropodist, chiropody, clyster, clysterize, demulcent, dinic, dolorifuge, donepezil hydrochloride (HCL), effleurage, embrocation, emollient, epulotic, euthermia, Exelon®Patch, exungulate, gelotripsy, geriatric care manager/geriatric case manager, gerocomical, gerontocomium, gerontogenes, gerontotherapeutics, gerontologist, gerontology, gray tech, hartshorn, holagogue, illinition, insanable, laparoscopy, malactic, Medea's cauldron/caldron, neopharmaphobia, nepenthe, neuraminidase inhibitors, nostologist, nostology, orthosis, orthotic, palliative, panacea, panpharmacon, Paro, pharmacomania, pharmacophobia, phrontifugic, physagogue, podiatrist, podiatry, polypharmacy, prevenient, probiotic, prosthesis, prosthodontics/prosthodontia, QALYS, Rember®, retinol, resveratrol, rhytidectomy, rhytidoplasty, roborant, robotic surgery, *Schlimmbesserung*, sclerotherapy, -scopy, subvention, succursal, sulforaphane, telepresence robots, tendsome, tripsis, tutelage, tutelary, viparious, walking speed, xeniatrophobia.

therapy: Subcategories

I. <u>In General</u>:
1. A formula for deciding the worthiness of treatment: **QALYS**
2. A form of Care: **tutelage**
3. Care giver: **geriatric care manager/geriatric case manager**, **CCRC**, **tutelary**
4. Effective treatment:
    a. state of being restored or saved: **apocatastasis/apokatastasis**
5. Fear of therapy:
    a. morbid fear of going to a new doctor. **xeniatrophobia**
6. Giving of help, aid, support, especially financial: **subvention**
7. Medicine or drugs: morbid fear of medicine or drugs: **pharmacophobia**
8. Morbid fear of new medicine or drugs: **neopharmaphobia**
9. Providing subsidiary help, support: **succursal**
10. Robotic: **telepresence robots**
11. Use of many drugs: **polypharmacy**

II. <u>General therapy</u>:
1. All purpose medicine: **panpharmacon**, **catholicon**
2. Cure-all removing all trace of a disease: **holagogue**, **panacea**
3. Having healing power: **epulotic**
4. "Improvement" that makes things worse: ***Schlimmbesserung***
5. Improves lean body mass and physical functioning: **capromorelin**
6. Incurable: **insanable**
7. Institution for care of the aged, nursing home: **gerontocomium**.
8. Large metal pot containing a putative rejuvenating potion: **Medea's cauldron/caldron**
9. Life-restoring, -renewing: **viparious**
10. Predictive of the need for physical activity, diagnostic evaluation: **walking speed**.
11. Prophylactic, coming before, anticipatory: **prevenient**
12. Requiring considerable attention: **tendsome**

III. <u>Ignoring, casting off cares and thoughts</u>: **phrontifugic**.
IV. <u>Science & treatment of the aged</u>:

    1 Medical study and treatment of the aged: **gerontology, nostology**

    2. Robotic "caregivers": **bots**

    3. Science of treating the aged: **gerontotherapeutics**

    4. Treatment of the aged: **gerocomical, gray tech**

V.   Suffix:

    1. Examining for possible treatment: **-scopy**

VI. Symptomatic treatment: **palliative, hartshorn**

VII. Uncontrolled desire to take or administer medication: **pharmacomania, polypharmacy**

VIII. In Particular:

    1. Alzheimer's treatment: anti-Alzheimer's disease drugs: **Aricept®, donepezil hydrochloride(HCl), Exelon®Patch, Rember®**

    2. A stimulant for fainting: **hartshorn**

    3. A treatment for dementia: **Paro**

    4. Injecting a chemical into a vein to destroy it: **sclerotherapy**

    5. Re: a remedy for dizziness: **dinic**

IX. Artificial body part: **prosthesis**

X.   Baths:

    1. Of baths and bathing: **balneal**

    2. Study and practice of using baths and bathing in treatment: **balneology**

XI. Cicatrisation & healing: **epulotic**

XII. Computer-controlled surgery: **robotic surgery**

XIII. Doctors:

    1. Cares for the elderly: **gerontologist, nostologist**

    2. Foot doctor: **chiropodist, podiatrist**

    3. Scientific study and treatment of the elderly: **gerontology, nostology**

    4. Study and practice of foot doctoring: **chiropody, podiatry**

XIV. Drugs, therapeutic agents:

    1. Drugs for treatment of influenza: **neuraminidase inhibitors**

    2. Enema, injection into the rectum: **clyster**.

    3. Grief -relieving agent: cures or alleviates grief: **dolorifuge**

    4. Heat induction: **euthermia**

    5. Longevity agents: **resveratrol, gerontogenes**

6. Nausea, anorexia; pain; decrease or eliminate narcotic use: **cannabanoids**
7. Prevention and treatment of flatus and farting: **carminative**, **physagogue**, **probiotic**
8. Refreshing, invigorating drug, physical agent: **roborant**
9. Softening, soothing or something doing this **demulcent**, **emollient**, **malactic**
10. Tranquilizer: **nepenthe**
11. Treat with enemas or injections into the rectum: **clysterize**
12. Treatment for relieving flatulence, constipation: **probiotic**
13. Wrinkle prevention: **retinol**

XV. False-teeth dentistry: dentistry using false teeth: **prosthodontics/prosthodontia**

XVI. Immune response: improves the immune response: **sulforaphane**.

XVII. Massage:
1. liquid used for rubbing and lubricating the body: **embrocation**
2. nerve-point massage; rubbing away tenderness due to neuralgia: **gelotripsy**
3. rubbing +/- lubricating as therapy; gentle rubbing as therapy; rubbing and lubricating as therapy; rubbing with liniment, massage: **anatripsis**; **effleurage**; **embrocation**; **illinition**, **tripsis** (See **gelotripsy** above.)

XVIII. Nails: trim, cut or cut off the nails (or hooves): **exungulate**

XIX. Orthopedic device: orthopedic appliance or apparatus: **orthosis** (pertaining to an orthosis, orthopedic appliance: **orthotic**)

XX. Scoping:
1. Computer-controlled endoscopic surgery: **robotic surgery**
2. Insertion of an examining endoscope into the abdomen's interior for examination and possible surgery: **laparoscopy**

XXI. Surgery:
1. computer-controlled endoscopic surgery: **robotic surgery**
2. plastic surgery, etc.: **aesthetics/esthetics**

3. surgical removal of wrinkles: **rhytidectomy**. **rhytidoplasty**
XXII. Tiredness: relieving tiredness: **acopic**
XXIII. Wrinkle prevention: **retinol**

thersitical (ther-sit'ti-kəl) adj. verbally abusive, loud and foul-mouthed; hurling curses. [<Thersites in Homer's Iliad: At the siege of Troy, Thersites (thur-sī'teess) was an ill-tongued G soldier notorious for his very loud-mouthed ugliness]. See **talk**.

thetic (the'tik) adj. 1. declared dogmatically; imposed arbitrarily. (2. relating to or having stress in classical poetry.) [< G *theticos* < *thetos* placed, stressed < *tithenai* to place]. adj. **thetical**. adv. **thetically**. Cf. **apodictic**, q.v. Cf. **ipsedixitism**, q.v. See **talk**.

thewless (thyoo'les) adj. 1. lacking bodily strength; without vigor or spirit. (2. cowardly; timid.) • Old age rendered him *thewless*. [< thew— usually pl.: thews, i.e. sinews, muscles; muscular strength; fig., mental or moral vigor—< OE *theaw* = OS *thau*, OHG *dau* usage, custom + -less, suff., free from, devoid of < OE *leas*, adv.]. See **tiredness, weakness**.

thixotropy training (thik-sot'trōp-pee) n.phr. inspiratory-muscle training for patients with COPD (chronic obstructive pulmonary disease) in order to improve their respiratory effort and oxygenation. (Thixotropy itself is the property exhibited by certain gels of becoming fluid when shaken or stirred, and then becoming semi-solid again at rest.) [< G *thixis* touch + *tropos* a turning]. alt. **thixotropism**. adj. **thixotropic** (-ō-trop'pik). See **therapy**. See **breathing**.

thrasonical (thra-son'i-kəl) adj. boastful, bragging, blustering, puffed up, overweening; self-congratulatory. [< L *Thraso*—< G *Trasonos*—the braggart soldier in *"Eunuchus"* (the Eunuch), a comedy by the Roman playwright Terence (c.190-c.159 B.C.)]. adv. **thrasonically**. syns. **braggadocio, fanfaronade, gasconade, rodomontade**, q.v. See **talk**.

thrombophilia (throm"bō-fil'lee-ə) n. a tendency to the occurrence of a hypercoagulable state, thrombosis, i.e., clotting of the blood. • *Thrombophilias*, which are often associated with thrombotic events, are usually acquired rather than inherited in the elderly. [< thrombo-, pref., meaning relationship to a clot or thrombus < G *thrombos* clot + < G *philein* to love]. See **blood, circulation, glands**.

tilmus (til'muss, -məss) n. floccillation, or picking at bedclothes, as may occur in the course of a severe fever; a sign that a person is approaching death. [< G *tilmos* plucking, tearing < *tillein* to pluck, tear]. syns. **carphology/carphologia, crocidismus, floccilegium, floccillation**, q.v. See **mentality, mentation, behavior**. See **end-of-life, death**.

tinnitus (tin-nīt'tuss, -təss) n. perception of a sound in one or both ears without an external stimulus; it may be objective or subjective; it results most commonly from hearing loss. [L, a jingling < *tinnio*, pp. of *tinnitus* to jingle, click]. alt. **tinnitus aurium**, whidh is in contrast to **tinnitus cerebri**, a subjective sensation of noise in the head. See **ear**.

tiredness, weakness: *abus de faiblesse*, **acopic, amyous, asthenia, asthenophobia, atony, attenuate, caducity, decrepit, decrepitude, delassation,** *éboulement*, **effete, elumbated, enervate, epicene, exinanition, forfoughen, forjesket/forjeskit, inanition, jacent, kopophobia, labefaction, labent, languescent, languid, languish, languorous, lassipedes, lentor, moribund, nazzard, recubation, senium, thewless, torpid, wan**.

tiredness, weakness: Subcategories

tiredness

I.   Becoming faint or tired: **languescent**.
II. Exhausted:
    1. Due to lack of food or water as a result of disease: **inanition**
    2. Morbid fear of exhaustion, overwork: **kopophobia**
    3. Tired out; extreme fatigue: **forfoughen**; **exinanition**
III. Fatigue, tiredness, lethargy, worn out:
    1. Fatigue: **delassation, wan**
    2. Lacking in vitality, strength; worn out, spent, lethargic: **effete, epicene, languid, thewless**; **torpid**
    3. Sluggishness: **lentor**
    4. Worn out, extremely tired; worn out, old, and in poor working order: **forjesket/forjeskit, decrepitude**

IV. Old age & its detriments:
1. Exploiting frailty, weakness of the aged: *abus de faiblesse*
2. Old age with its detriments: **senium**
3. The condition of being old, undergoing hardship due to deprivation: **languid**
V. Relief:
1. Relieving tiredness: **acopic**
VI. Tired Feet: **lassipedes**
VII. Recumbent; lying down on one's back: **jacent**; **recubation**

weakness

I. Feeble or insignificant person: **nazzard**
II. Fear of weakness: **asthenophobia**
II. In poor condition, old, not working efficiently: **decrepit**
III. Loss of strength, vitality:
1. Crumbling of a wall, or of physical strength: *éboulement*
2. Decline steadily in vitality, strength, success: **languish**
3. Decrepitude, feebleness, weakness of old age; droopiness: **caducity**
4. Lazily or pleasantly lacking vigor, vitality: **languorous**
5. Listless, slow moving, sluggish, indifferent, sullen: **languorous**
6. Loss of strength, weakness: **amyous**, **asthenia**, **thewless**. without strength; lack of muscular tone, strength; abnormally relaxed: **atony**
7. Make thin, weaken: make thin, slender; make less strong, weaken: **attenuate**
8. Recumbent: **jacent**
9. Weak: **wan**
10. Weak in the loins (the back between thorax and pelvis: *lumbus*) **elumbated**
IV. Near death, having lost all purpose or vitality, ineffective: **moribund**
V. Old age with its detriments: **senium**
VI. Slipping, falling: **labent**
VII. Weaken:
1. To weaken, take energy away from: **enervate**

　　　　2.　Weakening, undermining, overthrowing, especially morally: **labefaction**

titubation (tit-yoo-bay'shen) n. an unsteady, lurching, staggering, tottering, or stumbling gate, sometimes with shaking of the head and trunk, and due especially to neurologic, particularly cerebellar, disease or disorder. **lingual titubation** = stammering, stuttering. [< L *titubo*, pp. of *titubatus* to stagger]. adj. **titubant** (tit'yoo-bent). See **standing, walking, wandering**. See **talk**.

togetherness: commensal, commorant, commorient, comploration, compotation, contesseration, contubernial, *tessera hospitalis*, tontine.

togetherness: Subcategories

I.　Drinking:
　　1.　Drinking together: **compotation**
II.　Dying:
　　1.　Dying together: **commorient**
III.　Friendship:
　　1.　Making friends:
　　　　a.　as attested by a shared token of friendship: **contesseration**
　　2.　Pertaining to companionship: **contubernial**
　　3.　Something divided between two friends in attestation of their friendship: *tessera hospitalis*
　　4.　The act of making friends: **contesseration**
IV.　Living:
　　1.　Living and eating together: **commensal**
　　2.　Living together familiarly: **contubernial**
V.　Residing:
　　1.　A fellow resident: **commorant**
VI.　Survivor reward:
　　1.　Something of value owned by a group, but ultimately owned by the last surviving member: **tontine**
VII.　Sorrowing:
　　1.　Wailing and weeping together: **comploration**

TOMM40 n. a gene linked to APOE—See **ApoE4**. Individuals with a large number of extra copies—the "long repeat" version of TOMM40—coupled with ApoE3 develop Alzheimer's disease several years earlier—around age 70—compared to individuals with a "short repeat" version of TOMM40. See **Alzheimer's disease**. See **intelligence**.

tomophobia (tōm'mō-fōb'bi-ə) n. morbid fear of surgery. [< G *tomos* cutting + *phobos* fear]. adj. **tomophobic**. n. **tomophobe**. See **phobias**.

tontine (ton-teen') n. originally an investment or insurance or annuity scheme in which contributors pay equal amounts into a common fund, after which it is closed to new investors. Contributors receive equal dividends and benefits from it, with the final surviving contributor receiving everything. By extension, something of value, e.g. a bottle of precious liquor, a painting, etc., can be the prize won by the survivor. [F, < Lorenzo *Tonti*, a Neapolitan banker, who originated the tontine in France c. 1653]. See **togetherness**.

tootlish (toot'lish) adj. childish; muttering, babbling unintelligibly, as a senile old person might do; tooting in a gentle, continuous manner— toot, v.i., = make sound in short blasts. [Du or LG *tuten* < a Gmc. echoic base—tootling = pr.p. (freq. of toot); tootle = v.i.)]. vi. **tootle** = to mutter incoherently or like a child. See **talk**.

toper (tōp'pər) n. (arch., lit., or inf.) a heavy and habitual drinker of alcoholic beverages. [mid-17th C.?]. v.i. **tope** (**toped**, **toping**, **topes**) to drink liquor heavily and habitually. See **role**. See **drink, food**.

tophaceous (tō-fay'shəss) adj. hard or gritty; of the nature of or characterized by a **tophus**, q.v. [L *tophaceus* < *tophus* porous stone]. See **health, illness**. See **joint, extremities, back**.

tophus (tō'fus), pl. **tophi**, n. a chalky deposit of sodium urate occurring in gout. Tophi form most often around joints in cartilage, bone, bursae, and subcutaneous tissue; in the external ear, they produce a chronic, foreign-body, inflammatory response. [L, porous stone]. See **health, illness**. See **joint, extremities, back**.

torpid (tawrp'pid) adj. 1. sluggish and inactive, lacking physical energy; lethargic. 2. in a dormant state. 3. of a part of the body that is numb. [< L *torpere* to be stiff].

n. **torpidity** (-pid'di-tee). n. **torpor**. n. **torpidness**. adv. **torpidly**. See **tiredness, weakness**. See **nerve, muscle, movement, touch**.

Torschlusspanik (tor'schloos-pən"nik) n. a sense of panic brought on by the feeling that life is passing one by. [Ger. < *Tor* door + *Schluss* closing + *Panik* panic < the G god *Pan*, known for causing terror]. See **mentality, mentation, behavior**.

totter (tot'tər) vi. 1. to stand or walk unsteadily; wobble as if about to fall. 2. ({fig.} be shaken, unstable, on the point of falling, e.g., a state, system, etc.) [13th C. <?]. n. **totterer**. adj. **tottery**. adv. **totteringly**. See: **standing, walking, wandering**. See **role**.

tracasserie (traкasri) n. a sense of annoyance. • To his surprise, the **beldam**, q.v., quoted, "Life seems to me empty of all but *tracasseries*."—A citation in the OED from 1879. [F, < *tracasser* to worry, bother oneself]. See **mentality, mentation, behavior**.

traditionaliste (tradisjɔnalist) nm.&f. a conservative. [F, traditionalist]. adj. ***traditionaliste*** = conservative. See **role**.

traduce (trə-dooss') vt. to say very critical or disparaging things about someone, to abuse someone. • Seniors are the most traduced, i.e., abused, mistreated group, in America. [< L *traducere* convert, transfer, scorn, disgrace < *trans-* across, over + *ducere* to lead]. syns. abuse, calumniate, castigate, rail, revile. n. **traducement**. n. **traducer**. adj. **traducible**. Cf. slander. See **talk**. See **mentality, mentation, behavior**. See **role**.

tralatitious (tral-ə-tish'us) adj. traditional, handed down from one generation to the next. [< L *tralaticius* customary]. See **past, time**.

tremor (trem'mor or treem'mor) n. an involuntary trembling or quivering. One division of tremor is into involuntary and volitional types, but numerous special tremors exist, e.g., arsenic ~, coarse ~, essential ~, familial ~, passive ~, senile ~, etc., and the intriguing opiophagorum (ō"pi-ō-fə-gō'rəm) ~ that is found in opium users. • A senile *tremor* is one resulting from the infirmities of age. [< L *trememe* to shake]. See **nerve, muscle, movement, touch**.

tresayle (tres'sayl) n. a great-great-grandfather or grandfather's grandfather. [< OF *trei(s)* < L *tres* three + -ayle < F *aïeul* grandfather]. Cf. **quatrayle**, q.v., quintrayle. (The number of "grates" = one less than the number of "-ayles".) See **role**.

tripsis (trip'siss) n. 1. massage, rub down. (2. trituration: grinding into a powder.) [G, a rubbing]. See **therapy**.

troglodyte (trog'lō-dīt, -lə-dīt) n. (1. a cave dweller, especially one belonging to a prehistoric cave-dwelling community.) 2. (fig.) a person living in seclusion; a hermit; a recluse. [< G *troglodutes* < *trogle* cave + *duo* enter]. adj. **troglodytic(al)** (trog'lō-dit'tik{-əl}). See **loneliness, solitude, silence**. See **role**.

trophic (trōf'fik) adj. of or pertaining to nutrition. [< G *trophikos* nourishing]. suff., **–trophic, -trophin**. Cf. **dystrophic**, q.v. See **drink, food**.

tropophobia (trō"pō-fōb'bi-ə) n. morbid fear of making changes. [< tropo-, pref., 1. turning, change. 2. tropism < G *trope* turn (from the ancient belief that the sun "turned back" at the tropics of Cancer and Capricorn) + *phobos* fear]. adj. **tropophobic**. n. **tropophobe**. Cf. **centophobia**, **kaino(to)phobia** or **caino(to)phobia**, **neophobia**, q.v. See **phobias**. See **innovation, misoneism**.

truculent (truk'yə-lənt) adj. 1. aggressively or sullenly refusing to accept something or do what is asked. 2. displaying great anger or aggression. 3. pugnacious. (The current connotation is a mitigated, less harsh one even compared to the Concise Oxford 1929 ed.: "Of or showing bellicose aggressive merciless temper.") [< L *truculentus* savage, grim, fierce, cruel < *trux* savage, grim, fierce, wild]. adv. **truculently**. n. **truculence**. n. **truculency**. See **mentality, mentation, behavior**.

trumpery (trum'pə-ree) n. nonsense, gibberish, twaddle, rubbish, junk.
• The old cogger's *trumpery* was disregarded. [< LME *trompery* deceit < MF *tromerie* < *tromper* to deceive]. adj. **trumpery** = worthless, trashy, showy. See **talk**. See **physique, appearance**.

trypanophobia (tri-pan"nō-fōb'bi-ə) n. morbid fear of injections or inoculations. [< G *trypanon* an auger (a hand tool with a corkscrew-shaped bit for boring holes) + *phobos* fear]. (Note: A trypanocide is an agent for killing trypanosomes, parasites that can infect humans, cause sleeping sickness, and have a corkscrew-like motion, but have nothing to do with trypanophobia, although the word would seem to be applicable.) adj. **trypanophobic**. n. **trypanophobe**. See **phobias**. See **health, illness**.

tutelage (toot'tə-lij, toot'lij, tyoot'lij) n. 1. instruction and guidance provided by someone such as a tutor; guardianship. 2. the condition of being supervised or protected by a tutor or guardian. (3. the condition of being a tutor.) [< L *tutela* guardianship < *tut-* pp. of *tueri* to watch over]. See **health, illness**. See **therapy**.

tutelary (toot'tə-lair-ee, tyoo'-) adj. 1. acting in the role of a protector or guardian. 2. relating to or belonging to a guardian. [< L *tutelarius* < *tutela* guardianship < *tut-* pp. of *tueri* to watch over]. n. **tutelary**, pl. **–ies**, (lit.) a tutelary being, guardian or protector, especially a saint or deity. See **health, illness**. See **therapy**. See **role**.

twaddleize (twod'dəl-īz) vt. to speak or write twaddle; to talk in a silly or pretentious manner, or to prattle, gabble about something, someone. [late 18ᵗʰ C. <?]. vi. **twaddle**. n. **twaddle**. n. **twaddler**. adj. **twaddly**. See **talk**. See **role**.

twichild/twychild (twī'chel) n. 1. an elderly man or woman. 2. a **dotard**, q.v., or someone who has lost mental sharpness and is approaching or in "a second childhood", dotage. [< "twice a child", < *twy* twice, & inspired by Shakespeare's description in *As You Like It* of the concluding stage of the "seven ages" of man: "Last scene of all,/ That ends this strange eventful history,/ Is second childishness, and mere oblivion,/ Sans teeth, sans eyes, sans taste, sans everything." In *Paradise Regained* John Milton concludes with "The child is father of the man." Jeffrey Kacirk]. See **old man**. See **old woman**.

tyloma (tī-lō'mə, -maa) n. See **clavus**.

typhlology (ti-fol'lə-jee, -lō-jee) n. the scientific knowledge relating to blindness. [< G *typhlos* blind + -logy, suff., science of < *logos* word, reason]. See **eye**.

U

"Anyone who stops learning is old, whether at twenty or eighty. Anyone who keeps learning stays young. The greatest thing in life is to keep your mind young."
—Henry Ford

ubiation (yoo-bee-ay'shən) n. the act of occupying a new place. • The *ubiation* of living in a **geriatric center**, q.v., was unsettling. [< L *ubi* where + -ation, suff., an action or process or the result of it < L *-ation-*, forming nouns from verbs in *-are*]. Cf. n. **ubication** = the condition of being in a certain place; n. **ubity** (yoo'bi-tee) = place; n. **ubiety** (yoo-bī'ə-tee) = placement, position, locale; being in a certain place. See **retirement**.

ubication (too-bee-kay'shən) n. See **ubiation**.

ubiquarian (yoo-bi-kwair'ee-ən) n. a person who goes everywhere. [< L *ubique* everywhere < *ubi* where + -ian, suff., belonging to, coming from, being involved in, or being like something, directly; or via F *-ien*, < L *-ianus* or *-anus*]. See **mentality, mentation, behavior**.

umbratile (um'brə-til) adj. spent inside or indoors; private, not public. [< L *umbratilis* remaining in the shade; private; retired. Or < *umbraticus* too fond of the shade, lazy]. n. **umbratile** = 1. a person who spends his time indoors. (2. a person who spends his time in the shade—with the connotation of lazy.) • The pallor of the **gerontocomium's**, q.v., *umbrtatiles* could be arresting. See **mentality, mentation, behavior**. See **role**.

umbrageous (um-bray'jəss) adj. (1. creating or providing shade.) 2. easily offended; inclined to be irritated or take umbrage for little cause. [< L *umbratus*, pp. of *umbrare* to shade or overshadow < *umbra* shade]. adv. **umbrageously**. n. **umbrageousness**. n. **umbrage** (um'brij) = a feeling of offence, resentment, and annoyance; usually used with take: to take umbrage. See **mentality, mentation, behavior**.

unwitting (un-wit'ting) adj. 1. unaware of what is happening in a particular situation. 2. said or done unintentionally. [< OE *unwitende* < pres.p. of *witan* become aware of, learn]. See **mentality, mentation, behavior**.

uratic arthritis (yoo-rat'tik aar-thrīt'tiss) n.phr. gouty **arthritis**, q.v. (Primary gout affects mainly middle-aged men and post-menopausal women.) [< urate, a salt of uric acid, < L *urina* urine + < G arthr(o)-, pref., q.v., + -itis, suff., inflammation < G *-ites*, suff., inflammation]. See **joint, extremities, back**. See **health, illness**.

urceolate (ur'see-ə-lit, ō-layt, ə-layt, -ō-lit) adj. pitcher shaped: swollen at the bottom and contracted at the upper part. ● Her shape became increasingly *urceolate* with old age. [< L *urceolus*, dim. of *urceus* pitcher + -ate, suff.]. See **physique, appearance**.

urethremphraxis (yoo-reeth"rem-frak'siss) n. obstruction from any cause to the free flow of urine through the urethra, e.g. from benign prostatic hypertrophy. [urethr(o)-, pref., denoting urethra < G *ourethra* urethra + *emphraxis* a stoppage]. See **genitourinary**.

urination (yoo"ri-nay'shən) n. the discharge or passage of urine; pissing (an offensive term); peeing (indelicate); voiding. [< L *urina* < G *ouron* urine]. n.phr. **precipitant urination** = a sudden and strong, urgent desire to urinate. n.phr. **stuttering urination** = an intermittent flow of urine due to vesicle (urinary bladder) spasm, due to, e.g., prostatic obstruction, bladder infection, etc. See **genitourinary**.

uropathy (yoo"rop'pə-thee) n. any affliction involving the urinary tract. [uro-, pref., relating to urine < G *ouron* urine + *pathos* suffering]. See **genitourinary**.

usufruct (yooz'zə-frukt, yoos'sə-frukt) n. the legal right to use and enjoy the advantages or profits of another's property—the property owner is legally termed the "**naked owner**". [< L *usufructus*, variant of *ususfructus* use (and) enjoyment < *usus* pp. of *uti* to use + *fructus* enjoyment]. See **finance**.

usufructuary (yooz'zə-fruk'choo-air-ee, yoos'sə-), pl. = **-ies**, n. a person who is entitled by usufruct, i.e., legally, to the use and enjoyment of another's property. [< L *usufructus*, variant of *ususfructus* use (and) enjoyment < *usus* pp. of *uti* to use + *fructus* enjoyment + -ary, suff.]. adj. **usufructuary**. See **finance**. See **role**.

UVA & UVB rays (rayz) n.phr. ultraviolet A rays are those sun's rays that are primarily responsible for wrinkling and ageing of the skin. Both ultraviolet A and B rays can cause wrinkling and skin cancer, but UVB rays primarily cause sunburn. New sun-protection-factor (SPF) labeling, required by the Food and Drug Administration in 2012, indicates protection against both types of ultraviolet rays. Dermatologists recommend an SPF of at least 30. See **skin**.

uveitis (yoo-vee-ī'tiss) n. inflammation of the uvea, i.e., the middle coat (uveal tract) of the eyeball; the uvea consists of the iris, ciliary body, and choroid. [< L *uva* grape + < G -*itis*, suff., inflammation]. See **eye**.

V

Senectus insanabilis morbus est. [L] (Old age is an incurable disease.)

vade mecum (vaa'day may'kum) n.phr. handbook or other thing carried constantly about the person. [L, go with me]. Cf. **enchiridion**, q.v. See **mentality, mentation, behavior**.

vagarious (və-gair'ree-uss) adj. erratic and unpredictable in behavior or direction. [< L *vagari* to wander]. See **mentality, mentation, behavior**.

vagary (vay'gə-ree), pl. -ries., n. an unpredictable or eccentric change, action, or idea. [< L *vagari* to wander]. See **mentality, mentation, behavior**.

valetudinarianism (val"lə-too-dən-air'ree-ən-iz"zəm) n. a weak, sickly, or convalescent state; thinking only of one's illness; tendency to hypochondria. [< L *valetudinarius* in ill health, sickly < *valetudo* state of health; good or ill health; illness < *valere* to be well]. n. **valetudinarian/valetudinary** (-tood'-) someone with chronic ill health; an invalid; someone obsessed with his/her own health; a hypochondriac. (In contrast to hypochondriacs, and those with **Munchausen syndrome**, q.v.—a chronic factitious disorder with physical symptoms—valetudinarians do have something physically wrong with them.) adj. **valetudinarian** (or **valetudinary** (-tood'dən-). See **health, illness**. See **role**.

Valhalla or **Walhalla/Walhal** (val-hal'lə, vaal-haal'lə/vaal-hal') pn. in Norse mythology, the great hall where the souls of heroes killed in battle spend eternity. The word can be used fig. [late 17th C. via modern L < ON *valhall* hall of the slain < *valr* those slain in battle]. See **end-of-life, death**.

vaticinate (va-tis'si-nayt) vt. & vi. to predict events; speak as a prophet—chiefly ironical or connoting contempt. [< L *vaticinatio* prophesying; prediction, soothsaying < *vaticinatus*, pp. of *vaticinari* to prophesy; a *vaticinator* = a prophet. (The papal palace, the Vatican, gets its name from Vatican Hill, the home of the Roman *vaticanitores*, soothsayers)]. adj. **vaticinant** = prophesying. adj. **vatic** (va'-tik) or **vaticinal** = prophetic, oracular, inspired. n. **vaticinator** = a prophet. See <u>talk</u>. See <u>role</u>.

vecordious (ve-kor'di-əs) adj. (rare) mad, obsessive, senseless: the general sense is of folly, dotage rather than insanity. [< L *vecordia* < *vecors* senseless, foolish + -ous, suff., full of, having the qualities of, characterized by < L -*osus* abounding in]. n. **vecordy** (vek'kor-dee). See **mentality, mentation, behavior**.

veilleuse (vɛjøz) n. 1. a small and highly decorated nightlight, lamp. 2. a bedside food warmer. (3. an automobile sidelight. 4. a pilot light as on a water heater.) [F]. See **sleep**.

velitation (vel-i-tay'shən) n. (arch.) a minor conflict, slight skirmish, controversy. • In nursing homes, such *velitations* between residents are not unusual. [< L *velitatio* skirmishing < *velitari* to skirmish < *veles* light-armed foot soldier]. See **mentality, mentation, behavior**. See **work, activity**.

venerable (ven'nər-ə-bəl) adj. 1. worthy of respect as a result of great age, wisdom, remarkable achievement, or similar qualities. 2. revered for qualities such as great age or holiness. 3. extremely old. 4. used by the Roman Catholic church to describe somebody who has died and attained the first of three degrees of canonization. (5. used as a title to describe an archdeacon in the Church of England.) [< L *venerabilis* < *venerari* < *vener-*, stem of *venus* love, desire]. adj. **venerability** (ven"ner-ə-bil'li-tee). adv. **venerably**. vt. **venerate**. n. **veneration** (ven"ner-ay'shən). See <u>old</u>.

venous ulcer n.phr. cutaneous ulceration resulting from venous insufficiency: incompetent superficial and perforator veins, and post-phlebitic syndrome, i.e., complications associated with deep vein thrombosis, which are caused by greatly increased pressure in the deep and communicating veins, and characterized by persistent edema (swelling), pain, purpura and increased cutaneous pigmentation, eczematoid dermatitis, pruritus (itching), ulceration, and indurated cellulitis. [< L *vena* vein and < L *ulcus* < G *helkosis* ulcer]. See **skin**.

ventoseness (ven-tōss'nəss) n. windiness; (fig.) puffed up, pompously conceited, bombastic; (arch.) flatulence. [< L *ventosa*, f. of *ventosus* windy, full of wind; of the wind, wind-like < *ventus* wind + -ness, suff.]. adj. **ventose** (ven'tōss) = prone to vain, empty talk. (n. *ventouse*, F, a cupping glass.) See **talk**. See **gastrointestinal**.

ventricous/ventricose (ven'trə-koss/ -kōss) adj. 1. swelling out, especially on one side, or one direction, or unequally; protuberant. 2. big-bellied; abdominous; having a protruding belly. [< L *venter* paunch; protuberance; womb; appetite, gluttony + –ose or -ous, suffs., both forming adjs. meaning abounding in, characterized by, & both < L –*osus* abounding in]. syn. = **abdominous**, q.v. See **physique, appearance**. See **gastrointestinal**.

ventripotent (ven-trip'pə-tent, -pō-) adj. taking a greedy delight in eating. [< L *venter* paunch; protuberance; womb; appetite, gluttony + *potens*, pres.p. of *posse* to be able]. adv. **ventripotently**. See **drink, food**.

verbal apraxia (vur'bəl ay-praks'si-ə) n.phr. a type of speech disorder characterized by difficulty in initiating speech and inconsistent articulation errors. The cause is lesions, damage in the parieto-occipital (side-back) area of the brain. Cf. **aphasia**, **dysarthria**, q.v. See **talk**.

verbiage (vur'bee-ij) n. 1. an excess of words, especially in writing or speech with little or no meaning. 2. the style of language in which something is expressed. [< L *verbum* word]. syn. **verbosity**, **verboseness**, q.v. See **talk**.

verbigeration (vər-bij"jər-ay'shən) n. senseless, meaningless reiteration of clichés; repetition of the same words or phrases; if done obsessively, it can be a symptom of a psychiatric disorder. [< L *verbigerat-*, pp. of *verbigerare* to chat, talk < *verbum* word + *gerare* keep carrying on + -ation, suff.]. vi. **verbigerate**. n. **verbigerator**. syns. **battology, obganiation**, q.v. See **talk**. See **role**.

verbomania (vurb"bō-mayn'ni-ə) n. morbid talkativeness; a psychotic flow of speech. [< L *verbum* word + < G *mania* frenzy]. adj.

verbomaniacal (–mə-nī'ə-kəl). n. **verbomaniac**. See **logomania**. See **manias**. See **talk**.

verbose (vər-bōs') adj. expressed in or using excessive or too complicated words. [< L *verbosus* < *verbum* word]. n. **verbosity** (-bos'i-tee). adv. **verbosely**. n. **verboseness**. See **talk**.

verjuice (vur'joos) n. 1. ({lit.} the sour, acidic juice of unripe fruits, especially that of crab apples and grapes.) 2. (fig.) sourness of temperament. ● *Verjuice* is the hallmark of a **curmudgeon**, q.v., (N.W. Schur). [ME < OF *verjus* < *vert* green + *jus* juice]. adj. **verjuice** = sourness of temperament, disposition, or expression; bitter feelings, thoughts; attitude. See **mentality, mentation, behavior**.

versute (vər-soot') adj. crafty, wily. ● The old professor of Greek was as *versute* as Odysseus. [L *versute* (adv.) cunningly]. adv. **versutely**. n. **versuteness**. See **mentality, mentation, behavior**.

vertiginous (vər-tij'in-əs) adj. revolving, dizzy, suffering from vertigo; vacillating, inconsistent; causing dizziness; unstable, suddenly changing. [L *vertigo* turning, whirling, dizziness < *vertere* to turn, turn around + -ous, suff., full of, having the qualities of < L -*osus* & -*us*]. n. **vertigo** (vur'ti-gō). adv. **vertiginously**. Cf. **vortiginous**, q.v. See **standing, walking, wandering**.

vetust (vee-tust') adj. old, ancient, antique. [< L *vetustus* old; ancient, old times, old-fashioned; good-old-days; antiquated]. See **old**.

veuf (vœf) n.m. widower; *veuve* (vœv) n.f. widow. [F]. adj.m. *veuf* (vœf) widowed; adj.f. *veuve* (vœv) widowed; (fig.) bereft, deprived. See **marriage**. See **role**.

veuvage (vœvaʒ) n.m. widowhood or widowerhood. [F]. adj. syns. (widowhood only) **viduage** (vid"u'age), **viduation** (vid"u-ay'shən), **seneucia**, q.v. See **marriage**.

veuve (vœv) n.f. widow. (Swedish divers exploring a shipwreck off the Finnish coast in 2010 found several bottles of Veuve Clicquot, the most venerable and prized champagne. The bottles dated back to the early 1800s and were said to be more than drinkable.) [F]. See **marriage**. See **role**.

viaggiatory (vee-aj'ji-ə-tawr'ee) adj. traveling frequently, given to traveling about. [< It *viaggiare* to travel]. See **work, activity**.

viaticum (vī-at'ti-kum) n. 1. communion (Eucharist) given to someone dying; a portable altar. 2. provisions for a trip. 3. state expense account; money for a journey; travel allowance. [< L *viaticus* (adj.) for a trip, for traveling, travel. (n.) travel allowance, provisions for the journey < *via* way]. pl.n. **viatica/viaticals** = baggage. See **end-of-life, death**. See **work, activity**. See **religion, theology, morality**.

vibrissa (vī-bris'sə), pl. **vibrissae** (-ī/-ee) n. a bristle, hair, as in the nostril—growing in the anterior nares (vestibulum nasi)—or as a cat's whisker. • Nasal *vibrissae* are, regrettably, unusually prevalent in elderly men. [L, hair in the nostril, found only in the pl., < *vibro* to quiver]. See **physique, appearance**. See **nose, smell**.

vicissitude (vi-sis'si-tood), pl. **vicissitudes**, n. the fact of being variable; unexpected change of circumstances affecting one's life, fortunes. • The more aged one is the more *vicissitudes* one is apt to encounter. [< L *vicissitudo* change, alteration < *vicissim* or *vicissatim* by turns < *vic-* change, place (The E word "vicar" is derived from the L vic-: a vicar acted routinely as a substitute for, i.e., changed places with, a rector.)]. adj. **vicissitudinary** (-tood'də-ner"ree). adj. **vicissitudinous** (-tood'də-nəs). See **innovation, misoneism**.

vidua (vi-doo'aa) n.f. widow; spinster. [L]. See: **marriage**. See **role**.

viduage (vid'dyoŏ-aaj) n. (obs.) widowhood, state of being a widow, viduity; widows in general. [< L *vidua* widow; spinster < L *viduus* deprived, bereaved. *viduitas* = widowhood; bereavement < *viduare* to deprive, bereave]. n. **viduity** = the state or period of being a widow, widowhood. adj. (rare) **vidual** = pertaining to a widow. adj. (rare) **vidual, viduous** = widowed. syns. **seneucia**, *veuvage*, viduation, *viduité*, q.v. See **marriage**. See **role**.

viduation (vi-dyoŏ-ay'shən) n. (rare) widowhood, state of being a widow; widows. [< L *vidua* widow + -tion, suff., an action or process or the result of it, via F < L *-tion-*]. See **marriage**. See **role**.

viduité (vidüite) n.f. widowhood. [F]. syns. **viduity**, & *veuvage*, **viduation, seneucia**, q.v. See **marriage**. See **role**.

viduus (vi'doŏ-oŏss) n. widower; unmarried. [L]. syn. *veuf*, q.v. See **marriag**e. See **role**.

vieil (vjɛl)/*vieux* (vjɛ), q.v.

vieillard (vjɛjar) n.m. an old man. [F]. See **old man**. **(les) vieillards** (vjɛjar) n.m. old people. [F]. See **old person(s), people**.

vieille (vjɛj)/*vieux* (vjø), q.v., adj. aged; out of date, dated; antiquated. (*vieil* is used before *voyelle* or an h mute rather than *vieux*.) [F]. n.m., f. 1. an aged man (*un vieux*) or woman (*vieille*). 2. *les vieux* (le vjø) = the old, the elderly. 3. *un petit vieux* (œ̃ pəti vjø) = a little old man; 4. *mon vieux* (mɔ̃ vjø) = old chap, old buddy; *ma vieille* (ma vjɛj) = old girl; *une vieille* (yn vjɛj) = an old woman. [F]. See **old**. See **old man, woman**.

vieillerie(s) (vjɛjri) n. old thing(s), old idea(s). [F]. See **old age**.

vieillesse (vjɛjɛs) n. 1. old age; oldness. 2. *la vieillesse* (la vjɛjɛs), old people = *vieillards* (See *vieillard*.) [F]. See **old age**. See **old person(s)**.

vieillir (vjejir) vt. to age; to make someone look older. vi. to age, to grow old; ref.v. to make oneself look older. [F]. See **Old**.

vieillot, **-otte** (vjejŏ, -ŏt) adj. oldish, quaint, old fashioned. [F]. See **old**.

vieux (vjø)—*vieile* (vjɛj) is used in place of *vieux* (vjø) before a vowel or *h* mute—n. old man; often *mon vieux*. • *Pas si vite, mon vieux* = Not so fast, old man (lit.), or my friend (fig.). adj. *vieux* = old. [F]. See **old man**.

villeggiatura (vi-lej'ji-ə-toor'ə) n. a rural extended holiday, stay, or retirement. [It]. See **retirement**.

viparious (vī-par'ri-əss) adj. life-renewing. • Regular physical exercise can be *viparious* for the aged. [< L *vivus* alive + *parere* to bear]. See **therapy**.

vir magno jam natu (wir maag'nō jam naa'toŏ) n.phr. an impressive or great man advanced in years. [L, *vir* man + *magnus* big, large, great, impressive + *jam* now, already, long since + *natus* born, made, destined]. See **old man**.

virago (vi-raa'gō) n. a turbulent woman; an insulting term that disparages a woman's temperament or behavior; (arch.) a woman of masculine strength or spirit. [L, female warrior < *vir* man]. syns. **termagant**, etc., q.v. See **old woman**.

viripause (vir-i-pawss) n. the time of life when a man loses interest in sex or loses the ability to perform sexually (said by C. H. Elster to be used in a 1993 TV show, but not recorded in any dictionary.) [< L *vir* man, husband + *pausa* pause, stopping, cessation < G *pausein* to stop, cease]. Cf. **andropause**, **libidopause**, q.v. See **sex, love**.

virtual visit n.phr. a recent term applied to a patient visiting a "virtual office" of a physician by means of email, the Internet, i-Pad, or a **telepresence robot**, q.v., in place of physically visiting a doctor's office. The physician, if agreable to these methods, assesses the patient's texted complaint or image, then texts him/her online in return with recommendations for treatment, which may include a prescription, the need for an actual (physical) office visit, etc. A variation is to include real-time interaction between patient and doctor by means of Web video. Several commercial concerns, e.g. Skype, offer formats for conducting virtual visits. (Medical insurance can now be purchased online, and a site for comparative evaluation of policies is: www. Ehealthinsurance.com.) • The elderly, because of their difficulties in getting to a doctor's office, may find a *virtual visit* helpful. syn. = **online** or **digital visit**. See **health, illness**.

vitilitigate (vit"ti-lit'ti-gayt) vi. to be particularly quarrelsome. • *Vitilitigating* among geriatric-center residents seems to erupt periodically. [< L *vitiare* to corrupt, spoil, violate, mar; to falsify + *litigare* to quarrel, squabble; to go to court]. adj. **vitilitigous** (vit"ti-li-tig'gəs). n. **vitilitigator** (-lit'ti-gayt"tor). n. **vitilitigation** (-gay'shən). See **talk**.

vituperate (vī-toop'pə-rayt", vi-toop'pə-) vi.&vt. to attack somebody in harshly abusive or critical language. [< L *vituperari* to spoil (omen), render void; blame < *vitium* fault, defect, sin, vice + *parare* to make ready]. adj. **vituperative** (vī-too'pə-rə-tiv). adj. **vituperatory**. adv. **vituperatively**. n. **vituperativeness**. n. **vituperator**. See **talk**. See **role**.

vixen (viks'ən) n. (1. a female fox.) 2. an offensive term that deliberately insults a woman regarded as vindictive and bad-tempered; it is frequently preceded by *old*. [15th C. variant of *fixen* < OE *fyxe*, f. of fox]. See **old woman**.

void (voyd) vi.&vt. to empty, cast out as waste matter, either feces (excrementitious matter) or urine. [< OF *voide* empty < assumed Vulgar L *vocitus*, alteration of L *vocivus*, replacing L *vacuus* empty, clear, free]. adj. **voidable**. n. **voidableness**. n. **voider**. See **gastrointestinal**. See **genitourinary**. See **role**.

voluble (vol'yoo-bəl) adj. 1. talkative, loquacious—voluble connotes an enthusiastic, friendly talker, while **garrulous**, q.v., connotes over-talkativeness. (2. twining or turning.) adv. **volubly**. n. **volubility** (vol"yoo-bil'li-tee). n. **volvubleness**. [< L *volubilis* turning, spinning, revolving, swirling; voluble, rapid, fluent; changeable < *volvere* to roll, roll along, turn about; read (books); utter fluently; consider, weigh; under go; to bring on (of time), bring around]. See **talk**.

vortiginous (vawr-tij'jin-əs) adj. whirling around a center; vertical. [< L *vertigo* turning, whirling; dizziness < *vertere* to turn, turn around + -ous, suff.]. Cf. **vertiginous**, q.v. See **nerve, muscle, movement, touch**.

vulvar dystrophies (vul'vaar dis'trō-feess) n.phr. These are vulvar non-neoplastic epithelial disorders: 1. **lichen sclerosis** = a dermatosis of unknown cause, characterized by epithelial thinning, swelling, fibrosis of the skin, and labial shrinkage. 2. **squamous hyperplasia** = a dermatosis characterized by vulvar patchy pruritus with thickened and raised skin. 3. **other dermatoses**: such as **lichen simplex chronicus, lichen planus, psoriasis, chronic eczematous dermatitis**. These dermatoses are particularly found in the elderly. n. **vulva** = external female genitals—see **vulvitis**. adj. **vulval**. adj. **vulviform** (vul'və-fəwrm). See **genitourinary**.

vulvitis (vul-vīt'tiss) n. superficial inflammation, irritation, and dermatitis of the vulva, i.e., the region of the external genital organs of the female, including the labia majora, labia minora, greater and lesser vestibular glands, and vaginal orifice (*pudendum femininum*). ● Agents such as deodorants soaps, etc., used to mask the odor associated with urinary incontinence—not unusual in elderly women—can cause *vulvitis.* [L, *vulva* + G, *-itis* (a f. adjectival termination, agreeing with *nosos* disease, understood) inflammation]. See **genitourinary**.

vulvovaginitis (vul"vō-vaj"ji-nīt'tiss) n. inflammation of the vulva and vagina, or of vulvovaginal glands. Candida (monilial) vulvovaginitis is especially common in elderly women, especially if they are diabetic or obese. [L, vulva, + *vagina* vagina + -itis, suff., < G -*itis* inflammation]. See **genitourinary**.

W

"Wrinkle, wrinkle, every day,/We passulate*, then pass
away."—Prunella Croon

*passulate, v. = to dry up as grapes do into raisins. Prunella paronomastically suggests a prune as her image, i.e., a passulated, dried up plum.

waffle (wof'fel) n. 1. a heartily disliked old person. 2. speech that is indecisive, vague, nonsense; incessant talk. (3. yapping of a small dog.) [1.U.S. slang. 2. & 3. British slang; late 17th C. < waff to yelp or bark, onomatopoeic]. vt. **waffle** = to talk nonsense; to talk incessantly. See **old man**. See **old woman**. See **old person(s)**. See **talk**.

walking speed n.phr. the speed at which the elderly walk has been studied recently, and has been found useful in determining how long and well they can live. It's an inexpensive, safe, simple way of measuring physical performance and using it as an aid in predicting health problems, suggesting treatments, and improving well being. The walking-speed difference of 3mi./hr. vs. 3.5 mi./hr. in a 70-year-old man has been found, on average, to be 4 years of life. For a woman of that age, the difference is 6 to 7 years. The expected longevity of a 70-year-old man walking at 2.5mi./hr. wound be on average 8 years longer than if he walked at 1 mi./hr.; in the case of a woman of that age, the expected difference would average 10 years. More research on walking speed is needed, but its usefulness looks quite promising. syn. **gait speed**, q.v. See **health, illness**. See **therapy**.

wallflower (wawl' flowr") n. (1. a spring-blooming garden plant with fragrant yellow, orange, or brown flowers. 2. a fragrantly flowering wild plant often found growing on walls, rocks, and cliffs; it's native to southern Europe.) 3. (informal) a shy or retiring person who remains unnoticed at social events, especially a woman without a dance partner. • The mage of an elderly widow sitting unattended at a party is as suggestive of a *wallflower* as is that of a young maiden sitting out a dance. [< wall + flower. Equating a woman who sits by a wall— the same site on which wild flowers grow—at a social gathering, unaccompanied by anyone, is equated with a wallflower. First recorded in 1820]. Cf. **burdalone**. **See loneliness, solitude, silence**. See **role**.

wallydrag (waal'li-drag)) n. an unkempt, disreputable woman, often preceded by *old*. [Sc]. See **old woman**.

wamble (wamb'bəl, waamb'bəl) vi. 1. to move unsteadily or stagger about; twist or turn. • The cogger *wambled* into the room. 2. to rumble from the stomach; to be nauseated. [< M E *wamelen* to feel nausea. Ultimately < the I-E root *wem-* to vomit]. n.pl. **wambles** (waam'bəls) = milk sickness; nausea. vbl.n. **wambling**. adv. **wamblingly** (-bling-lee). See **standing, walking, wandering**. See **gastrointestinal**.

wan (wan) adj. 1. pale, sickly looking. 2. dim, faint, feeble or weak. 3. bland, uninterested. [OE wann dark, dusky, gray <?]. adv. **wanly**. n. **wanness**. See **color**. See **health, wellness**. See **physique, appearance**. See **tiredness, weakness**.

wanze (wanz) vi. to wither, fade, waste away, to become emaciated. • One can see him *wanze* as his cancer progresses. [OE *wansian* to diminish]. pres.p.adj. **wanzing** = evanescent. n. **wanzingness**. See **physique, appearance**. See **health, illness**.

waspish (woss'pish), **waspy** (wos'pee) adj. 1. of or like a wasp in behavior (stinging), or of slender form. 2. sharp in retort; easily irritated or annoyed. 3. ill-tempered, irascible, petulant; showing spite. (4. of or pertaining to WASP, i.e., white Anglo-Saxon Protestant, an acronym). • The irascible old **mossback**, q.v., did not know whether to be pleased or offended when she called him *waspish*. [OE *wæsp* < I-E weave]. adv. **waspishly**. n. **waspishness**. See **physique, appearance**. See **mentality, mentation, behavior**. See **talk**.

wastrel (ways'trəl) n. (insult) 1. somebody regarded as a spendthrift, a wasteful, prodigal, profligate spender. 2. someone who is lazy, non-contributing. • The elderly, i.e., those > 65 yeas of age, may, in a sense, be considered *wastrels* in the sense that they consume a mighty one-third of all medical spending in the U.S. [late 16th C. via ONF < L *vastus* empty + *-rel*, suff., indicating "little" or a derogatory sense]. See **mentality, mentation, behavior**. See **role**.

wattle (wot'təl) n. fleshy appendage hanging from the throat of animals: turkeys, other birds, lizards, and, by (improper) extension, humans. [OE *watul* <?]. syns. (as applied to humans) **buccula**, **dewlap, jollop**, q.v., See **physique, appearance**.

wellderly (wel'dər-lee) n. a neologism indicating collectively those elderly who live the longest, i.e., 100 years or more. • The *wellderly* are "living test tubes in which nature has concentrated a vital essence of longevity."—R. L. Hotz, the Wall Street Journal, 9/19/'08, "Secrets of the 'Wellderly'". [a portmanteau word combining well and elderly]. Cf. **supercentenarians**, q.v. See **health, illness**. See **old man**. See **old woman**. See **old person(s)**. See **role**.

welkin (wel'kin, -kən) n. (archaic or literary) the sky; the vault of heaven, empyrean; the air above. • The grandma vaguely indicated the *welkin* as her ultimate goal. [OE *weolcen, wolc(e)n* < cloud, firmament < Gmc.]. syn. **empyrean**. See **end-of-life, death**.

wheeze (weez, hweez) vi.&vt. 1. vi. to breathe with an audible expiratory whistling sound and with expiratory difficulty, usually due to respiratory disorder, e.g., asthma. • The old **codger**, q.v., *wheezed* as he ascended the stairs. 2. vt. to say or express something while breathing noisily and with difficulty. 3. vi. to make a noisy whistling or puffing sound that resembles wheezing. [15th C. <?]. adj. **wheezy.** • The **wheezy geezer**, q.v., had difficulty making himself understood. n. **wheeze** = 1. noisy and difficult expiratory breathing or the hoarse whistling sound of this. 2. (inf.) a hackneyed, trite story, joke, or saying. n. **wheezer** = one who wheezes. n. **wheeziness**. adv. **wheezily**. See. **breathing**. See **talk**. See **role**.

whiffle (whif'fel) vi.&vt. (1. {of wind} to blow lightly, shift about, drive {a ship} in varying directions; {of flame, leaves, & **fig.**} to flicker, flutter wander.) 2. to vacillate. 3. to make the sound of a light wind in breathing. [< whiff perhaps imitative, perhaps partly an alteration of ME *weffe* foul smell + -le verbal < ME *(e)len* < OE *–lian* < Gmc. *–ilojan*, with frequentive or diminutive sense (wrestle, twinkle, nestle, dazzle, crumple)]. n. **whiffle** = a slight movement of air. See **mentality, mentation, behavior**. See **breathing**.

whilom (wil'ləm) adv. (arch.) formerly; once. [OE *hwilum*, dat. pl. of while]. adj. **whilom** = former. syn. **quondam, erst, erstwhile**, q.v. See **past, time**.

whinge (hwinj, winj) n. a whining complaint; a peevish grumbling. [OE *hwinsian* < Ger.]. n. **whinger**. adv. **whingingly**. adj. **whingy**. v.i. **whinge** = whining, grumbling peevishly. syn. gripe. See **talk**. See **role**.

whitebeard (wīt'beerd) n. a white-bearded old man. [a portmanteau word]. See **old man**. See **color**.

widdendream (wid'ən-dreem) n. (obs.) in a state of confusion or mental disturbance—often used in the phrase "*in a widdendream*". [an obs. Sc word < an OE phrase meaning "*in mad joy*"]. See **mentation, mentality, behavior**.

withered (with'ərd) adj. having lost freshness, vitality; shriveled, dried up, shrunken, passulated. [probable variant of E weather, expose to the elements < OE *weder* < IE to blow]. vi.&vt. **wither**. syns. **gnarled, passulated, shriveled up, shrunken, wrinkled, wizened**, q.v. See **physique, appearance**.

wizened (wiz'ənd) **wizen** (wiz'ən), **weazen** (wee'zən) adj. of shriveled or dried-up appearance (chiefly of someone or of his/her face or look). [pp. of *wizen* to shrivel < OE *wisnian* < OHG *wesanen* < ON *visna*]. syns. **wrinkled, shrunken, shriveled up, withered; gnarled**, q.v. See **physique, appearance**.

WOG a chat and text-message initialism = <u>w</u>ise <u>o</u>ld <u>g</u>uy. [NetLingo. com]. See **old man**.

wonted (wawn'ted) adj. customary, likely to do something; habitual; usual. [12th C. < pp. of OE *wunian* be accustomed]. n. **wont** = (form.) a habit or custom followed by a particular person or group. (vi. {archaic} **wont** or **wonted, wonting, wonts** = to have or give somebody the habit of doing something.) See **innovative, misoneism**.

wooly (woŏl'lee) adj. fuzzy, vague, disorganized; rough. (The physical, material definition is not considered.) [OE *wull* wool. The metaphysical

meaning is probably derived from the feel of the material]. See: **talk**.
See: **mentality, mentation, behavior**. See: **intelligence**.

word salad: See **schizophasia**.

work, activity: agathobiothik, androgogy, aponia, diremption, disability measures, diurnal, durance, dyslexia, *fainéant, -e*, feckless, *floruit*, gawkocracy, geriatric care manager, geriatric case manager, gerontarchical, gerontarchy, *hors de combat*, *hors de concours*, ignavy, itinerant, latibulize, lentor, mah-jongg, motatorios, omniana, otiant, otiose, parergon, perseverate, philobat, piddle, ponophobia, recubation, renidification, *shpilkes*, Sisyphean, spry, superannuated, tai chi, velitation, viaggiatory, viaticum.

work, activity: Subcategories

activity

I.   <u>Avoidance or, lack of activity</u>:
      1. Ineffective or worthless labor; unwilling or uninterested in being active or in working: **otiose**
      2. Lack of exertion, abstention from labor: **aponia**

II.   <u>Competition</u>:
      1. Beyond competition: *hors de concours*
      2. Disabled, out of action: *hors de combat*

III. <u>Disinterest in food</u>: Pick at one's food: **piddle**

IV. <u>Disability scales</u>: **disability measures**

V.   <u>Elder-care management</u>: **geriatric care manager, geriatric case manager**

VI. <u>Exercise</u>: A form of Chinese physical exercise characterized by balletic body movements: **tai chi**

VII. <u>Fidgeting, inability to sit still</u>: **shpilkes**

VIII. <u>Game (Chinese) with tiles</u>: **mah-jongg**

VIII. <u>Government</u>: Re: government by old men; government by old men: **gerontarchical; gerontarchy**

IX. <u>Ineffective</u>:
      1. Idling, doing nothing, lazy: *fainéant, -e*
      2. Unsuited, unable, unwilling, or too disorganized to do anything useful or to succeed: **feckless**
      3. Work, act in a trifling way: **piddle**

X.   <u>Intensity</u>:

1. Constantly active: **motatorios**
2. Markedly brisk and active: **spry**
3. Sluggish, lethargic, slothful: **ignavy**
4. Those that look at television frequently or for long periods: **gawkocracy**
5. To continue an action for an unusually long time: **perseverate**

XI. Making a new nest, home: **renidification**
XII. Minor conflict, slight skirmish, controversy: **velitation**
XIII. Notes, jottings, writings, scraps of information: **omniana**
XIV Period when most active: *floruit*, **diurnal**
XV. Reading difficulty: **dyslexia** XVI. Teaching: The science of teaching adults: **androgogy**
XVII. The good life: **agathobiothik**
XVIII. Travel:
1. One who loves to travel widely: **philobat**
2. Provisions for a trip; money or expense account for traveling: **viaticum**
3. Traveling frequently; given to traveling about: **viaggiatory**
4. Wandering from place to place: **itinerant**
XIX. Unsuited: Unable, unwilling, too disorganized to do anything useful or to succeed: **feckless**
XX. Violent or final separation: **diremption**

inactivity

I. Avoidance of work:
1. Ineffective; worthless; unwilling or uninterested in being active or working: **otiose**
2. Lying down: **recubation**
II. Confinement: Long or forcible confinement or imprisonment: **durance**
III. Out of work:
1. Disabled, out of action: *hors de combat*
2. Dormant, unemployed, idle, resting: **otiant**
3. Retired, laid off due to old age: **superannuated**
4. Unable, unwilling, too disorganized to do anything useful or to succeed: **feckless**
IV. Sluggishness: **lentor**
V. To hibernate: **latibulize**

work

I. Avoidance of work: Ineffective; worthless; unwilling or uninterested in being active, working: **otiose**

II. Disqualified:
    1. Made obsolete, disqualified due to old age: **superannuated**

III. Fear:
    1. Morbid fear of becoming overworked, or fatigued: **ponophobia**

IV. Ineffective:
    1. Endless labor at a fruitless task: **Sisyphean**
    2. Unsuited, unable, unwilling, too disorganized to do anything useful or to succeed: **feckless**
    3. Work, act in a trifling way: **piddle**

V. New:
    1. Making a new nest, home: **renidification**

VI. Out of work:
    1. Disabled, out of action: *hors de combat*
    2. Dormant, unemployed, idle, resting: **otiant**
    3. Retired, laid off due to old age: **superannuated**

VII. Secondary: Secondary work or business: **parergon**

VIII. Teaching:
    1. The science of teaching adults: **androgogy**

IX. Unsuited: Unable, unwilling, too disorganized to do anything useful or to succeed: **feckless**

wowser (wow'zər) n. (informal) 1. somebody with a puritanical disposition who disapproves of activities such a drinking and dancing. 2. a person who disrupts or ruins the fun of others. [< Anzac (a soldier who served in the Australian and New Zeeland Army Corps in World War I: an ANZ) late 19th C. <?]. See **mentality, mentation, behavior**. See **role**.

wraith (rayth) n. 1. a person's double or apparition seen as a premonition shortly before his/her death, or seen shortly after death. 2. a ghost or insubstantial apparition. [< Sc. of unknown origin]. Cf. **taisch**. See **end-of-life, death**.

X

"Advice is what older men offer to younger men when they
[older men] no longer can set them a bad example."
—Irvin Shrewsbury Cobb

xanthelasma (zan-thee-laz'mə), pl. **xanthelasmas**. n. (obs. term for **xanthoma**, q.v.) a slightly raised, yellowish, well-circumscribed plaque composed of lipid-laden cells (histiocytes) typically appearing along the nasal aspect of one or both eyelids in older persons; it may accompany lipid disorders, and is called specifically **xanthelasma palpebrarum** (pal-pee-braa'rum). [-xanth(o)-, pref., yellow or yellowish, < G *xanthos* yellow + *elasma* a beaten-metal plate. *palpebra*, pl. *palpebrae*, gen. pl. *palpebrarum*, eyelids]. syn. = **xanthoma**, q.v. See <u>eye</u>. See <u>skin</u>.

Xanthippe (zan-tip'pee)/**Xantippe** (zan-tip'pee) n. a shrewish wife; an ill-tempered browbeating woman. [< Xanthippe, who was Socrates's wife and apparently such a woman]. syn. **termagant**, etc., q.v. See <u>old woman</u>.

xanthodont (zan'thō-dont) n. a person with yellowish teeth—yellow teeth are an accompaniment of old age as enamel tends to wear thin and the yellowish dentin beneath shows through. [xanth(o)-, pref., yellow or yellowish < G *xanthos* yellow + *odous odontos* tooth]. adj. **xanthodont** (zan-thō-don'tik) or **xanthodontous** (zan-thō-don'təs)—leukodontous = white toothed? See <u>mouth, gums, teeth</u>. See <u>role</u>.

xanthoma (zan-thōm'mə) n. (fibroma lipomatodes or vitiligoidea) a yellow nodule or plaque, especially of the skin, composed of lipid-laden histiocytes (tissue cells).

Xanthoma palpebrarum = soft, yellow-orange plaques found specifically about the eyes, and the most common type of xanthoma. [< xanth(o)-, pref., yellow or yellowish < G *xanthos* yellow + *oma* tumor]. See **xanthelasma**. See <u>eye</u>. See <u>skin</u>.

xeniatrophobia (zen"nī-at"trō-fōb'bi-ə) n. 1. morbid fear of (going to) a foreign doctor. 2. morbid fear of foreigners, strangers. [< G *xeno*s stranger + *iatros* physician + -phobia, suff., fearing < G *-phobia* < *phobos* fear]. adj. **xeniatrophobic**. n. **xeniatrophobe** (-at'trō-fōb). See <u>phobias</u>. See <u>therapy</u>. See <u>health, illness</u>.

xenophobia (zen"nō-fōb'bee-ə) 1. n. an intense fear, dislike, or hatred, possibly irrational, of foreigners or strangers, their customs and culture. 2. an extension of this attitude to anything foreign, strange. [xeno-, pref., foreign, strange, different < G *xenos* stranger, foreigner + -phobia, suff., an exaggerated or irrational fear < *phobos* fear]. adj. **xenophobic**. n. **xenophobe**. Cf. **xeniatrophobia**, q.v. See **phobias**.

xeroderma (zer-ō-derm'mə) n. excessive dryness of the skin, common in the elderly, and due to a slight increase of the horny layer and diminished cutaneous secretion; it can be a mild form of ichthyosis (scaly skin). [xero-, pref., meaning dry, < G *xeros* dry, + *derma* skin]. syn. **dermatoxerasia**; **xerosis**, q.v. See **skin**.

xeronisus (zeer-on'i-səs) n. inability to reach orgasm. [xer(o)-, pref., dry < G *xeros* dry +? < L *nisus/nixus* effort; soaring flight; position]. See **sex, love**. See **genitourinary**.

xerophthalmia (zeer"rof-thal'mi-ə) n. dryness of the conjunctiva that can result in loss of its luster and can even become skin-like from a lack of intrinsic secretion; lachrymal (tear) gland activity is diminished. Xerophthalmia can be an accompaniment of aging, or can be due to other etiology, e.g., **Sjögren's syndrome** (an autoimmune disease), and be accompanied by decreased salivary gland activity, **xerostomia**, q.v., (sicca syndrome). [xero-, pref., meaning dry < G *xeros* dry + *ophthalmos* eye]. syn. **xerophthalmus = xerophthalmia**. See **eye**.

xerosis (zee-rōs'siss) n. 1. pathologic dryness of the skin, **xeroderma**, q.v., of the conjunctiva, **xerophthalmia**, q.v., or of stomatic mucous membranes, **xerostomia**, q.v. 2. the normal evolutionary sclerosis (hardening) of the tissues in old age. • The cause of *xerosis* in the elderly is unknown, but appears to be related to an alteration of lipid composition of the outermost layer of the skin, which contains cells that are dead and desquamating. [xero-, pref., meaning dry < G *xeros* dry + G -*osis*, suff., condition]. See **skin**.

xerostomia (zeer"rō-stōm'mi-ə) n. a dryness of the mouth as a result of decreased or arrested salivary secretion (asialism). [xero-, pref., meaning dry, < G *xeros* dry + *stoma* mouth]. adj. **xerostomic**. See **xerophthalmia**, **xerosis**. See **mouth, gums, teeth**.

Y

"Age, I do abhor thee. Youth, I do adore thee."
The Passionate Pilgrim, XII—William Shakespeare

yammer (yam'-mər) vi.&vt. to whine, complain; to talk loudly and incessantly. [< MDu *jammeren* to lament]. n. **yammer** = the act of yammering. See **talk**.

yatter (yat'tər) vi. to make idle chatter. [?]. See **talk**.

yesterfang (yes'tur-fang, yes'tər-) n. (chiefly poetic) that which was taken at some time in the past. [yester-, pref., a specified time period past, or indefinite past < OE *geostran*, *gystran dæeg* + fang <? Gmc. v. *fanhan* to catch]. See **past, time**.

<u>**youth, younger generation**</u>: **Calypso**, **epigone**, **epigonous**, **horaphthia**, **juvenescent**, **mammothrept**, **neanimorphism**, **nepimnemic**, **tetnit**.

> <u>**youth, younger generation**</u>: Subcategories

I. <u>Appearance</u>: Looking younger than one's years: **agerasia, neanimorphism**
II. <u>Childhood memory</u>:
    1. Childhood memory retained in the subconscious: **nepimnemic**
III. <u>Generational difference</u>:
    1. Follower of a later, and presumably inferior, generation: **epigone**
    2. Of a later generation: **epigonous**
IV. <u>Youth</u>:
    1. Becoming youthful: **juvenescent**
    2. Child born of elderly parents: **tetnit**
    3. Child raised by his/her grandmother: **mammothrept**
    4. Neurotic preoccupation with one's youth: **horaphthia**
    5. One who promises youth (and immortality): **Calypso**

Z

"Zhizn nasha v starosti—iznoshennÿi khalat: I sovestno nosit' ego, I zhal' ostavit." (Our old age is like a worn-out dressing gown; it shames us to wear it, yet we cannot bring ourselves to throw it away.) Vyazemsky [Rus].

zaftig (zaf'tik, -tig) adj. full-figured; pleasingly plump; buxom. • The old **satyr**, q.v., invariably sought a *zaftig* **dowager**, q.v., for his next conquest. [< Yid. *zaftik* juicy < MHG *saftec* juice < OHG *saf* sap]. See **old woman**.

zeigarnik (zī-gawr'nik) n. a tendency to remember an uncompleted task rather than a completed one. [< Bluma Zeigarnik, a German psychologist who recognized that people are easily distracted by too many variables, tasks, options, and when confronted with too many are unable to focus on those current until earlier ones have been explored or completed]. See **memory**.

zoara (zō-ar'ǝ?) n. (obs.) insomnia. [? etymology—an obsolete term for insomnia. Zozra is both a mythological goddess of love, and a Biblical town, but the connection of either to insomnia is obscure at best]. Syns. See **sleep, wakefulness**.

zoilism (zō'il-iz-ǝm) n. nagging, carping, destructive criticism. [< L *Zoilus*, the proverbial stern Alexandrine critic of Homer]. See **talk**. See **mentality, mentation, behavior**.

zoster (zos'tur, -tǝr) n. a rash commonly called **shingles** [L *cingulus* belt, sash]: a spreading painful eruption of deep-seated vesicles on erythematous bases on one side of the body, following the course of a nerve, frequently along the side or waist. It occurs in the elderly because of waning immunity and reactivation of dormant herpes varicella virus, type 1 or 2, acquired usually in childhood and manifested then as chickenpox, but chickenpox may have been subclinical, unrecognized; re-exposure to the virus is also a possibility. A frequently successful prophylactic vaccine is called Zostervax® (Merck). [technically, herpes zoster < G *herpein* to creep + *zoster*, girdle]. syn. **herpes zoster**, **shingles**, q.v. See **skin**. See **nerve, muscle, movement, touch**. See **health, illness**.

zounds (zowndz) int. (archaic) a mild expression of surprise or annoyance that is often followed by an exclamation mark. [Late 16th C. contraction of "by God's wounds!"]. See **emotion**.

SENIOR TEXTING CODES (STC)
(SUGGESTED, UNORTHODOX,
AND UN-ATTRIBUTED)

ATD	=	at the doctor's	HGBM	=	Had good bowel movement.
BFF	=	best friend's funeral			
BTW	=	Bring the wheelchair.	IMHO?	=	Is my hearing aid on?
BYOT	=	Bring your own teeth.	LMDO!	=	Laughing my dentures out!
CBM	=	covered by Medicare			
CGU	=	Can't get up.	LOL	=	lots of Lipitor
CRAT	=	Can't remember a thing.	LWO	=	Lawrence Welk's on.
			OBA	=	old battle axe
CRS	=	Can't remember s—t.	OMRR	=	on my massage recliner
CUATSC	=	See you at the senior center.			
			OMSG	=	Oh my! Sorry, gas.
DWI	=	driving while intoxicated	ROFL!	=	Rolling on the floor laughing!
FWBB	=	friends with beta blockers	TTYL	=	Talk to you louder.
			WAITT?	=	Who am I talking to?
FWIW	=	Forgot where I was.	WOG	=	wise old guy
FYI	=	Found your insulin.	WTFA	=	Wet the furniture again.
GGLKI	=	Gotta go: Laxative kicking in.			
			WTP?	=	Where's the prunes?
GGPBL	=	Gotta go: Pacemaker battery low.	WWNO	=	Walker wheels need oil.
GHA	=	Got heartburn again.			

ALPHABETICAL LISTING OF FOREIGN HEADWORDS & PHRASES WITH THEIR DEFINITION, ETYMOLOGY, & CATEGORIZATION

Those words defined more fully as dictionary headwords in the main word list are indicated by "q.v.", which see, for further information. Pronunciation is often approximate at best.

A

Cineri gloria sera venit. (Fame is too late bestowed on a man's ashes.)—Martial. [L].

à l'ancienne (ã lãsjɛn) adj.phr. old fashioned; old style. [F].

A la Recherche du Temps Perdu (aa la ʀaʃɛʀs dy tã pɛʀdy) ɳ.phr. Remembrance of Things Past (the name of a novel cycle by Proust). [F].

à outrance (a utʀãs) adv.phr. to the extreme; to an excessive degree, excessively; to the death; a pun on death. [F].

abuela (aa-boo-ayl'laa, -lə), q.v., n. grandmother. [Sp].

abus de faiblesse (aby də fɛblɛs) exploiting frailty (of the aged), q.v., n.phr. [F].

aetate provectus (ī-taat'tay prō-wek'tuss), q.v., adj.phr. a collation meaning: of advanced age. [L].

agonistes (ag-ō-nis'teez), q.v., adj. pertaining to one engaged in a struggle—the adj. is placed *after* the noun modified, e.g., Moses agonistes. [L].

alieni juris (a la ay'nee yoo'riss), q.v., adj.phr. a term in law that literally means "of another's law". [L].

aide-mémoire (εd-memwar), pl. *aides-mémoire* (εd-memwar), q.v., n.phr. a document, memorandum, note written as an aid to the memory. [F].

alpha-omega (al'faa-ō-may'gaa) n.phr. first and last; beginning and end; whole. [G, first and last letters of the G alphabet].

alter Kocker (awl'tər kok'kər), q.v., n.phr. an old guy over the hill; canny, stubborn old man who is inept, forgetful. [Yid. < Ger.].

amaurosis fugax (am"maw-rōs'siss fyoog'gaks), q.v., n.phr. a transient episode of blindness. [L].

anilis -e (a-nee'liss -e) adj. of an old woman. [L[.

anilitas -atis (a-nee'li-taas -aa-tis) nf. old age (of women). [L].

aniliter (a-nee'li-ter) adv. like an old woman. [L].

apud se (aa'poŏd-say), q.v., adj.phr. in one's senses. [L].

arcus corneae/arcus cornealis (awr'koŏs kawr'nee-ī/ar'koŏs kor-nee-aa'lis), q.v., n.phr. a white or gray opaque ring in the corneal margin. It can be present at birth, or appear later in life; it becomes quite frequent in those over 50. [L].

arcus senilis (ar'koŏs sə-nee'lis) n.phr., q.v., an opaque, grayish ring at the periphery of the cornea just within the sclerocorneal junction; it occurs frequently in the aged, and results from fatty deposits or degenerative changes in corneal cells. [L]. See *arcus corneae*.

arrière-garde (arjεr-gard), q.v., adj.phr. old fashioned, old hat, *passé*. [F]

ars moriendi (aarz'maw-ree-en'dee) n. phr. the art of dying (well). [L].

B

Bis pueri senes. (Old men are children twice. Old men again are boys. In advanced age the aged become children.) [L].

babushka (bə-boŏsh'kə) q.v., n. 1. a traditional Russian grandmother figure, old woman. (2. a headscarf folded and tied under the chin.) [R, grandmother].

bien-pensant, e (bjɛ̃-pãsã, ãt = m. & f.), m.pl., **bien-pensants**, f.pl., **bien-pensantes** adj. & n., m. & f., conformist(s). [F].

C

Cineri gloria sera venit. (Fame is too late bestowed on a man's ashes). [L].

cacoethes carpendi (kaa-kō'ay-thees kawr-pen'dee) q.v., n.phr. a compulsion, ill habit, itch to criticize or find fault. [L].

cacoethes loquendi (kaa-kō'ay-thees lō-kwen'dee), q.v., n. phr. an irrepressible desire to talk. [L].

compos mentis (kawm'pos men'tis) sound of mind. [L]. syn. = **apud se**, q.v. See **mentality, mentation, behavior**.

compos sui (kom'paws soo'ee) having the use of one's limbs. [L].

coureur de veuves (kurœr də vœv) n.phr. one who runs after, hunts widows; a fortune hunter. [F] syn. = **coureur de dot** (kurœr də dɔt) n.phr. = a fortune hunter [*dot*, nf. = dowry].

D

Dum vita est, spes est. While there is life, there is hope. [L].

d'un certain âge (d' œ̃ sɛrtɛ̃ aʒ), q.v., adj. phr. elderly (lit. of a certain age); an extremely polite way of saying, indicating someone, especially a woman, is old, elderly. [F].

de bonne mémoire (də bɔn memwar) of good memory; of sound mind—mauvaise mémoire = bad memory. [F].

De mortuis nil nisi bonum. (day mawr'too-is nil-ni'si bō'num) About the dead nothing (should be said) except good. [L].

De Senectute (day sen-ek-too'tay) Concerning Old Age (Seneca). [L]

débrouillard, e (debrujar, ard), q.v., nm., nf. a capable, and self-reliant person not in need of help; follows up, and sees things through. adj. *débrouillard, e* = resourceful. [F].

démodé, e (demɔde), q.v., adj. old-fashioned. [F].

distrait, e (distrɛ, ɛt), q.v., adj. inattentive or absentminded. [F].

double entendre/double entente (dubl ãtãdr/dubl ãtãt), q.v., n.phr. an expression with two meanings—one often indelicate. [F].

doyen/doyenne (dwajɛ̃/dwajɛn), q.v., n. a man/woman who is the most senior or experienced and respected member of a group or profession. [F].

drame avec soi (dлam avɛк swa) dialogue with himself, talking to oneself; soliloquy. [F]

E

Dum vivimus, vivamus. While there is life, let us live. [L]

éboulement (ebulmã), q.v., n. the crumbling or falling of a wall, especially a fortification. Fig., a crumbling of physical strength, resistance, prowess. [F].

empressement (ãprɛsmã), q.v., nm. attentiveness, extreme politeness, display of cordiality; eagerness; in a hurry. [F].

enfin (ãfɛ̃), q.v., adv. finally; at last; in a word, in short. [F].

ennui (ãnчi) nm. 1. boredom, lassitude. (2. annoyance. 3. trouble.) • *Ennui* is a pervasive problem for residents in retirement homes. [F].

esprit de l'escalier/ esprit d'escalier (εspri də lεsκalje/εspʀi dεsκəlje) n.phr., lit., wit of the stairway, meaning fine rejoinders thought of too late, i.e., thought of after an encounter, e.g., as one is leaving, likely by way of a stairway. Such a circumstance is increasingly likely in old age when wit's acuteness is apt to be dulled. (The collocation is said to have first been used by Diderot.) [F].

Ewig-Weibliche (ay"vik-vīp'li-kə), q.v., n. "eternal-feminine character-
• istics". [Ger.].

ex capite (eks kaap'pee-tay), q.v., adv. from memory. [L].

extrema aetas (eks-tray'ma ī'taas) adj.phr. advanced old age. [L, *extrema* extreme, outermost, last + *aetas* age].

F

Eheu! fugaces labuntur anni! Alas! the fleeting years
glide away! [L]. (Horace).

fainéant -e, (fεneã, ãt), q.v., adj. lazy. [F].

fanfaron, onne (fãfarõ, ɔn) nm.&f. braggart. See **fanfaronade**. [F].

feuillemorte (fœjmɔrt), q.v., adj. having a yellow-brown, faded-leaf color. [F].

floruit (floruit), q.v., vi. flourished—said of an artist, sculptor, poet, musician, etc. [L].

G

Experto crede. Believe one who speaks from experience [L].

Gerousia (jer-roo'si-ə), q.v., n. Sparta's governing body of 28 old men, = or > 60 years of age and elected for life, plus Sparta's two kings. [G].

grisaille (grizɑj) n.f. one with grizzled hair, hair partly gray; black & white; grayness, dullness. vi. **grisaille** to turn gray (of hair, etc.). adj. **grisâtre** (grizaj) grayish. (se griser de {sə grise də} = to get drunk on) [F].

grognard (grɔɲar), q.v., nm. an old soldier, seasoned veteran [F].

H

Gaudeamus igitur. (Let us live then and be glad.)

habitué, -e (abitye), q.v., n. a person who frequents a particular place; a regular visitor or resident. [F].

hors de combat ('ɔr də kɔ̃ba), q.v., adv.phr./adj.phr. disabled; out of action. [F].

hors de concours ('ɔr də kɔ̃kur), q.v., adv.phr./adj.phr. beyond competition. [F].

I

Ho thanatos toioutos, hoion genesis, phuseos mustērion.
Death, like birth, is one of nature's secrets. [G]. (Marcus Aurelius).

idée fixe (ide fiks) pl. *idées fixes* (ide fiks), q.v., n.phr. an idea that dominates the mind; monomania. [F].

immortel (imɔrtɛl), q.v., n.m. immortality. 1. (fig.) an artistic image of remembrance after death. (2. a member of the French Academy; {pl.} the immortals, the gods. 3. n.f., *immortelle* (imɔrtɛl), or E, **immortelle** (im-mawr"tel'), everlasting {a plant}). [F].

impos animi (im'paws aa'ni-mī) adj.phr. not in control of one's mind. [L, *impos* without control, (with genitive) without control of + *animus*, mind, intellect (*animus*, -*i*, m., mind, as opposed to *anima*, -*ae*, f., soul; air; breath].

impotentia (im"paw-tayn'tee-aa), q.v., n. impotence, i.e., weakness, lack of power, or, specifically, in the male, inability to copulate, cohabit (*impotentia coeundi*), due to inability to achieve penile erection (*impotentia erigendi*), or to achieve ejaculation, or both. This may be due to neurological or psychological, emotional factors, and can imply inability to reproduce—*impotentia generandi* (gay-nair-aan'dee). [L].

in articulo mortis (in aar-tik'yoŏ-lō mawr'tees) n.phr. at the point of death. [< L *in* in, on, at, on the point of + *articul-us, -a, -um* joint; (grammar) clause; turning point + *mors* death].

in extremis (in ek-stray'mees) near death. [L, *in* at, on the point of + *extremis* extreme, near death].

incontinentia alvi (in"kawn-ti-nen'ti-aa, or –nen'shə, al'vī), q.v., n.phr. fecal incontinence. [L, *incontinentia* lack of self control & *alvus, -i* m. belly, bowels, stomach; boat; beehive].

incontinentia vesicae (in"kawn-ti-nen'ti-aa vay'si-kī) n.phr. (urinary) bladder incontinence. [L, *incontinentia* lack of self control & *vesica* bladder].

L

Jucundi acti labores. (The recollection of past labors is pleasant.) —Cicero. [L].

lao (low), q.v., adj. a respectful term, honorific used for older people. The term can apply equally to one's great-grandfather or the senior member of an assembly line or management team. [Chinese].

laolaiqiao/laolaiqiao Gaga (?), q.v., n./n.phr. a recent term found on Chinese video sites indicating old people "doing young things that even young people wouldn't do", even cross dressing. [Chinese].

lapsus calami (laap'soŏs kaa'laa-mee), q.v., n.phr. slip of the pen, or currently, of typing, texting. [L].

lapsus linguae (laap'soŏs lin'gwī), q.v., n.phr. slip of the tongue. [L].

laudator temporis acti (low-daa'tawr tem'paw-ris ak'tee) n.phr. one who is always extolling the good old days—Horace, *Art of Poetry*, 173. Cf. **nostomania, hesternopathia**, q.v. [L, *laudator* one who praises; eulogist; panegyrist + *tempore/tempori* in time, on time, in due time, at the right time + *act-a, -ae* deeds, actions, public acts].

lécheur (leʃœr), f., *lécheuse* (leʃøz), q.v., n. 1. a gourmand, gourmandizer. 2. a devotee of oral intercourse. 3. a licker. [F].

M

Juvenes dum sumus. (While young life's before us.) [L].

manqué -e (f.) (mãкe, -ə), q.v., adj. unfulfilled, might-have-been, missed, unsuccessful, abortive, frustrated in fulfillment of one's ambitions. [F].

megillah (mə-gil'ləh), q.v., n. any long-winded account, especially one concerning a minor matter benefiting from much greater condensation. [H. In Yid.,. *megillah* is usually preceded by *ganz* whole or complete, thus ***ganz*** (gaants) ***megillah*** = an exhaustive account].

memorabilia (mem"awr-aa-bil'i-aa) n.pl. things worthy of remembrance; things kept in memory of someone. [L, memorable things < *memorabilis* < *memorare* bring to mind < *memor* mindful].

modus vivendi (mawd'oŏs wee-wen'dee) n.phr. way or mode of living (together); practical method of getting along despite difficulties. [L, *modus* way, manner, mode; regulation; etc., & *vivere* to live].

mon vieux (mõ vjø) n.phr. old, boy (U.K., U.S.), old chap (U.K.), old buddy (U.S.). The feminine equivalent = *ma vieille* (ma vjɛj). *les vieux* (le vjø) = the old, aged; *les vieille* (le vjɛj) if all the aged are females. *un petit vieux* (œ̃ pəti vjø) = a little old man. *une petite vieille* (yn pətit vjɛj) = a liitle old lady, woman. *ses vieux* (se vjø) = his folks, her folks. [F].

morem gerere (maw'rem je-rer'ee) or *gerere morem* v.phr. to comply with or humor the wishes of a person. [L, < *mor-, mos* custom, humor + *gero, gerere, gessi, gestum* to display, exhibit; bear, carry; etc.].

N

(Les) bons souvenirs sont des bijoux perdus ({le} bõ suvnir sã de biʒu pɛrdy). (Good memories are lost jewels.)—Valéry. [F].

non compos mentis (nõn kwam'paws men'tis) not sound of mind; insane. [L, *non* not + *compos* (with genitive or ablative) in possession of, master of, having control over + *mens -tis* mind].

nunc dimittis (noŏnk dee-mit'tis), q.v., n.phr. indicating willingness, readiness to die; lit., Now lettest thou (thy servant) go (i.e., depart this life). [L,"*Nunc dimities servum tuum.*"].

O

Memento mori. (Remember you must die.) [L].

obiter dictum (aw'bi-ter dik'toŏm) any incidental or cursory remark not necessarily germane to the subject being discussed. pl = *obiter dicta.* • With increasing age, he was inclined in garrulous conversation to countless *obiter dicta.* (This would not be bad if his obiter dicta were *birrellisms*, i.e., thoughtful, but also good humored, comments tinged with irony, < Augustine Birrell {1850-1933}, professor of law at University College, London, who authored several essays published in 1884 entitled "Obiter Dicta", < N.W. Schur, q.v. [L, a thing said < *obiter*, adv., in passing, by way of, incidentally, < *ob-* toward + *iter* way + *dictum* neuter form of *dictus*, the pp. of *dicere* to say].

Opa Gefaengnis (ō-paag'e-fang'niss), q.v., n. a prison for old men [Ger.].

otium cum dignitate (ō'tee-oŏm koŏm di-nee-taa'tay) ease with dignity; ease with leisure. [L, *otium* leisure, free time, relaxation; freedom from public affairs, retirement; peace; quiet; ease, idleness, inactivity + *cum* with + *dignitatio* esteem, respect; dignity, honor— absence of financial concern is understood].

outrance (utrãs), q.v., n., utmost; excess. *à outrance* adv. = to the bitter end (a pun on a senior's life's end); excessively. [F].

outré (utre), q.v., adj. outside the bounds of what is considered usual, correct, proper, or generally acceptable. [F].

P

Mutare vel timere sperno. (I scorn to change or to fear.) [L].

passé-e (pɑse -ə), q.v., adj. out of fashion, old fashioned. [F].

R

Nos habebit humus. (Earth will slumber o'er us.)—N. W. Schur—A medieval student's song dating to 1626 with a liberal English translation. [L].

raconteur (rakɔ̄tœr), *-euse* (øz), q.v., n. a story teller. [F].

rente (rãt), q.v., n. 1. annual income; annuity. *Vivre de ses rentes* (vivr də se rãt) = to have a private income. *rente viagère* (rãt vjaʒɛr) = life annuity. [F]. n. *rentier* (rãtje) = one who receives or lives off of rents, an annuity, a financial portfolio.

retardataire (rətardatɛr), q.v., adj. behind the times, or characteristic of an earlier period—used mainly about artistic styles. n. one who is behind the times. nm&f. one who is late in arriving, a late-comer; loiterer, laggard. syn. *vieux jeu*. [F].

S

O tempora! O mores! *(*O the times! O the customs!)—Cicero denouncing the degenerate ways of his day. [L].

Schadenfreude (shaa'den-froy"də), q.v., n. taking pleasure in others' misfortune. [Ger.].

Schlimmbesserung (shlim-bes'ser-ung), q.v., n. an "improvement" that makes things worse. [Ger.].

senectus -a -um (sen-ek'-toŏs -aa -oŏm) adj. aged, old; nf. old age, senility. [L].

senectus -utis (sen-ek'toos, sen-ek-too'teess) nf. old age; old people. [L].

seneo -ere (say-nay'ō, say-ay'ree) vi. to be old. [L].

senesco -escere -ui (sayn-es'kō, -es'kay-ree, -oo-ee) vi. to grow old; to decline, become feeble, lose strength; to wane, draw to a close. [L].

senex -is (sen'eks -eess) adj. aged, old; nm. old man; nf. old woman. [L]. • *Senex psittacus neglegit ferulam* (sen'eks sit'ta-koŏs ne-gle'git fer-oo'lam) an old parrot does not mind the stick. See: **old as** or **as old as**. [L].

senilis -e (sen-ee-lis -e) adj. of old people, of an old man; aged; senile [L].

senior -us (sen-i-or' -us) adj. (comp. of **senex**, q.v.) older, elder; more mature (in years). **senior** nm. an elderly person, an elder (> 45 years of age {in Roman times}) [L].

Seniores priores. (see-nee-ō'rays pree-ō'rays) Elders first. [L, elderly persons + forefathers, ancestors, ancients].

senium -ii or **-i** (say'nee-um i or ee) n. feebleness of age, decline, senility; decay; grief, trouble; gloom; crabbiness; old man. [L].

sermunculus -i (ser-moŏn'koŏ-loŏs -ī), q.v., n. small talk, chit-chat. [L –i, nm.].

shibui (shi-boo'i), q.v., n. refers to beauty that only time can reveal: the impression—a distinct but ineffable sensation—that one gets from looking at the face of a certain kind of older person that reflects the person's personality and his or her experiences in life. [Japanese].

shpilkes (shpil'keeys), q.v., pl.n. an inability to sit still, fidgeting, ants in one's pants. Not sitting for long periods, moving, fidgeting is shown to prolong life. Sitting for long periods is unhealthy. [Yid.]. See **mentality, mentation, behavior**.

Struldbrug (stroold'broog), pl. **Stuldbrugs**, q.v., n. & adj. 1. an old, decrepit, shuffling person. 2. the term is applied recently to the difficulties governmental social programs have with the cost of providing continuing care to such individuals, or to the equivocal benefit of social planners' frantic efforts to prolong life in the very old by increasingly restricting many of life's enjoyments such as eating "unhealthy" foods, smoking, imbibing alcohol, etc. (Meltzer, P.E.) [Ger.].

sui juris (soŏ'ee joŏr'riss), q.v., adj.phr. legally competent to manage one's affairs or assume responsibility. [L, (*se*) *sui* of himself, herself, themselves + (*jus*) *juris* of law, justice, legal right, permission, prerogative, jurisdiction].

surdus (sur'dus) adj. & n. 1. deaf; deaf (person). (2. an irrational number. 3. voiceless, a voiceless sound.) [L, unable to hear or speak].

sussurator (soŏs'soŏ-ray-tawr) a whisperer, mutterer. [L].

susurrus aurium (soŏs'soŏr-oŏss aoŏ'ree-oŏm) n.phr. a whisper in the ear. [L, *susurrus* low gentle noise; whisper, murmur, buzz, hum + *aurium* in the ear].

T

Post jucundam juventutem, (After youthful pastime had) ***Post molestam senectutem***, (After old age hard and sad,) [L].

taedium vitae (tī'dee-oŏm wee'tī) n.phr. weariness of life; ennui or Weltschmerz. [L, *taedium* irksomeness, tediousness, weariness, boredom + *vitae* of life].

tempus edax rerum (tem'poŏs ay'daks ray'roŏm) time, the devourer of all things—"Metamorphoses", Ovid (43 B.C. – c. 18 B.C.) [L, *tmpus* time + *edax* gluttonous; (fig.) devouring, destructive + *res* thing, matter, affair]. (Time goes, you say? Ah no!/ Alas, Time stays, we go."—Austin Dobson, "The Paradox of Time", Proverbs in Porcelain, 1877. "But at my back I always hear/ Time's winged chariot hurrying near;/And yonder all before us lie/ Deserts of vast eternity."—Andrew Marvell, "To His Coy Mistress" (1650-1652). " Time's winged chariot is beginning to goose me." Noel Coward.)

tessera hospitalis (tes-ser'ra hos-pi-taal'liss), q.v., n.phr. a square tablet, which was divided as a tally or token between two friends in order that they or their descendants might thereby ever afterwards recognize each other. [L].

Torschlusspanik (tor'schloos-pan"ik, q.v., n. a sense of panic brought on by the feeling that life is passing one by. [Ger.].

tracasserie (traкasri), q.v., n. a sense of annoyance. [F].

traditionaliste (tradisjɔnalist), q.v., n., m. & f. a conservative. adj.
traditionaliste = conservative. [F].

V

quantum mutatus ab illo! (How changed from
what he once was!) [L].

veilleuse (vɛjøz), q.v., n. 1. a small and highly decorated nightlight. 2.
a bedside food warmer. [F].

veuf (vœf), q.v., n.m. widower. adj. *veuf* = widowed. [F].

veuvage (vœvaʒ), q.v., n.m. widowhood or widowerhood. [F].

veuve (vœv), q.v., n.f. widow. [F].

vidua (wi-doŏ'a), q.v, widow n.f. [L].

viduus (wi-doŏ'oŏs), q.v., n.m. widower. [L].

vieillard (vjɛjar), q.v., n.m. an old man. [F]. (*les*) **vieillards** (vjɛjar),
q.v., n.m. old people. [F].

vieille (vjɛj), q.v., n. (an) old woman; more formal: *une vieille* (yn vjɛj),
q.v., = an old woman. [F}.

vieillerie(s) (vjɛjri), q.v., n. old thing(s), old idea(s). [F].

vieillesse (vjɛjɛs) n. 1. old age; oldness. 2. *la vieillesse*, old people =
vieillards, q.v. [F].

vieillir (vjejir) vt. to age; to make someone look older. vi. to age, to
grow old; ref.v. to make oneself look older. [F].

vieux jeu (vjø ʒø) adj.phr. out of date, old fashioned, *passé*. syn.
retardataire. [F].

vir magno jam natu (wir maag'nō jam naa'toŏ) aged man, man
advanced in years. [L, *vir* man + magno great, aged+ *jam* now, already
+ *natu* born, age of, old—an idiom].

volventibus annis (wō-len'ti-boŏs aan'is) as the years roll by. [L, *volvere* roll, *annus* year].

See Index of Foreign Headwords & Phrases: Page 473

CATEGORICAL LIST OF
HEADWORDS & PHRASES
WITH PAGE NUMBER

INDEX OF
HEADWORDS & PHRASES

C

E

fustigate, 141
fustilugs, 141
fusty, 141

G

gadzookary, 141
gadzooks, 141
gaffer, 141
gait speed, 142
galimatias, 142
gammer, 142
garrulous, 142
gasconade, 142
gawkocracy, 144
geezer, 144
geezerhood, 144
geezersphere, 145
gelotripsy, 145
geniophobia, 145
gerascophobia, 147
geriatric care manager/geriatric
    case manager, 147
geriatric center, 148
geriatrics, 148
gero-, geron-, geront-, geronto-, 148
gerocomical, 148
geroderma, 148
gerodontic, 148
gerodontics/gerodontology, 148
geromarasmus, 148
geromorphism, 149
gerontal, 149
gerontarchical, 149
gerontic, 149
gerontiloquence, 149
gerontocomium, 149
gerontocracy, 149
gerontogenes, 149
gerontolagnia, 150
gerontology, 150
gerontophilia, 150

gerontophobia, 150
gerontopia, 150
gerontotherapeutics, 150
gerontoxon, 151
geroscience, 151
Gerousia, 151
glabrous, 151
gleet, 151
gloming, 151
glossolalia, 151
glusk, 152
gnarled, 152
gnoff, 152
gnome, 152
gnomic, 152
golden ager, 152
golden years, 153
Gompertz Law, 153
gormless, 153
grandam(e), 153
granocracy, 153
gray power, 153
gray rights, 153
gray tech, 153
graybeard, 153
great assize, 154
grimalkin, 154
grinch, 154
grisard/grizard, 154
grognard, 154
grouse, 154
gudgeon, 154
gynecomania, 155

H

habitué, -e, 155
Hadephobia, 155
hakam, 156
halcyon, 156
hamartithia, 156
hamartomania, 156

L

INDEX OF FOREIGN
HEADWORDS & PHRASES

THE END
